# THE PRACTICAL PLAYBOOK II
## Building Multisector Partnerships That Work

# THE PRACTICAL PLAYBOOK II
## Building Multisector Partnerships That Work

Edited by

**J. LLOYD MICHENER**

**BRIAN C. CASTRUCCI**

**DON W. BRADLEY**

**EDWARD L. HUNTER**

**CRAIG W. THOMAS**

**CATHERINE PATTERSON**

**ELIZABETH CORCORAN**

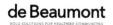

de Beaumont
BOLD SOLUTIONS FOR HEALTHIER COMMUNITIES

CDC
CENTERS FOR DISEASE
CONTROL AND PREVENTION

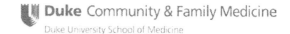

Duke Community & Family Medicine
Duke University School of Medicine

Oxford University Press is a department of the University of Oxford. It furthers
the University's objective of excellence in research, scholarship, and education
by publishing worldwide. Oxford is a registered trade mark of Oxford University
Press in the UK and certain other countries.

Published in the United States of America by Oxford University Press
198 Madison Avenue, New York, NY 10016, United States of America.

© Oxford University Press 2019

First Edition published in 2016
Second Edition published in 2019

Library of Congress Cataloging-in-Publication Data
Michener, J. Lloyd, editor.
Title: The practical playbook : building multisector partnerships that work /
edited by J. Lloyd Michener [and 6 others].
Description: Second edition. | Oxford ; New York : Oxford University Press,
[2019] | Includes bibliographical references and index.
Identifiers: LCCN 2018051629 | ISBN 9780190936013 (pbk. : alk. paper)
Subjects: | MESH: Public Health Practice | Primary Health Care |
Public-Private Sector Partnerships | Cooperative Behavior |
Community Participation
Classification: LCC RA418 | NLM WA 100 | DDC 362.1—dc23
LC record available at https://lccn.loc.gov/2018051629

3 5 7 9 8 6 4
Printed by Marquis, Canada

The mark "CDC" is owned by the U.S. Dept. of Health and Human Services (HHS) and is used with permission. Use of this logo is
not an endorsement by HHS or CDC of any particular product, service, or enterprise.

# Disclaimers

The findings and conclusion in this report are those of the authors and do not necessarily represent the official position of the Centers for Disease Control and Prevention (CDC) or the authors' institutions.

References to non-CDC Internet sites are provided as a service to readers and do not constitute or imply endorsement of these organizations or their programs by the US Department of Health and Human Services, the Public Health Service, or CDC. CDC is not responsible for the content of these sites. URL addresses were current as of the date of publication.

## NOTICE

This material is not intended to be, and should not be considered, a substitute for medical or other professional advice. Treatment for the conditions described in this material is highly dependent on the individual circumstances. While this material is designed to offer accurate information with respect to the subject matter covered and to be current as of the time it was written, research and knowledge about medical and health issues are constantly evolving, and dose schedules for medications and vaccines are being revised continually, with new side effects recognized and accounted for regularly. Readers must, therefore, always check the product information and clinical procedures with the most up-to-date published product information and data sheets provided by the manufacturers and the most recent codes of conduct and safety regulation. Oxford University Press and the authors make no representations or warranties to readers, express or implied, as to the accuracy or completeness of this material, including without limitation that they make no representations or warranties as to the accuracy or efficacy of the drug dosages mentioned in the material. The authors and the publishers do not accept, and expressly disclaim, any responsibility for any liability, loss, or risk that may be claimed or incurred as a consequence of the use and/or application of any of the contents of this material.

The Publisher is responsible for author selection and the Publisher and the Author(s) make all editorial decisions, including decisions regarding content. The Publisher and the Author(s) are not responsible for any product information added to this publication by companies purchasing copies of it for distribution to clinicians.

For additional copies, please contact Oxford University Press, or order online at www.oup.com/us.

# Contents

*Foreword by James B. Sprague*   **xiii**
*Foreword by J. Michael McGinnis*   **xv**
*Acknowledgments*   **xvii**
*Contributors*   **xix**

**SECTION I**   Introduction: Accelerating Partnerships for Health

1   **Overview: The Accelerating Movement of Partnerships for Health**   **3**
*J. Lloyd Michener, Brian C. Castrucci, Don W. Bradley, Edward L. Hunter, and Craig W. Thomas*

2   **On Health Equity**   **7**
*Viviana Martinez-Bianchi*

3   ***The Practical Playbook* in Action: Improving Health Through Cross-Sector Partnerships**   **15**
*John Auerbach and Karen B. DeSalvo*

4   **Insight from National Experts: From the Community-Based Organization Sector**   **23**
*Kim Foreman and Sandra Byrd Chappelle*

5   **Capitalizing on the Health Impacts of Improving Housing Conditions**   **35**
*Michael McKnight and Ruth Ann Norton*

6   **Partnering with Transportation Sector Actors and Advocates to Improve Health Outcomes**   **47**
*Teresa Wilke and Shawn Leight*

7   **Business and Public Health: Why Corporate America Will Soon Help Lead the Public Health Charge**   **61**
*Scott Hall*

8   The Path Forward: The Role of Hospitals and Health
    Systems in Advancing Health and Well-Being for
    Individuals and Communities                                  67
    *Jay Bhatt and Andrew Jagar*

9   Primary Care and the Social Determinants of Health:
    Lessons on Care Models, Capacity, and Culture for
    the Journey Upstream                                         75
    *Rishi Manchanda*

**SECTION II**   Collaboration: The Role of Multiple Sectors in
Improving Health

10  Overview—Collaboration: The Role of Multiple
    Sectors in Improving Health                                  89
    *Don W. Bradley and Brian C. Castrucci*

11  Engaging Residents for Health Transformation               93
    *Pedja Stojicic*

12  The Role of Primary Care in Population and Community
    Health: Pragmatic Approaches to Integration                 101
    *Julie Wood and Kevin Grumbach*

13  The Role of Elected Officials in Multisector Partnerships   109
    *Sylvia Garcia and Elsa Mendoza*

14  Engaging Elected Officials to Improve
    Community Health                                            113
    *Edward L. Hunter*

15  Working with the Faith Community to Improve Health          119
    *Richard Joyner and Alexandra Treyz*

16  Taking Collaborations to Scale                              125
    *Ahmed Calvo*

17  Case Study—Addressing Behavioral Health with a
    Multisector Approach: Why We Started Community
    of Solutions                                                137
    *Robert L. Phillips, Jr, Carol V. Davis, Ethan J. Phillips,*
    *Heather Davies, Valerie Flowe, Mary Beth Quick, and Lauren Terry*

18  Sustainability Through Accountability:
    The Accountable Community for Health Model                  149
    *Marion Standish, Bonnie Midura, Barbara Masters,*
    *Patricia Powers, and Laura Hogan*

**SECTION III** — Data: Finding and Using Information

19 Overview—Data: Finding and Using Information 161
Brian C. Castrucci and Don W. Bradley

20 All In: How and Why Communities Are Using Data
to Drive Community Health Improvement 163
Clare Tanner and Peter Eckart

21 Digital Data Exchange Between Health Care and
Public Health: Lessening the Burden 177
Jeffrey P. Engel and W. Edward Hammond

22 How to Draft Successful Memorandums
of Understanding and Data-Sharing Agreements 191
Matthew Penn and Rachel Hulkower

23 Is the Perfect the Enemy of the Good?
Using the Data You Have 205
Theresa Chapple-McGruder, Jaime Slaughter-Acey,
Jennifer Kmet, and Tonia Ruddock

24 Practical Lessons Learned from Baltimore's
B'FRIEND Initiative 219
Darcy F. Phelan-Emrick, Michael Fried, Heang Tan,
Molly Martin, and Leana S. Wen

**SECTION IV** — Innovation: Enhancing Coordinated Impact Through
New Roles and Tools

25 Overview—Innovation: Enhancing Coordinated
Impact Through New Roles and Tools 231
J. Lloyd Michener and Edward L. Hunter

26 Identifying and Addressing Patients' Social Needs
in Health Care Delivery Settings 235
Laura Gottlieb and Caroline Fichtenberg

27 The Role of Innovation in Improving Population Health 249
Jessica Solomon Fisher and Kellie L. Teter

28 Building an Agenda for Population Health from
the Grassroots Up 261
Tyler Norris and Ashley Hill

29    Case Study—The Alliance for Health Equity:
      Hospitals, Health Departments, and Community
      Partners Working Together for Health Equity
      in Chicago and Suburban Cook County                271
      *Jess Lynch, Megan Cunningham, and Julie Morita*

30    The Health System's Role in Community Health
      Improvement: The Work of Three Insurance Providers    283
      *Brian C. Castrucci, Elizabeth Corcoran, Loel S. Solomon,*
      *Caraline Coats, Alyse B. Sabina, Lamond Daniels,*
      *and Amy A. Clark*

31    Community-Centered Health Homes: Bridging
      Health Care Services and Community Prevention        291
      *Leslie Mikkelsen, Rea Pañares, and Larry Cohen*

32    Going Way Upstream: How One Foundation
      Redefined Its Work to Improve Population Health      301
      *Peter Long and Brittany Imwalle*

33    Case Study—Acting (and Funding) Locally:
      How One Virginia Foundation Is Changing the
      Way It Supports Communities                         315
      *Patricia N. Mathews*

SECTION V    Sustainability and Finance: Supporting Partnerships
             over Time

34    Overview—Sustainability and Finance: Supporting
      Partnerships over Time                              325
      *Craig W. Thomas and Brian C. Castrucci*

35    The Role of Community Development as a Partner
      in Health                                           329
      *Douglas Jutte*

36    Braiding, Blending, or Block Granting?
      How to Sustainably Fund Public Health
      and Prevention in States                            351
      *Amy Clary and Trish Riley*

37    Rethinking the Mission of Health Systems:
      Improving Community Health as Anchor Institutions   365
      *David Zuckerman, David Ansell, and Michellene Davis*

38    Case Study: BUILDing Ties with the
      Business Community                                375
      *Katherine Oestman, Rosalind Bello, Catherine Chennisi,*
      *and Anna Brewster*

## SECTION VI    Policy: Achieving Sustained Impact

39    Overview—Policy: Achieving Sustained Impact        385
      *Edward L. Hunter and Don W. Bradley*

40    Fighting Big Soda at the Local Level               389
      *Nikki Highsmith Vernick and Glenn E. Schneider*

41    Building Off of Evidence-Based Policies:
      The CDC's Health Impact in 5 Years (HI-5)
      Initiative and CityHealth, an Initiative of the
      de Beaumont Foundation and Kaiser Permanente       407
      *Elizabeth Skillen and Shelley Hearne*

42    The Impact of State and Territorial Public Health
      Policy: Interventions to Prevent Opioid Misuse
      and Addiction                                      425
      *Michael R. Fraser, Philicia Tucker, and Jay C. Butler*

43    Case Study: Nontraditional Partners in the Case
      of Kansas City                                     445
      *Scott Hall and Rex Archer*

## SECTION VII    Training and Workforce: Preparing for the Future That Is Already Here

44    Overview—Training and Workforce: Preparing for
      the Future That Is Already Here                    453
      *J. Lloyd Michener and Craig W. Thomas*

45    Shaping the Next Generation of Providers           457
      *Gerri Mattson and Karen Remley*

46    On the Synergies That Can Generate Excellence
      in Public Health Education                         465
      *Sandro Galea*

47    Case Study: State Innovations in Rural Training    471
      *Kristi Martinsen and Michelle Goodman*

48  **Better Together: Engaging Nursing Leaders in Community Collaborative Efforts**                483

*Anh N. Tran and Anne Derouin*

49  **Voices of the Next Generation**                491

*Elizabeth Corcoran, Sarah LaFave, Denny Fe Garcia Agana, Haleigh Kampman, John C. Penner, Margaret L. McCarthy, Katherine P. Mullins, Michelle Vu, and Ashten Duncan*

**SECTION VIII**  Conclusion: Taking the Next Steps Toward Population Health

50  **Conclusion: From the Edges Toward the Middle**                509

*J. Lloyd Michener, Brian C. Castrucci, Don W. Bradley, Craig W. Thomas, and Edward L. Hunter*

*Acronym List*                511
*Glossary*                515
*Index*                523

# Foreword

Public health and medicine have grown apart over the past century. The continuing separation and specialization of the two fields creates a harmful divide that keeps complementary practices from accomplishing their shared goal of healthy people. Today, if you asked the primary care department heads in hospitals and health systems the question, "Do you know the name of your health commissioner?" most of them will not know the answer. Similarly, the health commissioner might not know the name of the primary care and health system leaders. The first edition of this book, *The Practical Playbook: Public Health and Primary Care Together*, grew from a recognition of this divide and the hope of building a strong, permanent bridge to replace it.

We were delighted with the response to the first edition of the *Playbook*, initially conceived as an online resource and, since 2015, also published as a book. Practitioners came to us with copies that were dog-eared and worn. Health departments ordered copies for the entire staff. Medical schools use it as a supplemental textbook. It was encouraging to see the *Playbook* closing the divide that inspired it. In the past 4 years, all health disciplines have recognized and adopted strategies for improved population health. More collaborative partnerships of greater magnitude have emerged, and more attention is being given to local policies that create lasting changes in health. The first *Practical Playbook* facilitated the introduction and started the dialogue between public health and primary care. However, now there is a new call to action for health professionals, this time from outside the health system. The need for cross-sector partnerships that collaborate, innovate, and affect policy for improved population health is the work of the 21st century and the focus of the *Practical Playbook: Building Multisector Partnerships That Work*.

We are pleased to deliver this second edition into the hands of public health, primary care, business leaders, health system officials, community leaders, elected representatives, professors and trainers, transportation officials, housing authorities, students, and many more audiences that have a role to play in the health of their communities. Our noble partners at Duke University and the Centers for Disease Control and Prevention (CDC) have worked hard, in tandem with our incredible authors, to move the dialogue in the first *Practical Playbook* to a blueprint for action in the second. This time, the partners are not just primary care and public health, but partners from the multiple sectors and organizations that share the goal of healthier communities. The sections, chapters, and concrete examples in this volume go beyond a bridge between two disciplines, fostering action and shared responsibility for population health in all sectors, with all partners.

—James B. Sprague, MD
Chairman of the Board
de Beaumont Foundation
Bethesda, MD

# Foreword

Four years ago, the *Practical Playbook: Public Health and Primary Care Together*, was launched as an important new interactive online tool for improving the health prospects of individuals, communities, states, and the nation. Produced through a visionary initiative of the de Beaumont Foundation, in partnership with the Duke University Department of Community Medicine, the Centers for Disease Control and Prevention, and other national stakeholder organizations, the *Practical Playbook* provided a timely core resource for more effective engagement of pressing front-line challenges.

Those challenges are formidable, ranging from the visible and the immediate, such as obesity and opioids and their consequences, to those that lie beneath the surface, such as stigma, stress, and prejudice, to compound damage and render solutions more evasive. The first edition of the *Practical Playbook* took on squarely the challenge of the impractical: the notion that the most widespread and rapidly growing health threats could be engaged through separate and unconnected activities undertaken inside and outside the clinic doors.

Calling attention to the basic centrality of the linkages between public health and primary care and making more accessible evidence-based guidance and tools for facilitating those links, the *Playbook* has been used to forge active partnerships between state health departments and medical societies as they jointly fashion strategies, as well as to foster more effective management of multifaceted interventions by care delivery and public health workers in neighborhoods, cities, and counties. Both in its digital online format and through the application of well-worn hard copy pages, it is helping to change perspectives and capacities nationally.

This second *Playbook* volume offers a necessary complement for quickening the pace of progress in the journey to better health envisioned with the first. *Practical Playbook: Accelerating Multisector Partnerships for Health* takes the resource to the necessary next dimension of effective population health strategies—ensuring that strategies to mobilize community-wide initiatives for health action actively engage all sectors in the assessment and action.

For many people, the prospect for illness or injury is at least as much a product of their housing, transportation, job circumstances, school or work environment, and access to green space as it is to their biological predisposition to heart disease, cancer, stroke, addiction, or infectious agents. Whether on the basis of within-sector productivity or stakes in community-wide progress, health responsibilities cut across sectors.

Accordingly, the deep bench of leader-authors who lend their experienced voices as designers of the second *Practical Playbook* seek to enable communities in which the impact on health is a basic consideration for all areas of life, a genuine embodiment of the notion of health in all policies. Envisioned is a community culture in which the shared premium placed on health positions public health as the leader to an orchestra populated by expertise not only from medical care and epidemiology, but also from law and policy, employment and income, housing and transportation, and social services. As conductor to a community health orchestra, public health helps harmonize available strengths from different sectors to complement, inform, and empower each other, engaging each other in playing to respective strengths, finding a resonant frequency in a common goal of improved health.

Each of those involved in second *Practical Playbook*—the de Beaumont leadership and board, the editors, and the cadre of assembled experts—has produced a resource that engages the practical necessity of mobilizing multisector action against today's challenges. In addition, they have done so in a fashion that sets the stage for the second *Practical Playbook* to serve as a living document, amenable to revision and updating in real-time as lessons are gathered from its activation. If leadership from the many sectors involved in its design can be similarly enlisted to assure its use, the benefits will accrue widely to communities across the nation.

—J. Michael McGinnis, MD, MPP
Leonard D. Schaeffer Executive Officer of National Academy of Medicine
National Academy of Medicine
Washington, DC

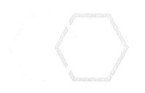

# Acknowledgments

The chapters, origin, and spirit of this text stemmed from the contributions of many, including and expanding far beyond the authors listed with each chapter. The gratitude of the editors extends to Dr. James Sprague, Courtney Simpson, Lauren Bodie, Deborah Thorp, Rachel Locke, Annie Patterson, Chad Zimmerman, Chloe Layman, and others across Duke University, the de Beaumont Foundation, Oxford University Press, and *Practical Playbook* teams, who were instrumental in bringing this book to life. Most of all, our gratitude goes to all who have tirelessly worked as part of local partnerships for health and whose experiences we have tried to capture here. We hope this book reflects both the wisdom shared and provides new insights and tools for the work ahead.

With thanks to all,
The Editors

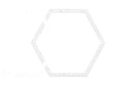

# Contributors

**Denny Fe Garcia Agana**
Epidemiology PhD Candidate
University of Florida

**David Ansell**
Senior Vice President for Community
Health Equity
Rush University Medical Center

**Rex Archer**
Director of Health
Kansas City Health Department

**John Auerbach**
President and CEO
Trust for America's Health

**Rosalind Bello**
Program Director, Office of
Health Policy
MD Anderson Cancer Center

**Jay Bhatt**
Senior Vice President and
Chief Medical Officer
American Hospital Association

**Don W. Bradley**
Consulting Professor, Department of
Community and Family Medicine
Duke University School of Medicine

**Anna Brewster**
Program Director
University of Texas MD Anderson
Cancer Center

**Jay C. Butler**
Chief Medical Officer and Director
Alaska Department of Health and Social
Services Division of Public Health

**Ahmed Calvo**
Director of National Leadership
Fellowship on Health Policy and Public
Service
Stanford University Haas Center for
Public Service

**Brian C. Castrucci**
Chief Executive Officer
de Beaumont Foundation

**Sandra Byrd Chappelle**
Founder and Principal
Strategic Solutions Partners, LLC

**Theresa Chapple-McGruder**
Former Senior Research and
Evaluation Officer
de Beaumont Foundation

**Catherine Chennisi**
Public Health Analyst
Harris County Public Health and
Environmental Services

**Amy A. Clark**
Managing Director of Community
Impact and Strategy
Aetna Foundation

**Amy Clary**
Senior Policy Associate
National Academy for State
Health Policy

**Caraline Coats**
Vice President
Population Health, Office of
the Chief Medical Officer at Humana

**Larry Cohen**
Founder and Executive Director
Prevention Institute

**Elizabeth Corcoran**
Special Assistant to the CEO and
Executive Leadership Team
de Beaumont Foundation

**Megan Cunningham**
Managing Deputy Commissioner
Chicago Department of Public Health

**Lamond Daniels**
Consultant, Healthiest Cities and
Counties Challenge
Aetna Foundation

**Heather Davies**
Department of Global and
Community Health
George Mason University

**Carol V. Davis**
Project Manager and Senior
Instructional Designer
Cybermedia Technologies (CTEC)

**Michellene Davis**
Executive Vice President and Chief
Corporate Affairs Officer
RWJBarnabas Hospital

**Anne Derouin**
Associate Professor
Duke University School of Nursing

**Karen B. DeSalvo**
Former Acting Assistant Secretary
for Health

**Ashten Duncan**
MD/MPH Candidate
OU-TU School of Community Medicine

**Peter Eckart**
Director of the Center for Health
Information and Technology
Illinois Public Health Institute

**Jeffrey P. Engel**
Executive Director
Council of State and Territorial
Epidemiologists

**Caroline Fichtenberg**
Managing Director, Social Interventions
Research and Evaluation Network
University of California San Francisco

**Jessica Solomon Fisher**
Chief Innovations Officer
Public Health National Center for
Innovations

**Valerie Flowe**
Senior Graphic Designer
American Trucking Association

**Kim Foreman**
President
Environmental Health Watch

**Michael R. Fraser**
Executive Director
Association of State and Territorial
Health Officials

**Michael Fried**
Chief Information Officer
Baltimore City Health Department

**Sandro Galea**
Dean and Robert A. Knox Professor
Boston University School of
Public Health

**Sylvia Garcia**
Texas State Senator

**Michelle Goodman**
Senior Policy Analyst, Division of Policy
and Shortage Designation, Bureau of
Health Workforce
Health Resources and Service
Administration

**Laura Gottlieb**
Associate Professor, Family and
Community Medicine
University of California San Francisco

**Kevin Grumbach**
Chair, Family and Community Medicine
University of California, San Francisco

**Scott Hall**
Senior Vice President
Kansas City Chamber of Commerce

**W. Edward Hammond**
Director, Duke Center for Health
Informatics

**Shelley Hearne**
President
CityHealth

**Ashley Hill**
Executive Fellow
Well Being Trust

**Laura Hogan**
Program Officer
California Accountable Communities
for Health Initiative

**Rachel Hulkower**
Public Health Analyst, Public Health
Law Program
Centers for Disease Control and
Prevention

**Edward L. Hunter**
Former CEO
de Beaumont Foundation

**Brittany Imwalle**
Chief Operating Officer
Blue Shield of California
Foundation

**Andrew Jagar**
Senior Program Manager, Center for
Health Innovation
American Hospital Association

**Richard Joyner**
Head of Hospital Chaplains
University of North Carolina Nash
Healthcare

**Douglas Jutte**
Executive Director
Build Healthy Places

**Haleigh Kampman**
MPH Candidate
IUPUI Richard M. Fairbanks School of
Public Health

**Jennifer Kmet**
Senior Epidemiological Officer
Shelby County Health Department

**Sarah LaFave**
MPH Candidate
Johns Hopkins University Bloomberg
School of Public health

**Shawn Leight**
Vice President and Chief Operations
Officer
CBB Transportation Engineers +
Planners

**Peter Long**
President and CEO
Blue Shield of California Foundation

**Jess Lynch**
Program Director
Illinois Public Health Institute

**Rishi Manchanda**
President and Founder
Health Begins

**Molly Martin**
Division Chief of Advocacy Services
Baltimore City Health Department

**Viviana Martinez-Bianchi**
Associate Professor, Department of
Community and Family Medicine
Duke University School
of Medicine

**Kristi Martinsen**
Hospital-State Division Director
Health Resources and Service
Administration

**Barbara Masters**
Program Director
California Accountable Communities
for Health Initiative

**Patricia N. Mathews**
President and CEO
Northern Virginia Health Foundation

**Gerri Mattson**
Adjunct Assistant Professor
University of North Carolina Gillings
School of Global Public Health

**Margaret L. McCarthy**
Population Health Scholar
Georgetown University School of
Medicine

**J. Michael McGinnis**
Executive Officer
National Academy of Medicine

**Michael McKnight**
Vice President of Policy and Innovation
Green and Healthy Homes Initiative

**Elsa Mendoza**
Staffer
Texas State Senate Office of Sylvia Garcia

**J. Lloyd Michener**
Professor, Department of Community
and Family Medicine
Duke University School of Medicine

**Bonnie Midura**
Senior Program Manager
The California Endowment

**Leslie Mikkelsen**
Managing Director
Prevention Institute

**Julie Morita**
Commissioner
Chicago Department of Public Health

**Katherine P. Mullins**
Population Health Scholar
Georgetown University School
of Medicine

**Tyler Norris**
Chief Executive Officer
Well Being Trust

**Ruth Ann Norton**
President and CEO
Green and Healthy Homes Initiative

**Katherine Oestman**
Program Coordinator
MD Anderson Cancer Center

**Rea Pañares**
Senior Advisor
Prevention Institute

**Catherine Patterson**
Managing Director, Urban Health
and Policy
de Beaumont Foundation

**Matthew Penn**
Director, Office of Public Health Law
Services
Centers for Disease Control and
Prevention

**John C. Penner**
Population Health Scholar
Georgetown University School
of Medicine

**Darcy F. Phelan-Emrick**
Chief Epidemiologist
Baltimore City Health Department

**Ethan J. Philips**
Student
Fairfax County Public Schools

**Robert L. Phillips, Jr**
Executive Director, Center for
Professionalism & Value
in Health Care
American Board of Family Medicine
Foundation

**Patricia Powers**
Program Officer
California Accountable Communities
for Health Initiative

**Mary Beth Quick**
Owner/Operator
Heart & Soul Yoga LLC

**Karen Remley**
Senior Fellow
de Beaumont Foundation

**Trish Riley**
Executive Director
National Academy for State
Health Policy

**Tonia Ruddock**
Maternal Child Health Epidemiologist
Georgia Department of Public Health

**Alyse B. Sabina**
National Program Director
Aetna Foundation

**Glenn E. Schneider**
Chief Program Officer
Horizon Foundation

**Elizabeth Skillen**
Senior Advisor
Centers for Disease Control and
Prevention

**Jaime Slaughter-Acey**
Assistant Professor
Drexel University College of Nursing
and Health Professions

**Loel S. Solomon**
Vice President of Community Health
Kaiser Permanente

**James B. Sprague**
Founding Chairman of the Board
de Beaumont Foundation

**Marion Standish**
Senior Vice President, Enterprise
Programs
California Endowment

**Pedja Stojicic**
Director of Resident Engagement
ReThink Health

**Heang Tan**
Deputy Commissioner: Aging and Care
Services
Baltimore City Health Department

**Clare Tanner**
Director, Center for Data Management
and Translational Research
Michigan Public Health Institute

**Lauren Terry**
Senior Designer
Hilton Creative Studio at Hilton

**Kellie L. Teter**
Maternal Child Health Manager
Denver Public Health

**Craig W. Thomas**
Director, Division of Population Health
Centers for Disease Control and
Prevention

**Anh N. Tran**
Assistant Professor, Department of
Community and Family Medicine
Duke University School of Medicine

**Alexandra Treyz**
Food and Faith Associate in Research,
World Food Policy Center
Duke University Sanford School of
Public Policy

**Philicia Tucker**
Research Associate
Association of State and Territorial
Health Officials

**Nikki Highsmith Vernick**
President and CEO
Horizon Foundation

**Michelle Vu**
Doctorate of Pharmacy/MPH Candidate
Mercer University Colleges of Pharmacy
and Health Sciences

**Leana S. Wen**
President
Planned Parenthood Federation of
America

**Teresa Wilke**
Strategic Consultant for
Generate Health
Silver Arrow Strategies

**Julie Wood**
Vice President, Health of the Public and
Science
American Academy of Family
Physicians

**David Zuckerman**
Manager for Healthcare Engagement
Democracy Collaborative

# Introduction: Accelerating Partnerships for Health

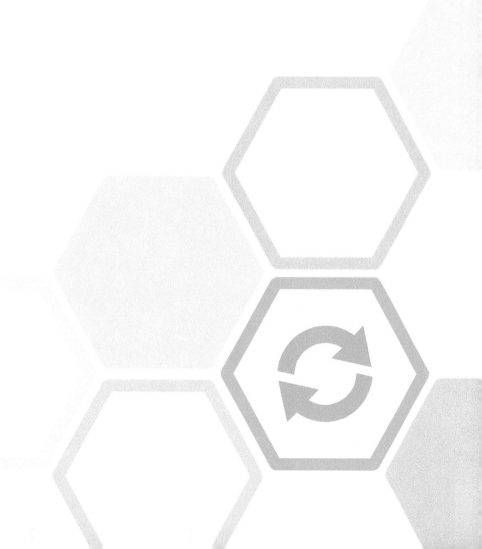

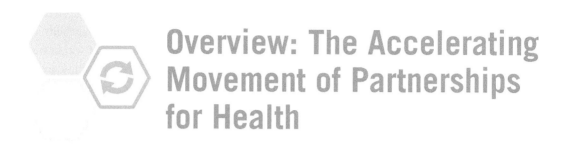

# Overview: The Accelerating Movement of Partnerships for Health

J. LLOYD MICHENER, BRIAN C. CASTRUCCI, DON W. BRADLEY, EDWARD L. HUNTER, AND CRAIG W. THOMAS

In 2010, the Centers for Disease Control and Prevention (CDC) and the Health Resources and Services Administration (HRSA) requested that the Institute of Medicine convene a committee to assess the opportunity for the agencies to improve population health through integration of primary care and public health. The Committee of Integrating Primary Care and Public Health released its report in 2012,[1] noting that communities across the country were already engaged in such partnerships and that there were steps the agencies could take that would accelerate and enhance these partnerships. With the leadership and support of the de Beaumont Foundation, that report spawned *The Practical Playbook*, an Internet-based initiative that sought to find, assemble, assess, and share stories of how communities and agencies across the United States were working together to improve health. The examples of collaborations quickly expanded to more than 1,000 web pages on the website (www.PracticalPlaybook.org), necessitating a restructuring of the site and, in 2016, a first hardcopy guide—*The Practical Playbook: Public Health and Primary Care Together*—on tools and technologies for collaboration. Since the first guide appeared, multisector collaborations that improve the health of communities and the individuals living within them have continued to expand, and there are currently more than 600 partnerships across the country. With this growth has come the realization that a completely new book was needed that would build on the experiences of the broadening array of sites and sectors and provide a concise set of tools, methods, and examples that support multisector partnerships to improve population health. That book is *The Practical Playbook 2: Accelerating Multisector Partnerships for Health*.

The reasons for this rapid growth of collaborations are need and timing. Rates of chronic disease across the United States have been increasing for decades, consuming an ever-increasing—and unsustainable—share of our economy. The medical model, which has been so effective in ameliorating acute illness, is, by itself, largely ineffective in dealing with underlying or "upstream" problems that have their roots in communities. The growing availability of data has made visible underlying patterns of differing outcomes within our communities. All too often, these patterns are worsening so that, in many areas, women are now living shorter lives than their mothers, rural men are living shorter lives than their fathers, and black men in inner cities have life spans more similar to those in Third World countries than to their neighbors a few miles away.[2] We are dying too soon of illnesses we know how to prevent and for which no country will ever have sufficient resources to effectively treat.

The powerful sense of the need for change, and the fact that the health system alone cannot drive it, is now driving communities to take the lead in finding solutions. Clinicians despair at the challenges of making a difference in the lives of their patients when the causes of illness are outside their ability to treat, public health officers and staff face funding cut after funding cut, and communities are increasingly suffering. Health is not something that any one person or group can achieve alone, but it is something that we can powerfully affect together.

Community partnerships for health are showing that health can be improved when we work across sectors. Often initiated by public health officials who have taken on the role of convener and leader, as described in Chapter 3, these health professionals help communities come together, organize, and implement local solutions to local priorities. They tackle long-neglected issues of health inequity (see Chapter 2), using data and graphics to raise awareness and advocate for programs that give everyone an opportunity for health. Community organizations become the source of and advocates for change, reflecting the historic role of community organizations in leading change (Chapter 4) while other sectors, such as housing (Chapter 5) and transportation (Chapter 6), reassert their roles as essential partners in making communities healthy and livable. And no sector of our economy is likely to have as much influence as the business community, as Chapter 7 powerfully reminds us.

Health care groups are increasingly part of the partnerships as well, as primary care returns to its roots of community engagement and advocacy (Chapter 13) and goes upstream to the social factors that powerfully affect health, linking its collaborative programs with community agencies that provide the services and supports that patients—people—need, in addition to meeting purely medical needs (Chapter 9). ("*Upstream determinants* are defined as features of the social environment, such as socioeconomic status and discrimination, that influence individual behavior, disease, and health status."[3])

Nursing, long active in providing services in rural and underserved communities, is increasingly engaged (Chapter 50), as are hospitals as they transform their business models and move from being sites of care to active partners in improving health and health equity (Chapter 8). Philanthropic foundations, long the support of programs for the underserved, are shifting upstream as well, realizing that addressing the roots of illness is critical if we are to become healthy and that foundations have a core role in leading that change (Chapter 26). And, most hopeful of all, students and trainees are articulating and advocating for a future that engages them in improving health in ways that reflect their values and preferences (Chapter 46).

But the barriers are formidable. Health care continues to take up a growing share of all funding, requiring the development of business models for shifting and sustaining investments in health (Chapter 34). Overall, coalitions are anecdotal, though programs to link and share them, such as *Practical Playbook 2* and the Robert Wood Johnson Foundation's Culture of Health, are under way. But the greatest barriers are cultural and lie in how we think about our work, what we are paid and expected to do, and what we are accustomed to doing. Working in multisector partnerships is new, complex, often unfunded, and anything but quick. Improving health through partnerships requires letting go of our traditional siloed mentality, engaging with others, and developing programs that are successful and sustainable together.

Culture can be a barrier in other more subtle ways. Improving health requires a shift from the concept of "best practice" to realizing that one size does not fit all and that different settings, with different priorities, strengths, and needs, require different solutions. We also need to abandon the proclivity for implementing "quick fixes." Improving health requires patience and a willingness to invest time and energy in creating new partnerships as well as in methods of working that weave together the frayed threads of our communities and programs that support health for all.

What is now needed—and what this *Practical Playbook 2* strives to provide—is a compilation of tools and methods that can be used by a variety of groups, in a variety of settings, and for a variety of issues as coalitions work together to improve health. We intend this to be a playbook not of *best practices*, but of *better practices* that can be adapted and shaped to build on local strengths and respond to local needs. The chapters that follow have multiple examples of successes and lessons learned along the way, which we hope you will find useful.

But beyond the tools and lessons, this book is intended as an invitation for all, young and old, and from all sectors, to join the movement for health. It is a call for action, for joining partnerships, for selecting among the wide range of tools and methods shared here and putting them into action to make a difference in the health of our diverse communities.

Our communities and the individuals living in them are dying of illnesses we know how to prevent, that have their roots in our communities, and that cannot be effectively treated by any one group alone. And, increasingly, communities are making a difference and leading the way to health. We hope you will use this book and these tools to join with our communities in the movement to health.

## REFERENCES

1. Institute of Medicine (IOM). *Primary Care and Public Health: Exploring Integration to Improve Population Health*. Washington, DC: The National Academies Press; 2012.

2. Murray CJL. The State of US Health, 1990–2016: Burden of diseases, injuries, and risk factors among US states. *JAMA*. 2018;319(14):1444–72. doi:10.1001/jama.2018.0158.

3. Gehlert S, Sohmer D, Sacks T, Mininger C, McClintock M, Olopade O. Targeting health disparities: A model linking upstream determinants to downstream interventions: Knowing about the interaction of societal factors and disease can enable targeted interventions to reduce health disparities. *Health Affairs (Project Hope)*. 2008;27(2):339–49. doi:10.1377/hlthaff.27.2.339.

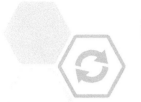

# Chapter 2

# On Health Equity

VIVIANA MARTINEZ-BIANCHI

Health equity is defined as the "attainment of the highest level of health for all people."[1] That "high level" of health is often determined by a mixture of personal responsibility, biology, and the options and possibilities for good health available to each individual (Figure 2.1). In equitable cultures, all persons can have similar choices. Health equity matters from many perspectives. At the highest level, health equity is rooted in the ethical principle of justice and requires providing everyone the opportunity to achieve good health. Pursuit of health equity requires addressing social factors that powerfully affect health, such as poverty, education, affordable housing, employment, wages, safe environments, discrimination, and racism, as well as access to health care. Importantly, access to health care alone is never sufficient to achieve health equity.

The economic survival of the entire community is affected by health equity; poor health is linked to absenteeism from school and work; chronic absenteeism from school contributes to school dropout and poor educational outcomes,[2] which in turn negatively affects health.[3,4] Healthy workers make healthy and productive workplaces and contribute to economically healthy communities, whereas absenteeism costs US employers more than $225 billion yearly in productivity losses.[5]

## PURSUING HEALTH EQUITY

Achieving health equity is not easy, and, in spite of long-standing multisector efforts to address avoidable health inequalities, we find ourselves in a world plagued by "differences in health status and in the distribution of health determinants between different population groups" (the definition of inequality in the *WHO Glossary of Terms*; http://www.who.int/hia/about/glos/en/

## Figure 2.1 ▾

Conceptual representation of multi-sector partnerships by Fer Miguez.

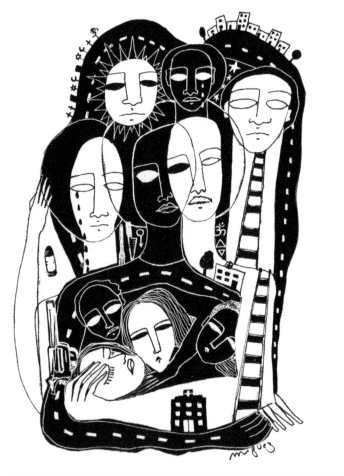

index1.html) and in differences in resource allocation between neighborhoods and communities. Improving health equity requires identifying the underlying factors that cause health disparities and working in multisector partnerships to improve health outcomes for those groups suffering the worst disparities. This work should be a manifestation of the social accountability of physicians and health systems.

The World Health Organization describes social accountability as "the obligation [of physicians and medical institutions] to direct their education, research and service activities toward addressing the priority health concerns of the community, region, and/or nation they have a mandate to serve."[6] For health care to be socially accountable, it must be equitably accessible to everyone and responsive to patient, community, and population health needs.[7] Social accountability in health care intentionally targets health care education, research, and services and addresses social determinants of health toward the priority health concerns of the people and communities served with the goal of achieving health equity.

Assuring conditions for optimal health requires academic health centers, health systems, industry, government, public health departments, nongovernmental organizations (NGOs), businesses, and large employers to demonstrate social accountability through engagement and investment in the local community. This upstream work requires multisector partnerships to improve health in organized approaches that do not leave vulnerable populations behind, value every member of a community, enhance services for those in most need, and engage all socioeconomic groups in the understanding that equity improves the lives of everyone in a community.

Multisector partnerships are highlighted in social obligation scales. Boelen[8] proposes social accountability as one of the most important criteria for excellence in medical education. Boelen suggests that to become *socially accountable*, academic medical centers must anticipatively adapt medical education to the local community's needs, define institutional objectives together with society, contextualize educational programs to improve local health outcomes, focus evaluations on impact, utilize partners as program assessors, and graduate true change agents. He proposes a social obligation scale (Table 2.1) that takes academic medical centers from "Responsible" through "Responsive" to "Accountable." He argues that most health care institutions are generally *socially responsible*; that is, these institutions identify social needs in an implicit fashion, and they are aware of their duty to respond to society's needs, but institutional objectives are defined by faculty, community-oriented programs and evaluations are focused on processes, and only internal assessors are used. These institutions graduate "good practitioners." Some academic institutions can be described as *socially responsive*. In these academic medical centers, the social needs of the community are identified in an explicit way, with institutional objectives inspired from data, educational programs that are community-based and have interventions to address these needs, evaluations that focus

| Table 2.1 ▼ The Social Obligation Scale | | | |
|---|---|---|---|
| | Responsibility ⇨ | Responsiveness ⇨ | Accountability |
| Social needs identified | Implicity | Explicit | Anticipatively |
| Institutional objectives | Defined by faculty | Inspired from data | Defined with society |
| Educational programs | Community-oriented | Community-based | Contextualized |
| Quality of graduates | "Good" practitioners | Meeting criteria of professionalism | Health system change agents |
| Focus of evaluation | Process | Outcome | Impact |
| Assessors | Internal | External | Health partners |

From Boelen C. Why should social accountability be a benchmark for excellence in medical education? *Educación Médica.* July–September 2016;17(3):101–105.

on outcomes, assessors that are external but not true partners, and graduates who meet criteria of professionalism. However, few are wholly accountable, thus recommending that, to make an impact on health, institutions need to have a positive impact with interventions that address political, economic, cultural, environmental, social, and health care inequities. Only solid multisector partnerships can achieve the goal of true accountability.

Access to health care is necessary but not sufficient to achieve health equity. Good health requires access to preventive and therapeutic health care services, from immunizations and prenatal care to treatments for chronic diseases. This in turn requires access to providers and health insurance coverage. Policies to make high-quality health care available to patients of all backgrounds are essential to health equity. However, even the best medical care cannot abolish health inequities; only 20% of health outcomes are determined by health care access and quality. Patients will continue to experience health inequities, even in health systems where all patients—regardless of race, ethnicity, or insurance status—have similar access to providers and services.

Multisector partnerships are valuable in advocacy and as allies against structural inequalities that marginalize people through power structures embedded in organizations. Effective allyship is a process of lifelong relationship building, where persons or organizations with positions of privilege and power work in solidarity with marginalized communities and groups of people. This relationship is based in comprehension, continuity, trust, education, consistency, and accountability. Allyship requires the ability to listen, humility, mutual understanding, community organizing, advocacy, collaboration, and the development of grassroots leadership to work toward economic, racial, ethnic, and gender justice (Figure 2.1).[9-12]

Improving health equity requires advocacy and advocacy planning and the use of an *equity and empowerment lens*, such as the one published by Multnomah County's Office of Diversity and Health Equity, when planning, allocating resources, and making policy decisions.[13]

Pursuing health equity requires the following:

- Addressing inequities
- Understanding the care of the individual patient in the context of his or her community
- Understanding, researching, and training to recognize the roles of bias and discrimination in systems and making needed changes to decrease their negative impact
- Looking at gaps in access or inadequate care for disadvantaged groups
- Addressing health determinants (negative and positive ones) using community health assessments that look at problems as well as social capital

- Paying attention to root causes of disease and wellness because it is through that knowledge that we will learn from our community how to make a positive difference
- Adopting practice models that include respect for the values and culture of the community, as well as those who work in health-related organizations
- Partnering with community organizations and respecting their history and leadership
- Engaging in cross-sector dialogue
- Ceasing to tolerate inequity

## TEACHING HEALTH EQUITY

The importance of health equity, awareness of bias and patterns of discrimination, and strategies for improving the health of groups that have been historically marginalized are issues that can be taught and role-modeled in all health-related educational programs and institutions. It has been the topic of multiple national and local programs.[12,13] One exemplar is the Institute for Health Care Improvement (IHI),[14] which states that health care professionals should play a major role in improving health outcomes for disadvantaged populations and that efforts should go beyond clinical work to leveraging the economic, social, and political power of the health care industry and of each organization within it. The IHI guide to achieving health equity has five key components:

1. *Make health equity a strategic priority that is leader driven and articulated by senior management.* Advancing equity is not a charitable afterthought but a critical component of the organization's mission.
2. *Develop structure and processes to support health equity work.* To advance equity, health systems must dedicate financial and information resources accordingly.
3. *Deploy specific strategies to address the multiple determinants of health on which health care organizations can have a direct impact,* such as health care services, socioeconomic status, physical environment, and healthy behaviors. Make sure research is done to identify the disparities existing in each community.
4. *Confront institutional racism within the organization,* addressing in particular any structures, policies, and norms that perpetuate race-based advantages.
5. *Develop partnerships with community organizations* to improve health and equity.

Similarly, the Robert Wood Johnson Foundation, in its Roadmap to Reduce Racial and Ethnic Disparities in Health Care, provides a six-step framework for health care organizations to reduce disparities and foster health equity. This comprehensive approach encompasses the following components:

1. Link quality and equity
2. Create a culture of equity
3. Diagnose the disparity
4. Design the intervention
5. Secure buy-in of partners
6. Implement and sustain change

## HEALTH EQUITY AS A PERSONAL VALUE

The principle of health equity attracted many of us to health fields. At the heart of our work is the desire to be of help to others, to care for people of all ages and in all life circumstances, to be accountable to our communities, to improve community and population health, to be engaged leaders, and to provide continuous, integrated, and whole person-oriented care. For many of us, our professions became our vehicle for social justice and health equity. To move the needle in health equity, we need to learn to look for the root causes of illness and to help advance whole communities toward equity in health. In the words of Rishi Manchanda, we must be true "upstreamists" in the delivery of health care if we want to improve health.

Finding passion in improving health for all and making a difference beyond the confines of the hallways of the hospital and the walls of the office—being active participants in true wellness in the community—can become a vehicle for personal resilience and prevention of burnout for members of the health care team. In working to make our communities healthy, we can find that we are often restoring meaning and health to our own lives.

### REFERENCES
1. National Partnership for Action to End Health Disparities' Federal Interagency Health Equity Team and Healthy People 2020, accessed 3.1.18 https://minorityhealth.hhs.gov/npa/files/Plans/NSS/NSS_05_Section1.pdf

2. State of Chronic Absenteeism and School Health A Preliminary Review for the Baltimore Community http://www.elev8baltimore.org/site/wp-content/uploads/2012/04/Absenteeism-and-School-Health-Report.pdf

3. The Causes And Costs Of Absenteeism In The Workplace https://www.forbes.com/sites/investopedia/2013/07/10/the-causes-and-costs-of-absenteeism-in-the-workplace/#3fc62e4e3eb6

4. Absenteeism Problems And Costs: Causes, Effects And Cures. Mehmet C. Kocakülâh, University of Southern Indiana, USA, Ann Galligan Kelley, Providence College, USA. Krystal M. Mitchell,Life Point Hospitals, Inc., USA Margaret P. Ruggieri, Providence College, USA International Business & Economics Research Journal—May 2009 Volume 8, Number 5 81 https://www.cluteinstitute.com/ojs/index.php/IBER/article/download/3138/3186

5. CDC Foundation, Business Pulse, Healthy Workers infographic https://www.cdcfoundation.org/businesspulse/healthy-workforce-infographic.

6. Boelen C, Charles, Heck, Jeffery E & World Health Organization. Division of Development of Human Resources for Health. 1995). Defining and measuring the social accountability of medical schools / Charles Boelen and Jeffery E. Heck. Geneva : World Health Organization. http://www.who.int/iris/handle/10665/59441

7. S Buchman, R Woollard, R Meili, R Goel: Practising social accountability: From theory to action Canadian Family Physician, 2016.

8. Boelen C. Why is social accountability a benchmark for excellence in medical education? *Educ Médica*. 2016;17:101–105 https://www.sciencedirect.com/science/article/pii/S1575181316300766#!

9. Guide to allyship http://www.guidetoallyship.com/

10. What is allyship? Why can't I be an ally? http://www.peernetbc.com/what-is-allyship

11. Ally Bill of Responsibilities, © Dr. Lynn Gehl http://www.lynngehl.com/uploads/5/0/0/4/5004954/ally_bill_of_responsibilities_poster.pdf

12. AAMC Health Equity Research and Policy https://www.aamc.org/initiatives/research/healthequity/

13. Multnomah county Equity and Empowerment Lens https://multco.us/diversity-equity/equity-and-empowerment-lens

14. https://catalyst.nejm.org/health-equity-must-be-strategic-priority/

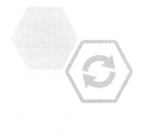

# The Practical Playbook in Action: Improving Health Through Cross-Sector Partnerships

JOHN AUERBACH AND KAREN B. DESALVO

The challenges of addressing the broad health issues facing our community require partnerships across sectors to create the conditions in which everyone can be healthy. As a result, working with and across multiple sectors to promote health is now a staple of public health conversation and action. Whether implied by such phrases as "a culture of health" or "health in all policies," virtually all public health officials and practitioners understand the concept and the need to develop the skills, teams, and resources to advance this model of health improvement. Many are gaining experience with practical efforts in the field.

The underpinning for this approach is the recognition that the most important factors influencing the public's health are not in the health sector per se but are rather a result of the impact of a multitude of factors at family, community, city, state, and federal levels. They include social and economic factors (e.g., poverty, racism, and other forms of discrimination), social isolation, and policies governing the environment writ large—that is, the social determinants of health. And the sectors that influence these factors include housing, education, transportation, economic development, city and county planning, and public safety.[1]

This widespread awareness of the importance of cross-sector work within the public health and health care sectors is a rather extraordinary development. The public health sector and, to a lesser extent, the health care sector have had a history of periodically recognizing the importance of the influence of factors outside their domains, such as the efforts to ensure clean water and air, to regulate the food industry, and to improve automobile safety. But the understanding of the importance of cross-sector work and the social determinants of health have gained greater currency only in the past decade.

This change represents nothing less than a cultural shift in public health practice. Not surprisingly, such a shift does not happen overnight. Due in part to the availability of discretionary funding, some public health and health care organizations have found it easier to change the larger social and political environment and/or the comfort level through change among leaders and practitioners.

Undeniably, there are success stories and model initiatives, supported by philanthropy and by government, that are pointing the way forward. The "early adopters" are role models for others who are interested in broadening their partnerships. Such efforts need to be brought to scale and supported by systematic policies and widespread practice. In summary, the interest in cross-sector work is widespread, but more attention, prioritization, and dedicated resources are needed if this interest is to be matched by action. This chapter briefly reviews the phenomena of growing awareness, innovation, and continued obstacles to near-universal implementation and concludes with some recommendations for further progress.

## INCREASING AWARENESS OF THE IMPORTANCE OF AND EFFORTS TO PROMOTE CROSS-SECTOR WORK

The writings and work of Sir Michael Marmot and the 2005 creation of the World Health Organization's Commission on Social Determinants established a framework for addressing the social and economic influences on health, which often involved the linkage of the health sectors to non-health sectors. Within the United States, the Robert Wood Johnson Foundation advanced this work with its County Health Rankings criteria, which heavily weighted the social determinants in such sectors as education, employment, and community safety. This was further enhanced with the Foundation's promotion of the notion of a "culture of health."

These public health and health care efforts to link with other sectors have received a fair amount of attention. *The Practical Playbook: Public Health and Primary Care Together* provided a single location for learning about those who were building these linkages and learning lessons. Its existence accelerated the uptake. While these "early adopters" demonstrated great promise, the most successful efforts have mostly been confined to a limited number of pilot or well-funded locations. The conditions to bring them to scale and accomplish national spread have not existed.

## THE PUBLIC HEALTH SECTOR'S POTENTIAL LEADERSHIP IN CROSS-SECTOR EFFORTS

The public health sector is well-suited to assume a leadership role in the promotion of cross-sector health-promoting initiatives. Unlike the health care sector, its focus is not on a patient panel but on the whole population within a jurisdiction, which draws it more frequently into contact with other sectors at the community level. In addition, there is a long, if uneven, tradition of public health cross-sector activity from the early 1900s, when the focus ranged from community sanitation in housing to collaboration with the transportation sector in addressing the needs of pedestrians and bikers and to partnership with the public safety sector in preventing and responding to emergencies.

Following the major budget cuts to public health in the Great Recession, many public health officials and advocates reflected on what was core to public health.[2] The rapid increase of chronic diseases with complex risk factors, such as obesity and diabetes, precipitated a growing recognition of the importance of work with the non-health sectors on such matters as addressing "food deserts" and the lack of available sites for physical activity. A few concepts provided guidance for the public health departments of the future, and these invariably identified a major role in developing cross-sector partnerships.

The first is the concept of the *chief health strategist*, which identified seven necessary characteristics for leaders of health departments of the future.[3] Two of these characteristics involved cross-sector work. The first prioritized a stronger partnership between the public health and the health care sectors, particularly in the context of expanded opportunities for health insurance coverage. The second characteristic prioritized additional cross-sector work with a wide array of non-health sectors, such as housing, transportation, and education.

A second widely disseminated concept (incorporating the chief health strategist model) was that of Public Health 3.0.[4] It framed "public health" as what society does to ensure the existence of conditions in which everyone can be healthy. It highlights the necessity of many sectors working collaboratively to achieve these conditions. The public health sector is singled out to assume a key role as a leader in partnering across multiple sectors and leveraging data and resources to address social, environmental, and economic environmental conditions. Since its launch in 2016 by the US Department of Health and Human Services, the Public Health 3.0 initiative has been a widely used guide for departments throughout the nation that are seeking to modernize their approach to public health and meet the emerging epidemiologic challenges underlying rising morbidity and mortality in the United States—the social determinants of health.

## OBSTACLES REMAIN IN ACHIEVING EFFECTIVE CROSS-SECTOR PARTNERSHIPS

A major obstacle has been the lack of resources. Relatively few public health agencies receive specialized funding or have the necessary training to work in authentic partnership with other sectors. The health care sector has a growing number of examples of formalized efforts, such as screening for social determinants, but its financial incentive to do so or the availability of specialized personnel familiar with other sectors is limited. And this is made all the more challenging by limited research regarding which cross-sector interventions work in meaningful and measurable ways.

Though there is a growing recognition of the importance of cross-sector partnership as an essential modern public health approach, there are obstacles to fully realizing the model and to sustaining it beyond focused projects or the tenure of charismatic leaders. Perhaps the primary obstacle is that there are few dedicated resources to support partnership work, and the cost is still poorly defined. Adding to this challenge is the fact that public health is primarily funded with governmental dollars that are restricted for specific purposes, usually to a specific health condition or programmatic effort. This structure of funding does not lend itself to work with another sector. Similarly, other sectors often lack the resources to dedicate to cross-sector health efforts. For example, health care providers and public health practitioners who identify the housing needs of their clients may establish partnerships with those in the housing sector. But the partnerships by themselves will not create additional housing and may in fact create additional pressures and frustrations for both clients and supportive housing agencies.

In addition, public health practitioners require training, skill-building, and support for some of the inter-sector work. For example, those interacting with the transportation sector would be more likely to contribute positively if they understood its decision-making, funding, and priority-setting rules and practices. Similarly, a lack of understanding of the community investment sector by public health officials proved to be a major barrier to partnership in a recent foundation-funded effort to bring the two sectors together.

Data sharing is a necessary element of successful public health interventions, including those that are multisectoral. Combining data sources can be a problem across some sectors for reasons of data confidentiality or privacy, particularly in the health care or educational systems. Though progress has been made, the data typically describing public health status, including social determinants data, are not timely and granular enough for action. In other situations, data sharing can be impeded by data-blocking practices as systems seek to deliberately restrict data access, failing to perceive the public good of making the data available and preferring to retain data to further their own organizational purposes. Perhaps the most significant challenge facing multisector partnerships is the limitation derived from the differing data infrastructures or the complete lack of a digital underpinning for many of the key social services partners needed to adequately address the social determinants of health.

Time is also needed to make a noticeable difference in health, particularly when those differences result from preventive measures. Often the impact of changes in other sector policies can take years to be noted. Over time, confounding variables interfere with definitive proof of impact, and often there is variability in the implementation of the efforts in the field, making for a mixed evidence base. In addition, our current actuarial and fiscal approaches in the United States do not provide for a means of appropriately estimating the impact of public health and preventive measures.

An investment in one sector may have results that impact another sector, but not its own. For example, paying for certain types of behavioral services by insurers may help with high school graduation or recidivism in the criminal justice system. But that likely will not motivate the insurers or other funders for whom success is often measured by controlling the costs of insurance premiums. This is the so-called *wrong pocket* problem, in which investments or savings in one sector are not easily accrued to another. This can hinder the sustainability of funding and partnerships.

In the current environment of declining federal, state, and local public health funding, it is unlikely that there will be a major infusion of new resources in the near future to address these obstacles. Progress needs to be made by directing funding to support multisector work that addresses the social determinants of health. We must also aggressively seek funding from philanthropies, insurance reimbursement, and innovative approaches to tapping targeted taxation, private funding, and social impact bonds.

## EXISTING MODELS OF EVIDENCE-BASED ACTION

Community-level cross-sector action is increasingly common across the nation regardless of the obstacles and unevenness of readiness for cross-sector action. There are many models of agencies that are leading the way and offering valuable lessons as well as of leaders driving this innovation. Many are highlighted in the later sections of this book.

The Public Health 3.0 report highlighted many such examples.[2] In some cases, the efforts are led by local public health, as in Healthy Allegheny, in Pittsburgh, Pennsylvania. In other cases, public health is an integral partner, but another sector is in the lead. For example, in Tennessee, the Nashville Health effort has been led by the business sector. Communities, such as Lawrence-Douglas County in Kansas, have forged a partnership led by public health and the local university that is focused on addressing substance use disorders.

Within the health care sector there have been positive examples as well, such as the Centers for Medicare and Medicaid Services (CMS) Innovation Center's groundbreaking Accountable Health Communities (AHC) initiative.[3] This model funds communities to assess the value of patient screening and linkage to housing and social service agencies. These efforts are raising the awareness of the health care sector to the importance and value of addressing all determinants of health. A number of organizations are emerging to provide support for health care organizations to bridge with community public health and social services organizations in addressing health-related social needs and to move more broadly to address the social determinants of health. The long-term partnership of Kaiser Permanente and Health Leads is an example of a successful model that connects patients to community-based resources.[4]

Other more recent efforts that have highlighted how to effectively design and/or implement partnerships between public health and health care and the work of other sectors include the Health Impact in 5 Years (HI-5) Initiative of the Centers for Disease Control and Prevention (CDC) (with 14 evidence-based policies, 6 of which involve sectors such as transportation, education, and others)[5]; the Camden Coalition of Health Care Providers (and its demonstrated connection between poor health and environment factors such as contaminated housing); and the UCLA Win-Win Project (which demonstrated that many public health interventions have positive implications for other sectors, such as education and crime).[6]

## RECOMMENDATIONS FOR FUTURE ACTION

Despite the potential challenges, cross-sector work is becoming increasingly common because such approaches are necessary to improve the public's health in an increasingly complex and resource-lean world. All of those engaged in this work—whether at the research, planning, implementation, or evaluation stage—are to be congratulated and encouraged. Their efforts—presumably your efforts, since you are reading this chapter—are important to advancing the field.

In consideration of the circumstances mentioned herein, we offer the following broad areas of necessary action to assure an inclusive and sustainable set of solutions:

- Develop leadership training for public health to develop chief health strategists
- Ensure specialized funding for staffing and infrastructure to support multisector partnerships
- Train and provide technical assistance to health department employees and key health sector leaders to build skills in multisector collaborative efforts
- Promote data liquidity and partnerships to mobilize and leverage data
- Expand research to show the return on investment of multisector collaboration

Multisector partnerships are complex but rewarding and can lead to significant and durable change. As public health transforms into a 21st-century model, communities will need to work together to create innovative and sustained organizational structures that include agencies or organizations across multiple sectors and with a shared vision. This will allow a blending and braiding of funding sources to capture savings for reinvestment over time and create a long-term roadmap for creating health, equity, and resilience in communities.

## REFERENCES

1. US Department of Health and Human Services. Healthy people 2020. https://www.healthypeople.gov. Accessed March 16, 2018.

2. DeSalvo KB, Wang YC, Harris A, Auerbach J, Koo D, O'Carroll P. Public Health 3.0: A call to action for public health to meet the challenges of the 21st century. *Prev Chronic Dis.* 2017;14:170017.

3. Accountable Health Communities Model. https://innovation.cms.gov/initiatives/ahcm/. Accessed 1/16/2019.

4. https://healthleadsusa.org/resource-library/roadmap/. Accessed 1/16/2019.

5. Camden Coalition of Healthcare Providers. https://www.camdenhealth.org/. Accessed 1/16/2019.

6. The WIN WIN Project. https://winwin.uclacha.org/. Accessed 1/16/2019.

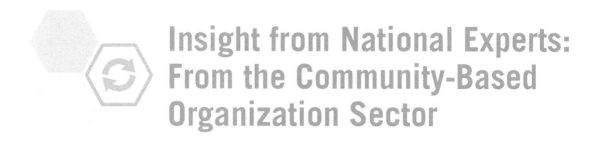

# Chapter 4

# Insight from National Experts: From the Community-Based Organization Sector

KIM FOREMAN AND SANDRA BYRD CHAPPELLE

A powerful paradigm shift is taking shape within the health sector. With an increasing understanding of the social determinants of health has come a growing understanding of the relationship (intersectionality) between human health and other leading indicators of well-being, from full employment to educational attainment and fair mortgage lending. Within the health sector, stronger ties are being forged between traditional health institutions, such as health departments and hospital systems, with community-based organizations (CBOs). In Cleveland, Environmental Health Watch (EHW), a small nonprofit with 35 years' experience in research and program development, is helping residents and institutions re-examine how they engage with one another to keep resident voices front and center in community development work. A number of annotated lessons were outlined during the local evaluation process of the Cleveland BUILD Health Challenge initiative, Engaging Communities in New Approaches to Healthy Housing (ECNAHH) (Figure 4.1). After 2 years, a growing network of residents and nongovernmental organizations (NGOs), together with public health officials and hospitals, attest to the value of having a local nonprofit serve as the backbone organization.

## ENVIRONMENTAL HEALTH WATCH

The role of EHW in the community has been twofold: (1) to align its technical and research capacity around environmental health issues, combined with (2) in-depth input from affected communities (those suffering from longstanding policies that have undermined the housing stock in low- to moderate-income, predominantly minority neighborhoods). Ongoing funding to sustain

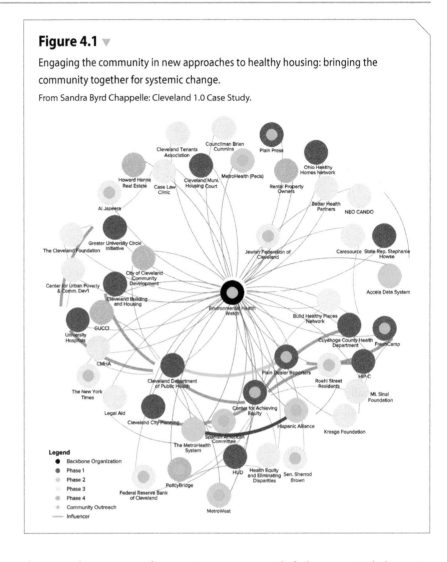

### Figure 4.1 ▼

Engaging the community in new approaches to healthy housing: bringing the community together for systemic change.

From Sandra Byrd Chappelle: Cleveland 1.0 Case Study.

**Legend**

- Backbone Organization
- Phase 1
- Phase 2
- Phase 3
- Phase 4
- Community Outreach
— Influencer

this critical community function is necessary to shift the power imbalances in the current system that maintains the status quo.

## A 35+ Year History: Healthy Homes Pioneer

The mission of EHW is to create healthy homes and sustainable communities by identifying and removing hazards, engaging people, and advancing equitable environmental solutions. Originally organized as a volunteer group known as the Council on Hazardous Materials in 1980, EHW is Northeast Ohio's longest standing environmental justice organization. This group of volunteers, consisting of concerned citizens and health professionals, began developing activities to educate the public about emerging concerns related to hazardous waste, pollution, and chemical accidents and how these impact human health and the overall environment. EHW positioned itself to be one of the first organizations to receive a Department of Housing and Urban Development (HUD) lead grant and a lead hazard control abatement training center for those hard to employ. Since its incorporation, the organization as a thought leader has engaged and convened concerned citizens and representatives regarding important and evolving environmental justice issues. EHW has partnered with numerous academic researchers throughout its history to further its understanding of environmental needs and develop new approaches to evolving environmental challenges. They continue to provide leadership and work alongside local, county, and state policymakers to address critical environmental justice and health concerns, develop policies, conduct research, and provide direct service to children and families.

The pioneering conferences convened by EHW, A Blueprint for a Healthy House, and produced jointly with the Housing Resource Center have taken place annually from 1985 to 1990. These were the first national meetings to bring together housing and health agencies and activists for an exchange on indoor pollution. In 1990, EHW published the Healthy House Catalog, the first national directory of residential pollution resources. In partnership with the Cleveland Department of Public Health (CDPH), EHW developed and operated the Cleveland Lead Hazard Abatement Center, a national model for addressing lead hazard control in low-income housing (1993–1995).

## EHW's Approach to the Work

Intersectionality has always been a part of how EHW models, pilots, and structures the projects. The Healthy Homes and Sustainable Communities projects, programs, and initiatives are core to our mission. EHW has evolved to include prioritizing and incorporating health equity and environmental justice as the foundation to its two program areas. Beginning with the Lead + Asthma Project with the City of Cleveland Health Department in 1998, EHW now continues its work with partners to build capacity and institutionalize healthy homes. In a leadership role, EHW is a neutral party that can bring sectors together, breaking down silos and reframing a disconnected approach to the work on the ground as well as with decision-makers. EHW is a small nonprofit in size, and collaboration has been embedded in the culture of the organization as regards its approach to the work and its position for success. During 35 years, EHW has worked intentionally to develop new relationships with strategic partners and has maintained many of the same partnerships through direct service projects, multisector collaboration, research, and advocacy efforts. To develop the correct set of partners, the expertise of the partner must be thoroughly investigated and the partner's role within the partnership must be defined. Leaders at EHW understand how to lead as well as follow. The approach has been very research-based, with EHW having the background to assist with technical expertise and possessing the understanding that fosters respect, as well as having the authority to lead. Having the research background and direct service experience, as well as the humility to listen and the willingness to continue learning from others, helps EHW bring a unique perspective to the table.

Sustainability: *How we define as an organization: We believe in promoting regenerative environments and communities by supporting continuous enhancement of health, justice, and prosperity while maintaining respect for the natural, social, cultural, and historic values of place and the people who live there.*

*In leadership, initiate
and ask the important
questions at the devel-
opment stage: Who is
sitting at the table before
the proposals and budgets
are created? Are we
moving the needle? Are we
profiting from unhealthy
communities? If we are
to thrive as a society, an
entire population suffering
from all types of social
factors that impact health
is unacceptable.*

## TACKLING THE ROOT CAUSE OF HEALTH INEQUITIES

Organizations, institutions, and decision-makers can't continue to write *about* impacted communities in their proposals, implement misguided projects, or have conversations focused solely on health disparity maps without actually hearing from, building authentic relationships with, and working with residents and leaders from the impacted communities. Health *as defined by impacted communities* has to be integrated into the initial development of projects, programs, initiatives, research, and conversations. Partnering in a different way will provide more authenticity, sustainability, and direction. Working this way is not a cookie-cutter process, and it can be messy. A true grassroots approach of equitable transition and application feels and looks different when we actually work toward shifting decision-making power to residents. From our perspective, the health equity movement is an extension of the environmental justice movement that began with the environmental racism conversation. The conditions haven't changed; they have just been repackaged and redefined. The US Environmental Protection Agency defines environmental justice as the fair treatment and meaningful involvement of all people regardless of race, color, national origin, or income with respect to the development, implementation, and enforcement of environmental laws, regulations, and policies.

Change to traditional leadership roles in community partnerships, such as who serves as the applicant organization and who gets invited to the table, inevitably causes shifts in ownership and participation while also generating power struggles, both subtle and pronounced. However, these partnerships are important and need to remain intact, continue to grow, and be responsive to the needs of the community; therefore, how conflict and issues are handled is important. Positive progressive change comes about when the affected group of constituents is properly represented at the table; this is well-documented in research, yet it can be hard to execute. In Cleveland, we have documented an initiative centered on how community-envisioned, community-led, and community-sustained work can be well executed and sustained when partners adhere consistently to this theory of change.[1]

Many CBOs, such as EHW, are designed with resident leadership in mind. They have the expertise to bring in those most affected by policies and/or program and system design to push past inertia and lead the way to the systemic change needed.

### Advancing Collaboration and Mitigating Power and Control: Examples from the Field

In any relationship, whether it is a marriage, business, or social alliance, miscues, miscommunication, and disagreements are bound to occur. How issues are handled is the key to whether a healthy, functioning relationship develops. To create the desired systemic change, new relationships must be formed among partner organizations and community members. Purposeful relationship-building increases the levels of trust and respect among network members. Recognizing when the use of old paradigms foster distrust and promote the perception of power and control is equally important. The following examples are illustrative of the type of power and control struggles that partners have identified and addressed; these are provided so that others in the field might be encouraged to identify and work through similar issues and increase their effectiveness in using equitable practices.

The following excerpt describes shared learning from Cleveland, Ohio, during the first round of the BuildHealth Challenge funding regarding building organizational and community trust.

## EXAMPLE 1: TRANSPARENT COMMUNICATION

In the early stages of the work, new personal and organizational relationships were being formed. One organizational representative was finding it difficult to grasp the details of the budding partnership and was ineffective in bringing back important details to their organization's chief executive officer, yet insisted on serving as the sole conduit to their organizational executive. This failure to communicate was preventing specific activities detailed in the organization's memorandum of understanding from moving forward.

*Solution.* After considerable efforts to work through the impasse with the agency representative failed, the backbone organization found it necessary to meet personally with the chief executive of the partner organization to communicate necessary information. An insignificant detail? The contrary is true. Bottlenecks often occur when a key staff person is not in agreement with organizational priorities and blocks progress. Senior leadership is generally never aware of what is happening. Often, the organizational representative is relying on his or her role within the organization to serve as a protective buffer between outside organizations and executive staff. Creating memorandums of understanding (MOU) related to partner roles early on made it possible to address these issues and sidestep the personal agenda of the organizational representative.

*Result.* In this instance, communication needed to be handled in such a way as to respect the organizational representative while resolving the issues creating the impasse. Using the commitments outlined in the MOU, the backbone organization arranged a friendly meeting to touch base with the executive officer of the partner organization. This action enabled forward movement on the original commitments.

## EXAMPLE 2: INCLUSION

As awareness of the partnership and its approach grew, several network members grew excited about the approach and began planning to replicate aspects of the work into other initiatives and partnerships. Contrary to expectations, a few organizations within the broader network made plans to seek funding to replicate key aspects of the work with other mainstream institutions with whom they had traditionally partnered. Left out of the budding replication process was the organization that had designed and piloted the initial approach. The mainstream organizations leading the replication process did not invite them to the partnership table, planning instead with partners with whom they had history.

*Solution.* Strategic Solutions Partners functioned as an intermediary in its role to create an ongoing learning community within the partnership and arranged a meeting with one of the lead organizations to raise awareness of how the planned replication was perceived. With newfound awareness and better understanding of local history, the planned replication was reworked to include the grassroots organization.

*Result.* With this small gesture, the excluded organization was brought to the table, their expertise included, and new opportunities to partner were cemented and continue to grow. As often happens, organizations gravitate toward those with whom they have shared experiences. It takes time and commitment, but new and more effective relationships can be created when we shift our thinking about who needs to be at the table.

## EXAMPLE 3: AMPLIFYING COMMUNITY VOICE

As community outreach efforts began, resident members of the partnership voiced concern over a major displacement effort happening within our targeted area. Area residents were living in poorly maintained rental properties owned by landlords with significant community clout. The tenants, all of whom were Latino, were being pressured to move through immediate, significant rent hikes. They did not have rental agreements and were paying cash on a month-to-month basis. Efforts to reason with the landlords were fruitless, and discussions with area nonprofits and community leaders had fallen on deaf ears. Some members of the team felt that this issue had nothing to do with our efforts and had no problem voicing this sentiment to residents. Housing displacement was an immediate crisis for these resident and superseded the work we were asking them to help lead. Their imminent displacement and the way in which the housing agreements had been set up left this close-knit group of residents with new stressors and little to no support from local CBOs. These types of issues contribute to the overall demise of community health due to the high stress levels and little ability to control what some would describe as unjust circumstances.

*Solution.* This circumstance became a teachable moment for ECNAHH community engagement partners: if ECNAHH expected residents to partner in identifying homes to remediate (one of our priorities), we needed to be attentive to related community conditions identified by residents as their priorities (imminent displacement). In fact, residents noted their frustration about well-intentioned groups that ask for support in carrying out work designed to help them only to retreat from the community—groups that have little interest in understanding how they might support the community in ways that matter to *them*. This might mean being prepared to delay a planned intervention until trust has been established by first attending to a community-identified priority. This attention to community priorities might mean in-kind planning, resource identification, or another action valued by community residents

*Result.* When all was said and done, one partner representative said they had gained a better understanding of the broader work related to the social determinants of health. Residents were displaced but were given time, with financial assistance, to relocate. The outcome was not what residents hoped for, but partnership intervention brought some relief to their situation and tangible evidence of mutual respect and concern.

## Strong CBO Leadership: Multisector Partnerships and Initiatives

Health is core to the mission of EHW and everything the organization does. It affects how the organization advocates, conducts research, and provides direct service. In addition, leadership and learning is always centered and grounded in human health. Using a broader definition of health than simply the absence of disease, it is important to recognize the social determinants as a precursor to full health. We can have a critical eye, but we can also sit at the table to participate in finding solutions that bring value while incorporating an equitable approach with health considerations. Partnership and the ability to convene multiple stakeholders and sectors for EHW is essential to our production. EHW cultivates authentic relationships with core partners and continues to engage with new sectors and stakeholders over time. Stakeholders also include residents and resident leaders, not just organizations and institutions. Partners have to establish a shared vision and values. Equity can be established and found within budgets and line items. Who decides whose expertise is more valuable? The grassroots and nonprofit communities are often devalued or not considered to be a necessary piece of the constructed plan or core team. Credible nonprofits can be a valuable asset to the development and execution of research projects, policies, and programs, but they need to be compensated fairly. Often, EWH is sought after to partner without pay, to volunteer, or to participate in a community engagement "check-the-box" exercise for the benefit of larger institutions with more power and funding. Now, opportunities are spearheaded by national foundations to create a new method and model of funding and leadership as it relates to multisector partnerships truly formed to advance equity (internal to the partnerships), as well as to focus on root causes and solutions that are community-led and sustainable.

In 2009, EHW was awarded an EPA Community Action for a Renewed Environment (CARE) grant. The partners, including Environmental Health Watch, Neighborhood Leadership Institute, the Cleveland Clean Air Century Campaign, and Earth Day Coalition, formed Neighborhood Leadership for Environmental Health (NLEH). This partnership brought together community stakeholders (residents, businesses, churches, institutions, and government agencies) in a collaborative process of data-gathering and education, followed by consensus priority-setting and action plan development, to address significant environmental concerns in Cleveland's east-side, inner-city neighborhoods. Our goal was to develop a sustainable environmental justice partnership.

One major turning point for EHW was leading the NLEH and having the opportunity to utilize the social determinants of health framing within our mission and direct service projects, which made sense and gave definition to what the organization was attempting to facilitate within communities of color. At the same time, the Centers for Achieving Equity (CAE; formerly Cuyahoga PlaceMatters) was at the forefront of the health equity movement, providing leadership and guidance for organizations, institutions, and policy- and decision-makers across the country. Since 2016, EHW has held a leadership role on the CAE team. Prior to joining, we were folding in and elevating the health equity frame and concepts into the organizational mission and vision of EHW.

The NLEH project was carried out in the context of an effort by Neighborhood Leadership Institute and EHW toward "greening the 'hood," aimed at bridging the divide between Cleveland's strong environmental organizations and people living in low-income, inner-city neighborhoods. In four targeted communities (Woodland, Buckeye, Central, and Fairfax), numerous problems exist (e.g., substandard housing, lack of access to fresh and high-quality food, air pollution, and high prevalence of lead poisoning and asthma), which can be improved by green approaches facilitated through collaboration between environmental organizations and neighborhood groups. This inclusive "green for all" strategy strengthens both. To date, we have built the capacity of four resident leaders who are still engaged as leaders and advisors in environmental justice- and health-related initiatives in the city of Cleveland and Cuyahoga County. We were able to implement several direct service and youth leadership projects focused in the city of Cleveland (Green Houses and Greenhouses; Easy Does It Cooking Classes I & II; Roots of Success Environmental Literacy Classes; Youth Farmers Leadership Project; and Race, Food & Justice Conferences, 2013–2018; and a Kresge Foundation FreshLo grant, 2017–2019). EHW continues to work with adult and youth leaders in different settings. Hunter Scott and Zri Hitchcock graduated from the Youth Farmers Leadership Project and currently contract with EHW on projects. EHW is the go-to environmental justice and environmental health organization in Cuyahoga County.

Developing and building the sustainable communities program in a grassroots fashion from the ground up led to partnerships with community development corporations, city planning, city council members, funders, and resident leaders. We expanded our community partners beyond the health departments, researchers, and institutions we were commonly affiliated with. Working within communities takes a lot of hard work, understanding, and flexibility. The planning team was willing to work on weekends and evenings, knocking on doors and passing out flyers, to build the base and truly partner with community.

The Healthy Eating Active Living (HEAL) Buckeye initiative demonstrated that residents can effectively envision, lead, and sustain efforts to create stronger communities through engaged residents.[1] It also illustrates the importance of sustained partnerships among communities, funding organizations, and policymakers and has demonstrated that it is possible to create shared visioning among people with diverse backgrounds and from different socioeconomic groups. HEAL is a community partnership working to make healthy eating and active living a part of the culture and everyday living in the Buckeye, Larchmere, and Woodland Hills neighborhoods. Together, families, friends, community groups, neighborhood organizations, and local businesses are working to transform the neighborhood into a place that supports healthy living, where options for healthy food and exercise are widely available, affordable, accessible, and desirable. EHW played a leadership role and leveraged funding from the Baldwin Foundation to implement cooking classes at Woodhill Homes as part of the technical assistance provided to residents. The HEAL initiative started within the same year that NLEH began, so we partnered and combined portions of the initiatives within the same service area, which strengthened both efforts. Guided by a council of community stakeholders consisting of residents, community organizations, and other neighborhood stakeholders, the HEAL initiative focuses on building strategies for and by the community in six areas: (1) affordable, accessible healthy food; (2) opportunities for exercise that build relationships; (3) opportunities to learn and practice healthy living skills; (4) communication and awareness about healthy living; (5) intraconnected and interconnected communities; and (6) healthy and safe community gathering spaces.[2]

## EHW LEADING SYSTEMS CHANGE: THE BUILD HEALTH CHALLENGE

The BUILD Health Challenge is creating a new norm in the United States by putting multisector, community-driven partnerships at the center of health to reduce health disparities caused by system-based or social inequity. This national program strengthens partnerships among CBOs, hospitals and health systems, local health departments, and others to cultivate a shared commitment to moving resources, attention, and action upstream to drive sustainable improvements in community health. BUILD Health Challenge–funded communities are required to have a local nonprofit organization to serve as the lead applicant. This requirement is a unique aspect of the BUILD Health Challenge framework and sets the stage to level power imbalances often found among residents, grassroots organizations, and traditional institutions. The requirement promotes authentic community-led visioning and gives residents a voice, essential components in effective local health and systemic change initiatives. EHW is the backbone organization for the partnership, and it works to ensure a culture of learning among partners. Much of the learning centers on authentic community leadership by ensuring that all levels of systems within the Cleveland housing sector are working together to foster sustainable, replicable systemic change. Identifying and addressing inequities related to power and control are integral components of the work. Staff from BUILD Health Challenge member organizations come with varying degrees of awareness related to the social determinants of health as well as how to apply an equity lens to planning and policy development. The CAE works with the partnership to identify and address partner activities that are leaning toward inequitable practices. CAE is also documenting local practices that build community capacity to advance equitable systemic change

## BUILD Health 1.0: Engaging the Community in New Approaches to Healthy Housing (2015–2017)

*The Center for Achieving Equity (CAE) equips affiliates to use an equity lens across multiple sectors, such as philanthropy, public health, city planning, environment, civic engagement, housing, and policymaking.*

Partners have aligned around creating a Healthy Homes Zone (HHZ) to tackle a root cause of local health issues—unhealthy housing. Goals of residents, MetroWest CDC, EHW, the CDPH, MetroHealth Hospital, the Hispanic Alliance, the Spanish-American Committee, and Cuyahoga PlaceMatters Community Health Equity Report converge around the health hazards associated with aged housing and blight. The partners envision achieving increased health equity by means of policies and strategies that engage the community inclusively and address prevention of home health hazards. Data systems managed by partner organizations along with established and planned relationships to share and evaluate the effects of interventions and policy/systems change will provide evidence of the efficacy of our approach.

### Community Impact and Outcomes of BUILD Health 1.0

The BUILD Health 1.0 project in Cleveland focused on policy efforts, code enforcement, and upstream approaches. In 2017, EHW integrated Public Health Department inspection/lead data into the City of Cleveland Accela data system, and the Building and Housing Department launched a proactive rental inspection program. The following results were also noted: (1) we expanded the City of Cleveland Accela data system, which includes a citizen access portal to integrate public health lead inspection data, allowing better workflow, efficiency, and communication between the CDPH and Building and Housing and Community Development department. (2) The initial goal for Building and Housing in 2017 is to inspect 2,500 units; 250 (25%) of the units will receive dust wipes. The city has set the following goals to reach the estimated 84,000 rental units: 2017: 50,000; 2018: 65,000; and 2019: 80,000. (3) The number of registered rentals increased from 35,000 to 42,309 in 2016. We estimate the City of Cleveland to generate $2.3 million/year in rental income. (4) The Hispanic Alliance Community-Based Organization organizers, who are educated in healthy homes, translated materials into Spanish, which allowed the delivery of healthy homes education to Spanish-speaking community residents. (5) We expanded the ability and skill set of MetroWest Community Development Corporation to provide home visits to families, identify hazards, and write intervention specs for contractor remediation services. (6) We are in the process of analyzing cost savings at MetroHealth Hospital system, based on utilization of the emergency room and admissions for patients with asthma and chronic obstructive pulmonary disease (COPD).

## BUILD Health 2.0: Cleveland Healthy Homes Data Collaborative (2017–2019)

The grant partners from BUILD Health 1.0, informed by community input, realized that the portal is only the starting point for a coordinated system for public access and use of healthy homes information. Although housing data from multiple sources is publicly available, systemic barriers limit access and use of the data. EWH will collaboratively develop a data system that shares data across sectors, includes two hospital systems, removes systemic barriers, and provides easy access to health-related housing data. A new healthy housing data system grounded in neighborhood community engagement will enable physicians, public health officials, and the public to easily access collaborative, useful information to address health disparities, with a focus on asthma and lead poisoning. Geocoded housing data relevant to determinants of health will be analyzed and prioritized to provide risk-stratified, place-based information. Value-added data from multisector sources will be used for identifying lead-safe housing, determining patient risk for asthma, supporting public policy, and targeting public health programs. Data will be disseminated through a smart-phone/web app, physician access tools with support for integration with medical records, and community outreach.

## Effectiveness of a Small Nonprofit Organization as Backbone and Intermediary Organization

The role of EHW in the BUILD Health work has demonstrated that smaller nonprofit organizations with the appropriate knowledge base have the capacity to lead major initiatives when properly resourced. In measuring the effectiveness of EHW as the backbone organization, several factors were identified, including the ability to execute, in a timely fashion, MOUs, manage finances, enact communications, promote data sharing and use within the partnership, leverage existing relationships, and engage key stakeholders. Partner observations included the ease of working with EHW, the high caliber of the staff, and the respectfulness and generosity of time, resources, and spirit with which they served community residents. Developing community nonprofits to lead major health programs is an essential element in improving the health of communities.

## REFERENCES

1. Gavin VR, Seeholzer EL, Leon JB, Chappelle SB, Sehgal, AR. If we build it, we will come: A model for community-led change to transform neighborhood conditions to support healthy eating and active living. *Am J Public Health.* 2015;105(6):1072–7. https://reducedisparity.org/research/publications/. Last accessed 1/16/2019.

2. BuildHealth. *Environmental Health Watch: Engaging the Community in New Approaches to Healthy Housing.* Cleveland, OH: BuildHealth. https://buildhealthchallenge.org/communities/engaging-the-community-in-new-approaches-to-healthy-housing/. Accessed 1/16/2019.

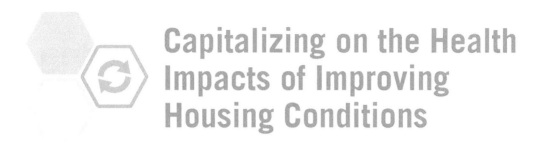

# Chapter 5

# Capitalizing on the Health Impacts of Improving Housing Conditions

MICHAEL MCKNIGHT AND RUTH ANN NORTON

The Green & Healthy Homes Initiative (GHHI) and its collective partners in government, the private sector, and philanthropy have embarked on a revolution in health and housing that is breaking the current link that exists between unhealthy housing and unhealthy families. GHHI is implementing integrative, holistic approaches to health, energy, and housing interventions so the public receives critical services and support in a more effective and efficient manner.

At its headquarters in Baltimore, the organization serves low-income families through an aligned delivery of case management, legal services, in-home environmental health education, and a comprehensive health, safety, and energy audit, as well as root-cause remediation of home-based environmental health hazards. GHHI has more than three decades of experience advocating for and delivering evidenced-based healthy housing services to thousands of families. Founded in 1986 to focus on eradicating lead poisoning, GHHI today has programs that encompass a wide range of services to address housing conditions and health, including lead poisoning, asthma, trip-and-fall injury, and energy efficiency. Based on its innovative, community-based approach to addressing asthma, GHHI was a proud recipient of the 2015 US Environmental Protection Agency (EPA) National Environmental Leadership Award in Asthma Management.

Families in poverty are at risk for eviction, foreclosure, and homelessness, and they often lack the resources, support systems, and connections needed to ensure safe and stable housing. From working with our clients, we were struck by the challenges that exist for families in navigating the significant number of services they may be seeking. For example, if they have an issue with mold in their apartment as a result of a leaky roof, whom should they call? The city's code inspector? A health department program that can address the mold? The

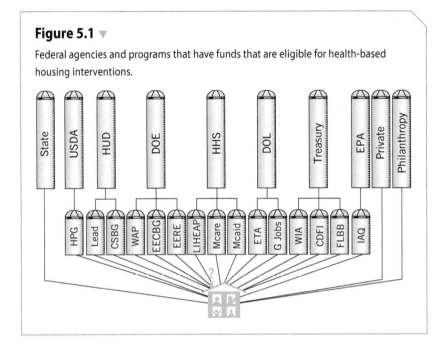

**Figure 5.1 ▼**

Federal agencies and programs that have funds that are eligible for health-based housing interventions.

housing department program with rehabilitation resources to fix the roof? An analysis looking at how a family could get all of their environmental home-based needs addressed found that it would require 23 days off work to meet with all of the various intake officials, inspectors, assessors, and contractors (Figure 5.1).

Dozens of programs and funding streams exist that may provide resources to improve housing conditions. But the local programs that implement those funding streams are rarely connected, and they tend to operate within their own silos.

The GHHI model works to integrate all of those resources to make services work for families. The organization utilizes housing as a platform to advance policies and investments in health, education, and economic mobility. GHHI works with its site partners to:

- *Align* programs and policies for federal, state, and local agencies to focus on integrated housing intervention strategies and standards across energy, health, and safety.
- *Braid* existing and new resources toward an integrated intervention. "Braiding" rather than "blending" refers to the fact that the model can be implemented while each funding stream retains its requirements for eligibility and services.
- *Coordinate* on-the-ground service delivery to better serve families and leverage the work of multiple partners (Figure 5.2).

Through establishing integrated housing programs, GHHI sites around the country are able to reduce energy consumption and costs, address home-based

**Figure 5.2** ▽

Process flow for Green & Healthy Homes Initiative (GHHI) standard practice.

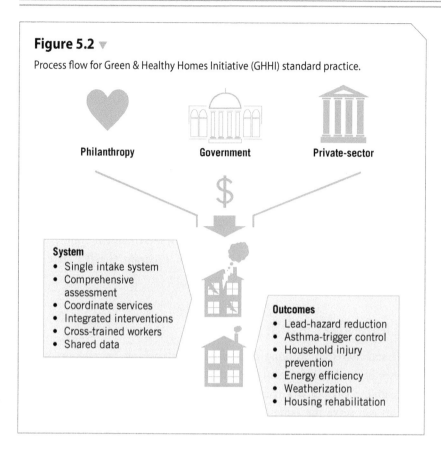

Philanthropy  Government  Private-sector

$

**System**
- Single intake system
- Comprehensive assessment
- Coordinate services
- Integrated interventions
- Cross-trained workers
- Shared data

**Outcomes**
- Lead-hazard reduction
- Asthma-trigger control
- Household injury prevention
- Energy efficiency
- Weatherization
- Housing rehabilitation

environmental hazards that cause asthma episodes, identify lead hazards that cause lead poisoning, and identify hazards that may cause household-related injuries, such as falls. Currently, more than 30 cities and counties are GHHI sites. To implement the model, GHHI staff work with the jurisdiction to execute the following aspects of the program.

## CROSS-SECTOR CONVENING

GHHI meets with stakeholders to develop a strategy to advance the greater integration of health, energy, and housing resources while expanding the capacity of services that can be offered to low-income residents. Stakeholders include but are not limited to the following:

- State, county, and city health departments
- State Medicaid offices
- Health care agencies, insurers, and providers
- State, county, and city departments of housing or environmental agencies
- Weatherization and energy-efficiency providers, including utility programs
- Other housing intervention and service providers or financing entities
- Community health workers, inspectors, and contractors

- Philanthropic, private, and public entities that may contribute resources to support the initiative

## ASSET AND GAP ANALYSIS OF LOCAL HEALTH, ENERGY, AND HOUSING RESOURCES

GHHI conducts an asset and gap analysis in each jurisdiction to identify specific health, energy, and housing resources that can be braided and coordinated. GHHI has developed templates and an effective methodology to identify existing resources as well as to identify community-wide funding gaps that need to be addressed. The organization develops strategies to secure new housing resources through nontraditional sources such as settlement funds, utility foundations, and Children's Health Insurance Program (CHIP) state plan amendments.

## COLLABORATIVE WORK PLAN

GHHI staff develops working collaborations at each site in support of the cross-sector model. The organization develops referral systems, opportunities to streamline eligibility, a triage methodology, a system by which multiple agencies can serve the same family in an efficient manner, and information about how data can be shared and utilized by multiple entities. An Outcome Broker—a person who is responsible for eliminating local service delivery silos by convening otherwise disconnected service providers, implementing coordination strategies, and closing funding and resource gaps—is typically identified in each community to help drive the collaboration.

## TRAINING

GHHI staff also train local partners about the integrated model of resident education, comprehensive assessment, and holistic, integrated interventions. Technical assistance staff also bridge sectors and support engagement between the local health, housing, and energy sectors and related associations.

## EVIDENCED-BASED MODEL

The data coming out of GHHI's work related to the impact in health outcomes, educational outcomes, and family stability have helped drive new partnerships with health care and the education sectors. In a study published in the journal *Environmental Justice*,[1] GHHI's work in Baltimore has shown that addressing housing conditions in a streamlined manner results in significant impacts to health. To date, Baltimore City residents served by GHHI have experienced the following:

- A 66% reduction in asthma-related hospitalizations
- A 62% increase in children not missing any school days due to asthma
- An 88% increase in parents not missing any work days due to their child's asthma

Similar results have been seen in work in Philadelphia (70% reduction in hospitalizations due to asthma, 76% reduction in emergency department visits) and Cleveland (58% reduction in hospitalizations, 63% reduction in emergency department visits) that follow GHHI's integrated approach.

The organization has also drawn on the strong evidence base in the literature around the impact of housing conditions. Existing research was compelling enough for the Surgeon General's Call to Action to Promote Healthy Homes[2] in 2009, which lays out the health and housing intersection. Multiple research studies have provided evidence that comprehensive asthma interventions inclusive of home-based environmental trigger reduction can improve asthma management. These services are included in the National Institutes of Health (NIH) National Asthma Education and Prevention Program (NAEPP) Expert Panel Report 3 (EPR 3).[3] The Centers for Disease Control and Prevention's Community Preventive Services Task Force implemented a systematic review of comprehensive asthma interventions and published results on the Community Guide website (Community Preventive Services Task Force 2011).[4]

- The Task Force recommends the use of home-based multitrigger, multicomponent interventions with an environmental focus for children and adolescents with asthma based on strong evidence of effectiveness in improving overall quality of life and productivity.
- The meta-analysis shows a median decrease of 0.57 acute health care visits per year, and cost-benefit studies also show a return of $5.30 to $14.00 for each dollar invested.

To further the evidence base for the specific GHHI model, the organization, in partnership with the US Department of Housing and Urban Development (HUD) and The Hilltop Institute at the University of Maryland, Baltimore County (UMBC), is conducting a Healthy Homes Technical Study using administrative data and a rigorous matched comparison group design to analyze the impact of GHHI's services on Medicaid claims and costs, school absences, and energy consumption and costs.

To turn positive outcomes into the basis of a stronger working relationship across sectors, GHHI has incorporated additional analysis to monetize the impact of healthy homes services for the entities that benefit from these services. In our case, this is Medicaid programs and health plans that avoid expenditures when their members stop going to the emergency department and the hospital once their homes are improved.

Often, housing programs do not have access to the relevant data to make a business case for their services. A health plan that GHHI works with in Maryland conducted an internal analysis using their claims data to report that, 6 months post intervention, their members who had received GHHI services had their average total cost of care lowered by one-third. This type of analysis is conducted routinely by health plans, and the data were aggregated and de-identified so that it could be shared with GHHI. Other programs could reach out to their local managed care organizations to conduct similar analyses.

Not only can the right data provide evidence for the value of a program that addresses social determinants of health to a particular health care payer, it can also be used to identify the right patient population for a contractual relationship between a payer and a provider. Patient-level data maintained by hospitals and health plans allow tracking of utilization, such as hospitalizations and emergency department visits, over time. These data can indicate which patients or members are ideal potential enrollees into a new program based on need and the potential impact on return-on-investment of these services.

The findings of the analysis can be used to develop enrollment criteria. In GHHI's asthma projects, this could be, for example, a Medicaid member who has had a hospitalization with asthma as a primary diagnosis. With managed care organizations, GHHI has often had actuarial analysis of claims across multiple years to help indicate to payers the potential impact in medical cost reduction of a comprehensive asthma intervention model. In Memphis, for example, Tennessee Medicaid (TennCare) provided GHHI's actuarial partner, Milliman, with data from statewide claims across 5 years. In New York State, GHHI analyzed the New York Medicaid population to determine the scale of members who would be potentially positively impacted by energy efficiency and healthy homes services.

Once the scale of the population is established, a critical issue is to assess how that potential set of patients will be referred into the new program. Will referrals come from the emergency department? An outpatient clinic? The health department? A health plan's disease management program? Often, "warm handoffs" from primary care physicians or clinical staff to the community-based program lead to higher enrollment rates. The information included in the referral can be important as well; the more information that can be shared by the health care entity, the better prepared a community-based program will be in delivering services. The information shared is usually set out in a business associate agreement.

## PROGRAM DESIGN

Designing a program model involves a collaborative effort between medical providers, healthy homes providers, and other social service providers. Programs need to ensure efficient delivery of services and avoid duplication of efforts. The scale is also critical to determine if the capacity exists among community-based providers to meet the need of potential patients who meet the eligibility criteria.

Another important aspect is performance management. Healthy homes providers and their local health care organizations utilize different data systems. Health care data are especially sensitive, given considerations related to receiving, storing, and transmitting protected health information (PHI). It is often easier to design a data management plan in which health care referral partners have access to a housing or social service data platform than one in which nonclinical providers receive access to PHI.

To accurately set costs and budget, begin with a good understanding of all program elements, including staffing, supplies, and services. If elements of the services are unknown, you can review similar models, either locally or nationally. Having partnerships with other organizations or programs that can also provide services to the patient, but that have resources from other areas, can help the program lower its average cost.

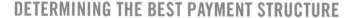

## DETERMINING THE BEST PAYMENT STRUCTURE

Services that address the social determinants of health are often considered apart from medical services but there are various pathways for bringing medical resources to bear. GHHI staff comprehensively assess a variety of potential payment and/or reimbursement mechanisms based on each state's Medicaid program structure and the preferences of health plans or hospital systems.

## COMMUNITY BENEFITS

The Internal Revenue Service (IRS) requires nonprofit hospitals to engage in community benefit activities to qualify for tax exemption. Acceptable activities have grown from charity/uncompensated medical care to include community-based services targeting community health. Every nonprofit hospital has to do a community needs assessment regularly as well as design community-benefit activities to address those needs. Health and safety improvements in housing conditions are eligible activities. In Chicago, working with Presence Health, GHHI identified a set of patients who were regularly receiving uncompensated care for asthma. Presence Health covers its losses from uncompensated care with community benefit funds. After conducting an analysis of potential savings through looking at Presence Health's charge records, GHHI, in partnership with Elevate Energy, designed a pilot that uses community benefit resources upstream. Environmental assessments and interventions for identified patients are being conducted to prevent future energy department visits and hospitalizations.

## VALUE-BASED PURCHASING

Current authority within Medicaid managed care allows for managed care organizations to implement alternative payment models or value-based purchasing arrangements to pay for outcomes rather than a fee for a service. These outcomes may be supported by interventions that address the root causes of many of the most costly medical conditions, such as remediation of mold that triggers asthma attacks. Working in partnership with a Medicaid provider, community-based providers can augment clinical services to help achieve an outcome that triggers a value-based payment to the Medicaid provider, such as a reduction in the total cost of care of a Medicaid member. In New York, the New York State Energy Research and Development Authority (NYSERDA) is working on developing partnerships with managed care organizations and health care providers for people who could benefit from home remediation services; a value-based payment arrangement would be shared with health plans that reduce medical costs for their members.

## PAY FOR SUCCESS FINANCING
## WITH VALUE-BASED PURCHASING

Pay for Success is a relatively new model that aims to shift the spending focus for government and other payers on the outcomes that they want to achieve, rather than funding services with the hope of getting to those outcomes. Private funders provide upfront resources to deliver services, and the end payer only pays if agreed-upon outcomes are met. This model is very much aligned with value-based payment arrangements in Medicaid. As providers enter into more value-based arrangements, Pay for Success financing can help spread the risk to other stakeholders and provide the upfront capital needed to deliver services. In the Memphis project that GHHI is developing, partners are seeking Pay for Success funding to support the high-risk asthma program that Le Bonheur Children's Hospital is implementing. Le Bonheur will be entering into value-based agreements with the Medicaid health plans in Tennessee (Figure 5.3).

## BUNDLED SERVICES

Another approach that makes it easier for nontraditional providers to partner with health care providers is bundling services as part of a payment arrangement. That allows a more comprehensive set of services to be cohesively delivered, rather than to only use specific codes for each specific measure that a holistic intervention will entail. For GHHI's asthma program in Maryland, a bundle for high-risk Amerigroup members was established. That bundle includes multiple home visits overseen by a Certified Asthma Educator, environmental supplies such as a hypoallergenic mattress and pillow covers, environmental assessment, and integrated pest management. A key consideration

**Figure 5.3** ▾

Model to use Medicaid-managed care resources under a value-based arrangement. Upfront capital to deliver services is provided by private funders.

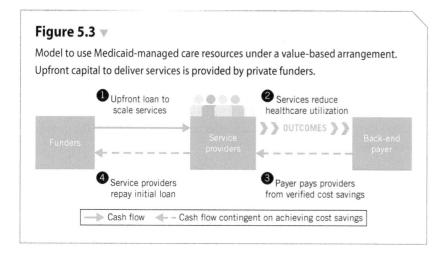

for designing bundles is to identify which services can be considered medical and which would normally have been paid for by the managed care organization out of the administrative portion of their budget.

## OTHER OPTIONS TO FUND HEALTHY HOMES

In 2017, CMS approved a proposal from the Maryland Department of Health to launch a $7.2 million initiative to address two conditions of home environmental health: (1) childhood lead poisoning and (2) asthma. The initiative leverages federal funds available through the CHIP under the authority of a Health Services Initiative (HSI) State Plan Amendment. GHHI is providing training to local health departments on implementing these programs. This arrangement is an example for other states of how to use CHIP to fund healthy homes services.

Other potential health care pathways to pursue coverage of healthy homes services include Medicaid state plan amendments, delivery system reform incentive payment (DSRIP) programs, Medicaid Section 1115 waivers, Medicare Advantage plans, and targeted or community-based care management programs.

## PILOTING SERVICES

Piloting a new partnership is the best way to uncover and solve the challenges of working across different sectors. When building a coordinated housing partnership in a new city, GHHI often works with partners to implement services in one area of the city as a pilot. The purpose of a pilot is to test the operational capacity to deliver services in a collaborative fashion. This can include data management and information sharing. Having strong metrics regarding performance management can make a pilot more worthwhile. It is also important to understand the limitations of pilots. They do not often offer the opportunity to perform academic research or capture statistically significant impact measures because of their small size.

Funding for pilots can come from a variety of sources, including existing operational funds, current grants, new grants, or sources such as hospital community benefits. Once funding is secured and a pilot launches, it is good to periodically review outcomes and adjust as necessary to improve the operation as services are scaled up.

As part of the Presence Hospital project for uninsured asthmatics in Chicago, a pilot includes home visits for asthma education, medication adherence, assessment and remediation of environmental triggers, and connection with primary care providers. The current pilot phase will test the service delivery model and identify areas for improvement. Philanthropic funding and hospital community benefit funds have been secured to pilot services for patients over 4 months. A completed pilot will demonstrate the viability of scaling these preventative services to broader patient populations.

## CONCLUSION

As GHHI has expanded its work to more than 30 cities and counties, along with 20 innovative financing and Pay for Success projects, some common themes have emerged. Operationalizing partnerships is a significant lift, but having a person in a role such as the Outcome Broker can be helpful to drive a collaboration. When measuring the impact of comprehensive services, access to data is critical. Providers can reach out to payers to work on direct access to data, access to de-identified data for cost-benefit analysis, and opportunities to pilot a combined set of holistic services. Armed with the information from robust analysis, providers such as GHHI and its partners are able to maximize program design and referral sources. Bringing suggested payment arrangements to Medicaid health plans can quickly determine if a payment structure and contract can be finalized, and under what terms.

### REFERENCES

1. Norton RA, Brown BW. Green & Healthy Homes Initiative: Improving health, economic, and social outcomes through integrated housing intervention. *Environ Justice*. 2014;7(6). https://www.liebertpub.com/doi/pdf/10.1089/env.2014.0033. Accessed on 1/16/2019.

2. United States Public Health Service Office of the Surgeon General. The surgeon general's call to action to promote healthy homes. Office of the Surgeon General (US). Rockville (MD): Office of the Surgeon General (US); 2009. https://www.ncbi.nlm.nih.gov/nlmcatalog/?Db=nlmcatalog&DbFrom=books&Cmd=Link&LinkName=books_nlmcatalog&IdsFromResult=2211852.

3. National Asthma Education and Prevention Program Expert Panel Report 3. Guidelines for the diagnosis and management of asthma. Summary Report 2007.

National Heart Lung and Blood Institute. NIH Publication Number 08-5846. October 2007. Bethesda, MD.

4. Crocker DD, Kinyota S, Dumitru GG, et al. Effectiveness of home-based, multi-trigger, multicomponent interventions with an environmental focus for reducing asthma morbidity. A community guide systematic review. *Am J Prevent Med.* 2011;41(2S1):S5–S32. https://www.thecommunityguide.org/sites/default/files/publications/Asthma-AJPM-evrev-homebased.pdf.

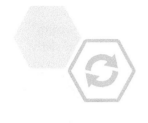

# Chapter 6

# Partnering with Transportation Sector Actors and Advocates to Improve Health Outcomes

TERESA WILKE AND SHAWN LEIGHT

Where we live, work, and play impacts our health, and how we move within and between our communities is critical to improving quality of life and fostering lifelong wellness. Safe, effective, and reliable transportation connects people to social and structural determinants of health, including employment, fresh food, stable housing, quality education, and health care services. The transportation industry is a complex network of agencies, organizations, and infrastructure that governs the physical assets, built environment, and movement patterns of people and goods throughout a community and region. Each plays a specific role in the regulation, planning, design, and operation of the transportation system. Given the interconnected nature of transportation, there is rarely a single entity or authority that governs all aspects of a transportation issue, be it bike lanes, rail lines, traffic patterns, or bus stops (Box 6.1).

The transportation profession has undergone major changes since 2008, and this change is ongoing. Industry actors have recognized the need for greater transportation choice and equity, as well as for incorporating performance outcomes related to health. Many transportation professionals are eager to work with health advocates to achieve these goals. Moreover, new technologies in the form of Smart Cities, Big Data, shared mobility, and connected and autonomous vehicles are presenting new opportunities to address community needs.

The St. Louis Multimodal Plan was undertaken to develop a robust transportation plan for Downtown St. Louis, providing a framework to coordinate and prioritize future projects as well as leverage future state and federal funding. The goal was to develop a transportation plan for Downtown St. Louis that supports a robust multimodal

system, where users of all ages and abilities feel safe, including pedestrians, bicyclists, transit users, and motorists and promotes economic growth, social equity, community development, better air quality, and improved public health. For details, please see http://www.downtownstltransportationstudy.com/.

## DEMONSTRATING THE CONNECTION BETWEEN TRANSPORTATION AND HEALTH

Effective transportation decision-making can improve access to healthy food, affordable housing, quality education, good jobs, and health care. The Centers for Disease Control and Prevention (CDC) Transportation and Health Tool (THT) outlines several ways that transportation decisions can improve and promote population health.[1] Examples include the following:

- *Active transportation*: Transportation systems and facilities can be designed in such a way that they encourage people to be more active by walking and biking instead of driving.
- *Equitable connectivity and mobility*: Well-connected transportation networks provide access to necessities such as jobs, healthy food, and health services. In fact, more than 3 million Americans miss or delay health care every year due to transportation issues.[2,3] Transportation planners and operators are responsible for designing connected, multimodal systems that serve all segments of a community, including low-income populations, people of color, children, the disabled, and the elderly.
- *Air quality*: Air pollution can contribute to heart disease and respiratory illnesses (such as asthma). Transportation emissions can be reduced by mitigating congestion, supporting cleaner vehicles, and promoting multimodal options that reduce driving. (See the Federal Highway Administration [FHWA] guidance at: www.fhwa.dot.gov/environment/air_quality/.)
- *Safety*: Road crashes continue to be a leading cause of death in the United States. The number and severity of roadway crashes can be lowered through improved transportation facilities, enforcement of traffic laws, and public education. (See the Federal Highway Administration [FHWA] https://safety.fhwa.dot.gov/ and Institute of Transportation Engineers [ITE] www.ite.org/visionzero/.)

- *Noise*: Noise impacts sleep and has an adverse impact on health. Transportation noise can be reduced through effective planning and design of transportation facilities. (See www.fhwa.dot.gov/environment/noise/ and https://www.fhwa.dot.gov/Environment/noise/regulations_and_guidance/.)

Several transportation design and operational strategies exist to benefit health outcomes, including these, compiled by the CDC and US Department of Transportation (USDOT):

- https://www.cdc.gov/healthyplaces/transportation/incorporate_strategy.htm
- https://www.cdc.gov/healthyplaces/transportation/hia_toolkit.htm
- https://www.transportation.gov/mission/health/strategies-interventions-policies

## STAKEHOLDERS, ACTORS, AND INFLUENCERS OF TRANSPORTATION POLICIES AND SYSTEMS

There are generally three levels of influence in the transportation system: (1) the built environment and physical infrastructure, (2) "rolling stock" (e.g., vehicles, buses, trains), and (3) regulatory policies and planning. Transportation planning is a *continuous* process that seeks to respond to shifts in the environment and dynamic customer needs. Do your homework before engaging transportation actors to determine the right individuals, timing, and tactics for partnering.

The first step is to identify the transportation organizations that "own" the issue you hope to influence. Like a team of multidisciplinary health providers who meet frequently to coordinate patient-centered care, transportation actors regularly collaborate across entities to ensure safe, efficient, and accessible transportation for their end users. The following describes the various players who constitute transportation industry actors and influencers:

- *Infrastructure owners* are the agencies that own, maintain, and operate transportation infrastructure, including roadways, sidewalks, and bicycle facilities. Examples are state departments of transportation (DOT), city and county highway and/or public works departments, and local elected officials (e.g., mayor, city council member).
- *Service providers* are the organizations that deliver transportation services directly to customers. Examples are transit agencies, cab companies, and shared mobility companies (e.g., Uber, Lyft, and bikeshare companies).
- *Regulators and policymakers* design and approve laws, regulations, and practice standards. Regulatory agencies are government officials and bodies such as state, local, and federal elected officials, Metropolitan Planning Organizations (MPOs), and federal agencies (e.g., FHWA and

USDOT). Standard-setting organizations are nongovernmental bodies that establish design and operational standards and guidelines. Examples are the American Association of State Highway and Transportation Officials (AASHTO), the Institute of Transportation Engineers (ITE), and the National Electrical Manufacturers Association (NEMA).

- *Professional training and education associations* provide professional development and training to transportation professionals. Examples are ITE, the Intelligent Transportation Society of America (ITS-A), the Transportation Research Board (TRB), and the AASHTO.
- *Advocacy groups* educate the public and champion specific transportation projects and policies. Examples are bike/pedestrian groups, Mothers Against Drunk Driving (MADD), and ITE's Vision Zero Network.
- *Employers/high-impact utilizers* include hospitals, universities, and other large-scale employers and entities that require high numbers of individuals to be moved to and from their site locations to promote robust commerce, education, health care, and other community services that compose a strong economic development infrastructure.

Transportation organizations often produce planning documents that are available for public review, including long-range transportation plans, transportation improvement plans, walkability plans, and technology/Smart City plans. These documents offer details about the actors and stakeholders who may influence your transportation issue. Carefully review these plans to learn how the authors incorporate health-related metrics and goals and how your advocacy partners can engage in the decision-making process.[4]

## HOMEWORK ASSIGNMENT 1: CLARIFY THE ISSUE OF CONCERN AND GATHER AVAILABLE DATA

The complexity of transportation policy, planning, funding, maintenance, and decision-making requires that advocates apply systems-thinking frameworks (e.g., identifying critical leverage points in which to exert influence) combined with community mobilizing tactics and principles to authentically co-create solutions with populations that are disproportionately impacted by social determinants of health. This requires engaging partners from a position of solidarity rather than authority and recognizing the interdependence and broad impact of unequal resource distribution in transportation and mobility access.[5]

First, identify the critical pathways by which the existing transportation system is impacting your population of focus. Engage affected populations to gather qualitative data in the form of personal experiences, perspectives, and first-hand narratives; then triangulate this information with aggregated data. Second, crosswalk available demographic, mobility, employment, transportation, and health data to create a holistic picture of how transportation might be impacting the health of your target population. Examples of readily accessible public data sets include US Census Bureau information regarding average of commute time to work and the percentage of households with vehicle access; Community Commons (http://communitycommons.org) public health data and mapping focused on behaviors, disease prevalence, and mortality; and community health needs assessments (CHNAs) that cite assets and barriers relating to health and health care access. Public health departments can request disaggregated patient data directly from hospitals when there is a population health concern to be addressed,[6] and community asset and gap analyses provide excellent assessments of community resources and perceived challenges.

A data inventory can also be used to assess what is known and what data are needed to better understand the target issue, influence additional stakeholders, and facilitate a shared vision for change.[7] Compare your community's existing assets and policies with best practices and metrics for examining transportation access, feasibility, efficiency, and racial equity found in the references at the end of this chapter (Box 6.2).[1,8–11]

---

### Box 6.2 | Generate Health St. Louis

Generate Health St. Louis evolved over 20 years as a vibrant, long-standing maternal and infant health consortium, and, in 2015, they formed the FLOURISH St. Louis initiative—a focused strategy that allowed its broad coalition of community organizations, from health systems to nonprofits—to come together to tackle the complex problem of racial disparities in infant deaths. Specifically, FLOURISH seeks to reduce the alarming rates of infant mortality experienced by the city's Black moms and babies. Learn more about FLOURISH at http://www.flourishstlouis.org.

In 2017, Generate Health St. Louis was selected to participate in the Bold, Upstream, Integrated, Local, and Data-driven (BUILD) Health Challenge 2.0, a national program that provides funding, technical assistance, and peer net-work support for multisector partnerships that work to address upstream social determinants to improve community health. St. Louis was selected be-cause of its BUILD strategy to improve maternal and infant health outcomes for Black moms and babies by targeting transportation access for pregnant women and new parents in the City of St. Louis. Infant mortality rates in the zip codes of focus (comprised primarily of Black residents) were three times the state average. FLOURISH held 17 community listening sessions attended by more than 350 community residents to identify the most pressing issues for improving maternal and infant health. Transportation was cited as a major barrier to meeting health care and social needs. Vision for Children at Risk, a community-based organization partner, facilitated parent cafés to take action on resident-identified priorities. This yielded a Transportation Community Café, which worked over 8 months to develop specific priorities and action items relating to transportation access, safety, and ongoing communications with the transportation sector.

# HOMEWORK ASSIGNMENT 2: IDENTIFY TRANSPORTATION INITIATIVE SCOPE AND FOCUS

Though your coalition can consist of a wide range of actors and interests, the initial vision of a transportation initiative should be clearly defined so that collective actions can be targeted toward specific, measurable, achievable, relevant, time-bound (SMART) objectives. Once you have identified how the transportation system is impacting the population of focus, you can present options regarding the scope and nature of the group's shared agenda.

Starting with your core group of established partners, consider whether the project should be focused at a tactical (project) or strategic (policy) level. A tactical level effort involves decisions under the control of infrastructure owners and service providers who are managing infrastructure and assets on a day-to-day basis. These project decisions are typically made by professional-level staff at these organizations. Examples include moving a bus stop to better serve a neighborhood or constructing bicycle facilities on a street. Strategic-level decisions influence broader transportation policy as set by *regulators and policymakers*, such as modifying roadway design standards that could impact all future projects. These efforts require a coalition of aligned stakeholders, so we suggest conducting an environmental scan to locate and engage advocates who may already be working on your chosen issue. Offer to speak with professional transportation training and industry associations, which often invite cross-sector experts to educate transportation professionals about new issues and techniques (Box 6.3). For example, ITE runs a podcast series to educate

---

**Box 6.3 | Transportation Decision-Making in the St. Louis Multimodal Plan**

The St. Louis Multimodal Plan took a tactical approach to transportation decision-making by focusing project-level decision-making within the control of infrastructure owners (e.g., the City of St. Louis Streets Department, Board of Public Service, and Missouri Department of Transportation) as well as service providers (e.g., Bi-State Development Agency/Metro). Note that both city and state agencies were involved in the process as infrastructure owners because roads in the downtown area are operated and maintained by both the City of St. Louis and the Missouri Department of Transportation.

Project outcomes include a hierarchy of streets (e.g., vehicle-, pedestrian-, bicycle-, and transit-focused streets) and a menu of treatments that support each street type. For example, pedestrian-focused streets are now prioritized for enhanced landscaping, pedestrian-scale wayfinding, high-visibility crosswalks, and lighting. The plan will ultimately promote more walking and biking by improving the physical infrastructure and safety of the built environment for those activities.

**Table 6.1 ▼ Tactical and strategic project examples**

| | Tactical example | Tactical partners | Strategic example | Strategic partners |
|---|---|---|---|---|
| Safety | Address a hazardous intersection | Infrastructure owners Service providers | Implement state seat belt laws | Regulators and policy makers Advocacy groups Professional training and education associations |
| Active transportation | Improve a sidewalk Construct path | | Establish regional biking plan | |
| Equitable Connectivity | Improve connection to bus stop | | Improve regional public Transportation | |
| Noise | Install sound wall quiet rail zone | | Implement regional noise controls | |
| Air quality | Electrify bus fleet | | Improve regional air quality | |

professionals about various issues, including how transportation decisions can improve health (http://www.ite.org/learninghub/podcast.asp). Table 6.1 illustrates tactical and strategic level examples, partners, and health connection points.

Tailor your transportation "ask" to the most directly involved transportation actor, but also remain open to a natural discovery process that will likely unfold as you partner with transportation actors and advocates who may already be deeply involved in the issue. For example, if you want to improve a bus stop shelter, start by targeting the entity that owns the streets or sidewalks rather than a state policymaker. Conducting due diligence about the processes, regulations, and planning systems in place will help you to determine the level of influence or authority, as well as regulatory constraints and incentives, that might be impacting system actors and influencers. Well-researched and supported rationale and data analysis will give internal transportation advocates the information they need to advocate for proposed changes to other actors within the transportation system. Tailored one-pagers or concept briefs (two to three pages) can be extremely helpful for engaging and mobilizing coalition actors, aligned advocates, transportation influencers, and actors across sectors and multiple levels of authority.

# READY FOR ACTION: PARTNERING WITH TRANSPORTATION TO ADDRESS POPULATION HEALTH AND EQUITY

## Prepare Established Coalition Allies

Though you likely have a long-standing coalition of stakeholders who are passionate about your health issue of concern, transportation may be an "upstream" issue that is new to these partners and allies. Take the time to prepare your constituencies by providing them with concept papers, briefings, and talking points that demonstrate how and why transportation is important to their own priorities and individual agendas, as well as how it promotes health equity and the shared vision of the health coalition. Leverage the expertise of regional academic institutions, graduate students, and city leadership program cohorts that might be able to offer unique perspectives for translating, interpreting, and amplifying the data you have collected about perceived needs and challenges.

### Engage Closest Transportation Sector Actor

Start with professional staff who are most closely associated with the issue, then engage in an exploratory dialogue. Questions to ask include the following:

- What constraints or challenges have you encountered in trying to address this issue?
- What other groups/agencies that you work with "own" this problem, in addition to you?
- What data do you need to help guide this issue or understand this problem?
- What can we do to work with you to solve this problem or improve circumstances?

Often the leverage point in a transportation system is influenced by a small, close-knit group of actors who are collaboratively responsible for the transportation component. The key is to find the right actors who can help you to navigate and expand your understanding of the issue and the broader system. These will become your most crucial allies for change and improvement, and these individuals will know exactly who else needs to be engaged in order to influence key leverage points in the system. Transportation infrastructure is a public asset, and investment decisions are normally governed by a public-facing, transparent process. There is a pervasive desire for "fairness" in resource allocation, so your internal transportation allies will likely appreciate best practices and information about how transportation can be used to improve health equity and how their policies impact the health of local populations (positively and negatively).

### Create a Flexible Blueprint for Change

Develop a draft logic model or driver diagram to help frame your efforts in terms of inputs, activities, short-term objectives, and long-term impact (Box 6.4).

Connect with other communities that are seeking to address similar issues and systems. For example, the health equity data system graphic in Figure 6.1 was adapted by Generate Health St. Louis and based on a framework shared by a peer Bold, Upstream, Integrated, Local, and Data-driven (BUILD) Health Challenge grantee in New Orleans.

**Box 6.4 | Racial Equity Lens to Identify BUILD Strategic Objectives**

Generate Health St. Louis used a racial equity lens to identify the following strategic objectives for their Bold, Upstream, Integrated, Local, and Data-driven (BUILD) project:

1. *Data*: Conduct quantitative and qualitative research and data analysis (centered in directly reported community experiences) to advise transportation policy, health sector planning, and population health strategies.
2. *Systems*: Promote institutional policies, planning methods, and coordinated local investments that create a more trauma-responsive system of transportation and health.
3. *Innovation*: Pilot, scale, and sustain innovative modes of delivering nonemergency medical transportation (NEMT).
4. *Policy*: Develop and activate a targeted health/transportation policy agenda.
5. *Community voices*: Cultivate authentic relationships, build trust, co-create resident-driven solutions, and establish accountability structures and pathways for local self-advocacy.

An overall project logic model and individual driver diagrams that reflected the coalition's racial equity framework were developed to facilitate team planning and to promote cohesive coalition communications.

## FOCUS ALLIES ON KEY LEVERAGE POINTS

Community members, nonprofit organizations, health providers, and public health entities each have unique spheres of influence and expertise. These stakeholders can take distinct leadership roles to target key leverage points within the transportation planning structure and transit system. Examples of these roles are shown in Figure 6.2.

### Integrate for Impact

Transportation and health have long been impacting one another, but only recently have the two sectors had the shared metrics, planning resources, and pragmatic tools needed to articulate and shape those connections in a coordinated way. Public health departments, hospitals, health systems, and health equity advocates can now partner directly with transportation allies to design durable structures and policies that promote population wellness and reduce health disparities over the long term (Box 6.5).

The transportation sector is uniquely transparent and solicitous of public engagement, but health advocates must identify the right actor(s) to engage based on the focus and scope of the transportation issue to be addressed.

## Figure 6.1 ▼

St. Louis Bold, Upstream, Integrated, Local, and Data-driven (BUILD) Health Challenge – Health Equity Data System Framework.

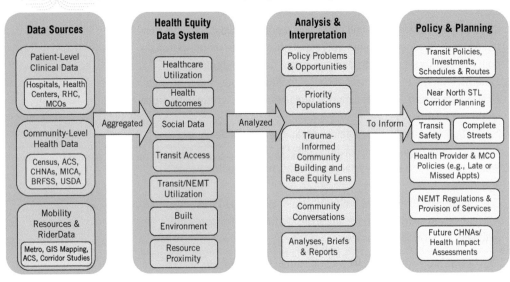

FLOURISH    BUILD Health Equity Data System Framework

**Data Sources**

Patient-Level Clinical Data

Hospitals, Health Centers, RHC, MCOs

Community-Level Health Data

Census, ACS, CHNAs, MICA, BRFSS, USDA

Mobility Resources & RiderData

Metro, GIS Mapping, ACS, Corridor Studies

→ Aggregated →

**Health Equity Data System**

Healthcare Utilization

Health Outcomes

Social Data

Transit Access

Transit/NEMT Utilization

Built Environment

Resource Proximity

→ Analyzed →

**Analysis & Interpretation**

Policy Problems & Opportunities

Priority Populations

Trauma-Informed Community Building and Race Equity Lens

Community Conversations

Analyses, Briefs & Reports

→ To Inform →

**Policy & Planning**

Transit Policies, Investments, Schedules & Routes

Near North STL Corridor Planning

Transit Safety | Complete Streets

Health Provider & MCO Policies (e.g., Late or Missed Appts)

NEMT Regulations & Provision of Services

Future CHNAs/ Health Impact Assessments

## Figure 6.2 ▼

Potential leadership and engagement roles for stakeholders.

**Community Residents and Grassroots Orgs** ⇒

- Appeal to local elected officials and policy makers
- Provide input in transportation planning forums and meetings
- Mobilize groups of parents, youth and other residents
- Provide first-hand reports of personal experiences to verify the aggregated public health and transportation data

**Hospitals and Health Providers** ⇒

- Leverage authority as major employer
- Collect and aggregate data re: patient experiences and challenges
- Correlate ED or other aggregated EHR data to demonstrate need
- Communicate with patients about advocacy priorities
- Disseminate need data to influencers and actors in health and managed care sectors

**Public Health Department**

- Stratify and interpret prevelance data to define hotspots and conduct root cause analyses
- Lend expertise of epidemiologists and public health educators
- Share shape files to inform GIS mapping of health indicators
- Contribute to legislative testimony
- Serve as convening authority for cross-sector dialogues

> ## Box 6.5 | Using Consultants in the BUILD Health Challenge
>
> To catalyze efforts under the Bold, Upstream, Integrated, Local, and Data-driven (BUILD) Health Challenge, Generate Health St. Louis hired two consultants to work in tandem with its existing staff and FLOURISH coalition: one focused on community mobilization and one focused on systems and policy change.
>
> The community mobilization strategist, Steve Parish, recommended a trauma-responsive, relationship-based approach focused on trust-building and community empowerment. "This effort is an opportunity for people of consciousness, sincere about saving babies, to build relationships with communities they have not traditionally had them with. We are using BUILD to give FLOURISH a greater chance to authentically become the type of partner people most affected by historic disparities need," he said.
>
> During the launch phase of BUILD, the systems and policy change strategist focused on data analysis and communications infrastructure, and the two BUILD consultants met weekly to ensure a braided approach that continuously re-centered the project on principles of racial equity while balancing the perspectives and priorities of the system and the individuals affected. This integrated approach also allowed the project to swiftly flex in response to dynamic community needs and remain nimble enough to influence policy shifts and impromptu advocacy opportunities.

Transportation actors may include (1) infrastructure owners who control the physical infrastructure (e.g., streets and sidewalks); (2) mobility operators who control rolling stock (e.g., buses, trains, cabs, and other vehicles) that operates on the physical infrastructure; and/or (3) regulators, standard-setting organizations, advocates, and researchers who influence transportation policy.

Doing your homework, engaging in an authentic discovery and relationship-building process, aligning efforts across your established health industry partners, and proactively integrating community perspectives will help bridge the divide between the health and transportation sectors. There is genuine desire among transportation industry actors to design responsive, health-promoting transit and transportation systems, and health advocates can provide a critical link between transportation actors and the constituencies they serve. It is truly "win-win" when health and transportation planning efforts are engaged collaboratively. Aggregated data and first-hand stakeholder perspectives translated across these sectors can improve health equity and reduce disparities by addressing multiple barriers to health and wellness assets.

Transportation sector planning, investment, maintenance, and governance directly influence population mobility, which can promote or inhibit reliable access to social determinants of health and opportunities to thrive across the lifespan.

## REFERENCES

1. Centers for Disease Control and Prevention. Transportation and health tool. Updated 2015. https://www.transportation.gov/transportation-health-tool Equity focused strategies; https://www.transportation.gov/mission/health/equity. Accessed on 1/16/2019.

2. Syed S, Gerber B, Sharp L. Traveling towards disease: transportation barriers to health care access. *J Comm Health*. 2013;38(5):976–3.

3. National Center for Mobility Management. Transportation to healthcare destinations. 2014. https://nationalcenterformobilitymanagement.org/wp-content/uploads/2014/09/NCMM_Healthcare_Business_Case_Context.pdf. Accessed on 1/16/2019.

4. ChangeLab Solutions. Getting involved in transportation planning: An overview for public health advocates. 2013. http://www.changelabsolutions.org/publications/getting-involved-transportation-planning. Accessed on 1/16/2019.

5. Ventres W, Dharamsi S, Ferrer R. From social determinants to social interdependency: Theory, reflection, and engagement. *Social Med.* May 2017;11(2):84–9.

6. Sharfstein JM, Chrysler D, Bernstein J, Armijos L, Tolosa-Leiva L, Taylor H, Rutkow L. Using electronic health data for community health: Example cases and legal analysis. December 2017. http://www.debeaumont.org/EHDforCommunityHealth. Accessed on 1/16/2019.

7. Nazaire JNQ. Living Cities Data Inventory. May 2016. Available for download under Creative Commons Attribution 4.0 license. https://www.livingcities.org/resources/313-data-inventory. Accessed on 1/16/2019.

8. Boisjoly G, El-Geneidy A. Measuring performance: Accessibility metrics in metropolitan regions around the world. Brookings Institution. August 2017. https://www.brookings.edu/wp-content/uploads/2017/08/measuring-performance-accessibility-metrics.pdf. Accessed on 1/16/2019.

9. National Academies of Sciences, Engineering, and Medicine. *Exploring Data and Metrics of Value at the Intersection of Health Care and Transportation: Proceedings of a Workshop.* Washington, DC: The National Academies Press; 2016. https://doi.org/10.17226/23638; https://www.nap.edu/catalog/23638/exploring-data-and-metrics-of-value-at-the-intersection-of-health-care-and-transportation. Accessed on 1/16/2019.

10. American Public Health Association and Urban Design 4 Health. The hidden health costs of transportation. February 2010. https://www.apha.org/~/media/files/pdf/factsheets/hidden_health_costs_transportation.ashx. Accessed on 1/16/2019.

11. Lee RJ, Sener IN. Transportation planning and quality of life: Where do they intersect? *Transp Policy (Oxf).* March 2016;48:146 55. https://www.ncbi.nlm.nih.gov/pubmed/27546998. Accessed on 1/16/2019.

## RESOURCES

The Annie E. Casey Foundation. Embracing equity: 7 Steps to advance and embed race equity and inclusion within your organization. Written in partnership with Terry Keleher. January 2015. http://www.aecf.org/resources/race-equity-and-inclusion-action-guide/.

The Annie E. Casey Foundation. *Trauma Informed Community Building Evaluation Infographic: A Formative Evaluation of the TICB Model and Its Implementation in Potrero Hill.* Baltimore: The Annie E. Casey Foundation; July 2015. http://www.aecf.org/resources/trauma-informed-community-building-evaluation/.

Benford, RD, Now DA. Framing processes and social movements: An overview and assessment. *Annu Rev Sociol.* 2000;26:611–39.

Health Research & Educational Trust and American Hospital Association. *A Playbook for Fostering Hospital-Community Partnerships to Build a Culture of Health.* Chicago, IL: Health Research & Educational Trust; July 2017. www.aha.org. https://www.aha.org/ahahret-guides/2017-07-27-playbook-fostering-hospital-community-partnerships-build-culture-health.

Health Research & Educational Trust and American Hospital Association. Transportation and the role of hospitals. November 2017. http://www.hpoe.org/resources/ahahret-guides/3078.

PolicyLink, Prevention Institute and Convergence Partnership. Healthy, equitable transportation policy: Recommendations and research. 2009. http://www.policylink.org/sites/default/files/HEALTHTRANS_FULLBOOK_FINAL.PDF.

Weinstein E, et al. *Trauma Informed Community Building: A Model for Strengthening Community in Trauma Affected Neighborhoods.* San Francisco, CA: BRIDGE Housing Corporation; May 2014. http://bridgehousing.com/PDFs/TICB.Paper5.14.pdf.

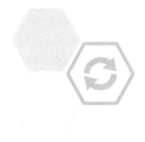

# Chapter 7

# Business and Public Health: Why Corporate America Will Soon Help Lead the Public Health Charge

SCOTT HALL

O n a hot July night in 1887, seven men gathered at the Brunswick Hotel in downtown Kansas City, Missouri, to advance the city's business interests. From that conversation the Commercial Club of Kansas City was formed to "[m]ake Kansas City a good place to live in." It wasn't the first organization of its type in Kansas City, but it was the one that endured, albeit with a different name and a different mission statement.

More than 130 years later, the Greater Kansas City Chamber of Commerce (KC Chamber) is "leading the way to the best KC region" on behalf of more than 2,000 members, representing several hundred thousand Kansas City area employees. The KC Chamber serves not only as the chamber of commerce for Kansas City, but also as the regional chamber of commerce serving all of Greater Kansas City, which comprises more than 2.1 million people, 120 municipalities, 14 counties, and 2 states.

While many things have changed over the past 130 years, the core of the KC Chamber's mission remains the same—to make Greater Kansas City a better place by promoting the growth of business. The KC Chamber takes a broad approach to this mission, tackling not just traditional business issues, such as business regulation and taxation, but also quality-of-life issues that impact our community.

The KC Chamber's current projects include efforts to advance the region's arts, urban redevelopment, life sciences, transportation, and, yes, even community health. In fact, we are proud to focus not only on the enterprise aspect of our mission, but also on the betterment of our entire community.

It is with these dual motivations in mind—the civic and the enterprise— that we launched "Healthy KC," a regional health and wellness strategy for Greater Kansas City.

## THE CIVIC: WHY THE BUSINESS COMMUNITY'S HEART SHOULD BE IN PUBLIC HEALTH

Chambers of commerce and many similar civic organizations are built on an almost instinctive feeling common to all of us about where we live, work, and play. You might call this feeling, "pride of place." We all want the place we call home to be a place that others envy. This civic pride, while changing in the new millennium, pushes people to action. Some run for elected office, others make philanthropic donations, and still others volunteer their time to improve community assets.

Similarly, there is an almost reflexive civic call to action whenever our community appears threatened. Such threats can be physical, like a natural disaster; economic, like a major employer leaving town; or emotional, like belittlement of our place by others. It was the last of these three threats, perhaps the least serious but nevertheless still painful, that inspired the KC Chamber to amplify its work in community health.

A high-profile fitness magazine published a list of the "fattest" cities in the United States. Kansas City was second on that list.

Admittedly, this was not what anyone would call a scientific study of the issue, and when your region's brand is built around barbeque and jazz, you begin such a cursory evaluation at a significant disadvantage. It was, nevertheless, an event that threatened our pride of place. A biting commentary on where our region stood in comparison to our peers and in the minds of others that, admittedly, struck a nerve.

We knew that, regardless of whether Kansas City really was the second fattest city in the country, we weren't as healthy as we needed to be, and that felt like a punch to the (flabby?) gut. So, the KC Chamber began work on a project that would later be named "Healthy KC," a regional initiative aimed at making Greater Kansas City a destination for health and wellness.

It is worth noting, though, that pride of place alone will not move enough people in any community, including Kansas City, to action. Of course, there will be some who are so passionate about a single purpose, in this case public health, that they will rally around the emotional cause without anything else. Others will have a particularly prideful sense of place because of their role in the community, which is the position that the KC Chamber was in. You might call these the "easy converts."

It will take something more, though, than just an appeal to emotion to elicit a widespread response to pressing issues of public health. In the case of the KC Chamber, and our membership, the second important piece of this puzzle was and remains the growing empirical case that healthy employees, companies, and communities will outperform their peers.

# THE ENTERPRISE: WHY THE BUSINESS COMMUNITY'S HEAD SHOULD BE IN PUBLIC HEALTH

The business case for public health is easy to understand. It can be simply summarized in "The Widget Story" (attributional disclaimer: "The Widget Story" was first told to me by Matt Condon, President and CEO of Bardavon Health Innovations, Chair of the KC Chamber Board of Directors, and one of our guiding lights in our health and wellness work).

You see, every one of the KC Chamber's members makes a widget—even those who don't "make" anything at all. Whether you are making greeting cards, like Hallmark, or offering engineering services, like Burns & McDonnell, you face fundamentally the same competition. Someone else, somewhere else, is offering to do essentially the same thing, which makes your good or service, to some degree, replaceable.

Every good and service offered by a KC Chamber member, or every business in your community, can then, for purposes of this conversation, be considered a widget.

If you make a widget and your competition down the street (they actually don't have to be down the street, they can be halfway around the world) also makes a widget, customers will be driven by a number of factors when deciding which widget to purchase. Assuming all else is equal, whichever widget costs the customer less will be the widget that is more often purchased. Alternatively, if the products are offered at the same price, then whichever widget maker controls internal costs more efficiently will make more money with each widget that is sold.

It follows, then, that the widget maker who offers the product for less (or at the same price with a higher profit margin) will outperform the other widget maker. And eventually the widget maker who outperforms the competition will put the widget maker down the street out of business.

This theory can be easily applied to employee and community health. Those businesses that are able to control their health care costs will, all other factors being equal, outperform their peers. In other words, if a business can save 1% on health care costs because they have a healthier workforce, they will eventually buy the competition "down the street." Moreover, if the loved ones of those employees are also healthier, then they will miss fewer days of work taking care of others and be able to focus more clearly on their work when present.

The principle illustrated in "The Widget Story" applies not only to individual businesses but also to communities. While one community will never buy another, it will outgrow others. For chambers of commerce, this speaks to the heart of our mission. We are charged to make our place the best place to grow a business. It follows, then, that this is only possible if we are promoting public health.

A growing body of data is accumulating that is beginning to demonstrate the principle in "The Widget Story."

First, the costs to employers associated with tobacco use are astounding. According to a study conducted by Ohio State University, the average annual cost to a private employer for *each* employee who uses tobacco is $5,816 per year. This figure takes into account the amount of extra spending for health insurance premiums, but also the amount of lost productivity due to smoking breaks and sick days as well as the cost of the inability to perform work due to tobacco addiction. This amount even includes a credit back to the employer for savings on pension payments, because the average smoker doesn't live as long.

The savings to business, though, don't stop with tobacco; they are also being demonstrated in other arenas of worksite wellness.

From 2009 to 2015, the S&P 500 index grew 159%. That is impressive growth, to be sure, until you consider that the growth of those S&P 500 companies that were high performers in the Health Enhancement Research Organization (HERO) Scorecard over that same period of time grew 235%, or that the stock appreciation for the C. Everett Koop Health Award Winners was 325%, or that the stock price increase for the Corporate Health Achievement Awards for High Performers was 345%.

These data are especially interesting because they show, at the very least, a correlation between the robustness of a wellness program in the workplace and stock price performance. Although this study stops short of concluding that excellent workplace wellness programs increase stock price, you can bet that CEOs for other S&P 500 companies are taking notice.

This appears to be "The Widget Story" in action.

These data, coupled with the pride of place, form the recipe needed to inspire chambers of commerce and their businesses to engage in public health discussions.

The next question, then, is how businesses properly engage in public health efforts. The answer is by understanding who they are and who they are not.

## WHAT ROLE CAN BUSINESS PLAY IN PROMOTING PUBLIC HEALTH?

Every time I talk about public health, I have to offer a very honest, but important, disclaimer: I don't know anything about public health. Moreover, the KC Chamber isn't a public health organization, and we don't have anyone on our staff who is a public health expert.

Chambers of commerce are business advocacy and enhancement organizations that are much more comfortable crafting policy positions that articulate the need for minimal business regulation than presenting information to groups about the need for trauma-informed care and resilience, for example.

These facts are incredibly important for all communities to remember as they approach their local chamber of commerce to engage in a dialogue on public health. Chambers of commerce are, largely, uninformed. We are well-intentioned, to be sure, but we don't have an MD, DO, or MPH. In fact, many of us don't even know what that last one stands for.

It is, then, incumbent on the public health community to engage the local chamber of commerce—and, really, the local business community—in a way that will empower them to be helpful as the converted advocate: the voice of the non-expert who hears the call to action coming from those who truly understand the issue in a deep way and can translate that as an independent authority into plain language, understandable by a broader audience.

When this is done, chambers of commerce and public health experts will stand together, implementing positive public health change that is inspired by what one feels in one's heart and reinforced by what one thinks in one's head. This change will lead our places to be stronger, more vibrant, more inclusive communities: destinations for profound community health and wellness.

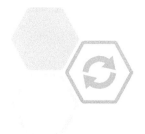

# Chapter 8

# The Path Forward: The Role of Hospitals and Health Systems in Advancing Health and Well-Being for Individuals and Communities

JAY BHATT AND ANDREW JAGAR

A great transformation is under way. For decades, hospitals and health systems in the United States have served as anchors during tumultuous times of disasters, outbreaks of disease, and tragedies; as employers and sources of learning and care in communities large and small; and as embodiments of technological wonder as the marvels of cutting-edge medical science extended lives and brought relief to the suffering—all of which they continue to do. However, as demographics change and disease burden shifts from acute to chronic, hospitals and health systems are also leading an unprecedented transformation to re-envision their role and extend their impact beyond the clinic walls. They are working to create new models of care that prioritize teaming and partnership with the aim of engaging in true population health: advancing health and well-being by bridging care and community. This transformation aims for no less than "a society of healthy communities where all individuals reach their highest potential for health."[1]

While these complex, crucial organizations work to have a greater impact on the conditions affecting today's patients and future generations, there is growing consensus that care delivery must be redesigned in a way that prioritizes value. Even as the rate of cost increases begins to slow, the imperative to enhance value is leading to new models of care delivery and reimbursement. In these new models, quality and efficiency are explicitly incentivized. But there is much more to the picture than payment models alone. American Hospital Association members have embraced the notion of "redefining the H," suggesting a substantive reimagining of accountabilities and roles that hospitals play in their communities. The "H" of the future encompasses hospitals, health systems, and health organizations that strive to advance health in America by leading changes to how people experience health and care, inside and outside hospital walls.

## PROMOTING AFFORDABILITY AND ENHANCING VALUE

Health care costs in the United States have increased, with $3.3 trillion, or more than $10,000 per person, spent in 2016, approximately one-third of that amount in the hospital sector.[2] Although these dollars support needful and urgent work, such as providing a lifeline to communities in times of disaster, outbreaks, and tragedies, the nation's hospitals and health systems are realigning resources to meet the evolving needs of the patients and communities they serve.[3] To do this, hospitals and health systems are taking multiple approaches. First, many have embraced the frameworks and objectives around value-based care. A shift toward value under these frameworks requires hospitals to not only consider the needs of communities and populations conceived broadly and work to address these needs, but also to actively engage those they serve.

At the same time, hardworking clinicians already struggling with damaging rates of professional burnout[4,5] cannot continue to do more with less. Instead, health care professionals should focus their efforts on those areas that have the greatest impact on advancing well-being. This shift in focus will require substantially reducing the unsustainable regulatory burden faced by hospitals and health systems.[6] For example, addressing the many federally mandated clinical quality measures, a 2016 National Quality Forum (NQF) report noted that "performance measures have proliferated across a diverse range of clinical areas, settings, data sources, and programs" decreasing the utility of quality data and "pos[ing] challenges for providers, patients, health plans, regulators, and others who use measures to assess performance."[7] To advance quality and enhance value, a streamlined set of measures focused on what matters most to clinicians and the patients they care for—and a sustainable set of regulations—must replace the overwhelming and at times contradictory framework used today.

To address challenges in a constantly evolving field, health care organizations need to reconceive their roles, and new partnerships must be developed. Many hospitals and health care systems are important employers and purchasers in their communities, so they are well suited to convene organizations and stakeholders that might otherwise not be willing to collaborate. One promising idea is developing "chambers of health," akin to local chambers of commerce, that represent local economic interests. Because health care is essentially local, hospitals and health systems are intimately familiar with local cultures and power dynamics, opening opportunities to bridge political and organizational gaps. Furthermore, this unique position could foster the creation of sustainable partnerships with a variety of organizations, including local governments, community-based organizations, and even multinational organizations with local economic interests. With the increasing recognition that the health needs of today require addressing upstream factors (e.g., social determinants of health and the role of place in well-being), such "chambers of health" could serve an important role as advocates for local health needs in partnership with and on behalf of communities.

## ADVANCING POPULATION HEALTH

While most acute care in the United States is outstanding,[8] and state-of-the-art interventions save untold numbers of lives that would have been lost in the past,[9] too many individuals and communities continue to lack access to needed care.[10–12] Or, when care is available, the quality of care in some communities may be uneven.[5–7] As hospitals and health systems continuously work toward increasing access and eliminating disparities in care quality, there is increased recognition that even the very best clinical care may be insufficient to promote the well-being to individuals and communities in light of the profound influence that social factors have on health, such as a lack of access to nutritious food, economic instability, and unstable housing.

A new model of care, one based on a broadly conceived framework of population health, is needed to enable individuals and communities to attain their highest potential for health. As with enhancing value, multisector partnership is key to extending health care's impact beyond the four walls of the hospital or clinic. Such partnerships bring great promise but also require careful coordination and thoughtful collaboration. As empirical evidence[13,14] and the experience of clinicians across the country attest, moving the needle on widespread conditions such as diabetes, hypertension, and substance addiction requires a variety of expertise, ranging from understanding local barriers and opportunities to coordinating clinical visits with medical specialists. Achieving success in reducing the prevalence of these conditions calls for sustainable partnership and coordination, so developing shared language and understanding is a necessary first step. Pathways to Population Health is a collaborative effort (supported by the Robert Wood Johnson Foundation) among five organizations—the American Hospital Association/Health Research & Educational Trust (HRET), the Institute for Healthcare Improvement, the Network for Regional Healthcare Improvement, the Public Health Institute, and Stakeholder Health—to "support health professionals in identifying opportunities for their organizations to make practical, meaningful, and sustainable advances in their population health journey."[15] The Pathways to Population Health model provides the framework for the journey to population health, starting with offering consensus definitions of key terms, including the key distinction between *population management*, which refers to provision of health care services to achieve specific health metrics for a defined population,[16] and *population health*.[15] A commonly accepted definition of population health has been provided by Kindig and Stoddardt, who define it as "the health outcomes of a group of individuals, including the distribution of such outcomes within the group. These groups are often geographic populations such as nations or communities, but can also be other groups, such as employees, ethnic groups, disabled persons, prisoners, or any other defined group."[17]

Pathways to Population Health includes four portfolios of work focused on (1) physical and/or mental health, (2) social and/or spiritual well-being, (3) community health and well-being, and (4) communities of solutions.[15] Broadly, these portfolios can be seen as two complementary paths—population management and community well-being creation—on the journey to achieving population health. This journey must link these two approaches with continued focus on equity achievement, delivery system and payment innovation, and patient and family engagement. This journey implies prioritizing "upstream" causes of illness; that is, addressing root causes of illness and social determinants of health. Engaging in this work also suggests accountability for the broad spectrum of what produces—and harms—health.

## EQUITY OF CARE: WELL-BEING FOR ALL

Health care disparities continue to exist for far too many racially, ethnically, and culturally diverse individuals. Disparities have been identified across individuals' life spans[18] and in a variety of clinical areas and conditions,[19] in access to and efficacy of treatment,[20] and in follow-up care.[21] Although a host of factors may contribute to disparities, such as individual behaviors, cultural and linguistic barriers to effective communication, and the way care is organized and financed, hospitals and health systems across the country are engaged in serious efforts to ensure that every person in every community receives high-quality, equitable, and safe care.

One concrete initiative involves increasing the collection and use of race, ethnicity, language preference (REAL) and other sociodemographic data. REAL and sociodemographic data, when collected accurately using patient report,[22] can be used to stratify patient outcomes to guide performance improvement.[23] The Institute for Diversity and Health Equity has guided organizations to achieve the promise of equity, ensuring that everyone has a fair and just opportunity to be healthier,[24] through its #123forEquity Campaign to Eliminate Health Care Disparities. A collaboration of the American Hospital Association, American College of Healthcare Executives, Association of American Medical Colleges, Catholic Health Association, and America's Essential Hospitals, this campaign asks organizations to pledge to increase collection and use of REAL and sociodemographic data, to conduct cultural competence training, to provide diversity in leadership and governance, and to improve and strengthen partnerships with communities. At the close of 2017, more than 1,700 hospitals had taken the pledge nationally, and 50 state hospital associations have entered in partnership, representing an 11% increase in pledges over the previous year.[25]

Taking the pledge to reduce disparities is a crucial first step, but data alone won't create equity if organizations do not act. To that end, in collaboration with the Institute for Diversity and Health Equity and the Disparities Solution Center, participating hospitals and health systems are developing diversity inclusion action plans and fostering cultural competence training via #123forEquity training symposiums across the United States. Notwithstanding these important steps, to achieve health equity, it is also necessary that incentives for and measures of care equity be aligned across payers, both public and private, to avoid further increasing the measurement burden of providers.[26] Organizations that have been at the forefront of advancing health equity have found that reducing disparities is the right thing to do, and it also pays dividends for communities as well as hospitals and health systems.[27]

## CONCLUSION

Hospitals and health systems play an important role in the health of communities across the country. While that role is changing and will likely continue to evolve, the importance of these institutions as anchors in their communities is likely to increase in coming years. Health and well-being is more than just the absence of illness and, as such, cannot be produced only within the walls of hospitals or clinics. Rather, there must be real integration with the communities and homes where people live, work, and play. Moving upstream from treating illness to advancing health and well-being involves productive partnerships between health care providers, community-based organizations, schools, faith-based organizations, municipal agencies and economic interests, and other stakeholders. Coordinating the activities in these partnerships calls for organizations that are influential and that understand local identities and cultures. Among this rich organizational mix, hospitals and health systems are uniquely positioned to promote the sort of advocacy and leadership required to align a wide variety of interests and stakeholders.

At the same time, as anchor organizations in many communities, hospitals and health systems have the clout to foster positive change in the community-level factors that drive health and well-being. Whether through convening stakeholders, engaging in community investment, or providing employment opportunities for individuals across the socioeconomic spectrum, hospitals and health systems will continue to play a vital role in their communities. As health needs change and demographics shift, one constant is that these organizations will continue to "redefine the H" while reimagining notions of value and care via the strategic vehicle of population health to create healthy communities in which all individuals can reach their highest potential for health.

## REFERENCES

1. American Hospital Association. Mission and vision. https://www.aha.org/about/mission-vision. Accessed March 12, 2018.

2. Centers for Medicare and Medicaid Services. NHE-fact-sheet. https://www.cms.gov/research-statistics-data-and-systems/statistics-trends-and-reports/nationalhealthexpenddata/nhe-fact-sheet.html. Published February 14, 2018. Accessed March 12, 2018.

3. The New York Times. The Hospital's Place in the New Health Landscape. https://www.nytimes.com/2018/03/04/opinion/hospitals.html. Accessed March 12, 2018.

4. Shanafelt TD, Hasan O, Dyrbye LN, et al. Changes in burnout and satisfaction with work-life balance in physicians and the general US working population between 2011 and 2014. *Mayo Clin Proc*. 2015;90(12):1600–13. doi:10.1016/j.mayocp.2015.08.023

5. Sinsky C, Colligan L, Li L, et al. Allocation of physician time in ambulatory practice: A time and motion study in 4 specialties. *Ann Intern Med*. 2016;165(11):753. doi:10.7326/M16-0961

6. American Hospital Association. *Regulatory Overload: Assessing the Regulatory Burden on Health Systems, Hospitals and Post-Acute Care Providers*. Chicago, IL; 2017. https://www.aha.org/system/files/2018-02/regulatory-overload-report.pdf. Accessed March 19, 2018.

7. Quality Forum. NQF: Variation in measure specifications—Sources and mitigation strategies final report. http://www.qualityforum.org/Publications/2016/12/Variation_in_Measure_Specifications_-_Sources_and_Mitigation_Strategies_Final_Report.aspx. Accessed March 19, 2018.

8. Health System Tracker. Measuring the quality of healthcare in the U.S. Peterson-Kais Health System Tracker. https://www.healthsystemtracker.org/brief/measuring-the-quality-of-healthcare-in-the-u-s/. Accessed March 12, 2018.

9. Walker N, Tam Y, Friberg IK. Overview of the Lives Saved Tool (LiST). *BMC Public Health*. 2013;13(Suppl 3):S1. doi:10.1186/1471-2458-13-S3-S1

10. Okoro CA, Zhao G, Fox JB, Eke PI, Greenlund KJ, Town M. Surveillance for health care access and health services use, adults aged 18–64 years—Behavioral Risk Factor Surveillance System, United States, 2014. *Morb Mortal Wkly Rep Surveill Summ Wash DC 2002*. 2017;66(7):1–42. doi:10.15585/mmwr.ss6607a1

11. Horner-Johnson W, Dobbertin K, Lee JC, Andresen EM. Disparities in health care access and receipt of preventive services by disability type: Analysis of the Medical Expenditure Panel survey. *Health Serv Res*. 2014;49(6):1980–99. doi:10.1111/1475-6773.12195

12. 2016 National Healthcare Quality and Disparities Report. Content last reviewed June 2018. Agency for Healthcare Research and Quality, Rockville, MD. http://www.ahrq.gov/research/findings/nhqrdr/nhqdr16/index.html. Published June 30, 2017. Accessed March 12, 2018.

13. O'Donnell MP. Can diabetes prevention improve health and save Medicare money, does Medicare care know, and why is this important? *Am J Health Promot AJHP*. 2016;30(6):412–15. doi:10.1177/0890117116658442

14. Koller EA, Chin JS, Conway PH. Diabetes prevention and the role of risk factor reduction in the Medicare population. *Am J Prev Med*. 2013;44(4 Suppl 4):S307–16. doi:10.1016/j.amepre.2012.12.019

15. Pathways 2 Population Health. https://www.pathways2pophealth.org. Accessed March 9, 2018.

16. Institute for Healthcare Improvement. Improving the health of populations. http://www.ihi.org:80/resources/Pages/Publications/Improving-the-Health-of-Populations.aspx. Accessed March 15, 2018.

17. Kindig D, Stoddart G. What is population health? *Am J Public Health*. 2003;93(3):380–3. doi:10.2105/AJPH.93.3.380

18. Singh GK, Siahpush M. Widening socioeconomic inequalities in US life expectancy, 1980–2000. *Int J Epidemiol*. 2006;35(4):969–79. doi:10.1093/ije/dyl083

19. Graham G. Disparities in cardiovascular disease risk in the United States. *Curr Cardiol Rev*. 2015;11(3):238–45. doi:10.2174/1573403X11666141122220003

20. Rangrass G, Ghaferi AA, Dimick JB. Explaining racial disparities in outcomes after cardiac surgery: The role of hospital quality. *JAMA Surg*. 2014;149(3):223–7. doi: 10.1001/jamasurg.2013.4041

21. Mead H, Ramos C, Grantham SC. Drivers of racial and ethnic disparities in cardiac rehabilitation use: Patient and provider perspectives. *Med Care Res Rev*. 2016;73(3):251–82. doi:10.1177/1077558715606261

22. Klinger EV, Carlini SV, Gonzalez I, et al. Accuracy of race, ethnicity, and language preference in an electronic health record. *J Gen Intern Med*. 2015;30(6):719–23. doi:10.1007/s11606-014-3102-8

23. Chin MH, Clarke AR, Nocon RS, et al. A roadmap and best practices for organizations to reduce racial and ethnic disparities in health care. *J Gen Intern Med*. 2012;27(8):992–1000. doi:10.1007/s11606-012-2082-9

24. Robert Wood Johnson Foundation. What is health equity? https://www.rwjf.org/en/library/research/2017/05/what-is-health-equity-.html. Published May 1, 2017. Accessed March 15, 2018.

25. Equity of Care. http://www.equityofcare.org/. Accessed March 15, 2018.

26. Chin MH. Creating the business case for achieving health equity. *J Gen Intern Med*. 2016;31(7):792–96. doi:10.1007/s11606-016-3604-7

27. Thornton RLJ, Glover CM, Cené CW, Glik DC, Henderson JA, Williams DR. Evaluating strategies for reducing health disparities by addressing the social determinants of health. *Health Aff Proj Hope*. 2016;35(8):1416–23. doi:10.1377/hlthaff.2015.1357

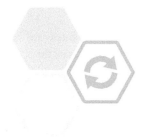

# Primary Care and the Social Determinants of Health: Lessons on Care Models, Capacity, and Culture for the Journey Upstream

RISHI MANCHANDA

What a difference a decade makes.

When I was working as a primary care physician at a community health center in south-central Los Angeles 10 years ago, few of us then would have predicted what is happening today. Now, more and more of us in health care, from health plan executives and hospital leaders to frontline clinicians, are coming to the same conclusion that our peers in public health have long understood: moving upstream to improve care and the social determinants of health is not only necessary, it's possible (Box 9.1).

This was not the case 10 years ago. In 2008, as a National Health Service Corps scholar with clinical and administrative responsibilities, it was my job not only to care for my patients but also to help navigate and implement major business changes for our practice. Many of these changes came with their own language of associated terms and acronyms, such as EMR (electronic medical record) implementation and PCMH (patient-centered medical home) transformation. On a daily basis, we responded to these changes and navigated the waves of programs and newly insured patients ushered in by the economic stimulus package of 2009 and the subsequent passage of the Patient Protection and Affordable Care Act (ACA) in 2010. At every level, our leadership meetings, our care team huddles, and our community work were consumed by these major changes and pressing questions of productivity, capacity, and coordination.

### Box 9.1 | Screening for Housing Insecurity

*Barbara Rubino*

Two years ago, I heard a keynote speech. The presenter—a primary care "upstreamist" with HealthBegins—spoke about screening patients for housing insecurity and dared the several hundred of us in the audience to try it. I thought there was no way we could do this at our hospital-based primary care clinic. But then, as the months passed, I kept recalling his charge. Maybe I'd be bold enough to try some of the work that could move us upstream.

With a lot of collaboration across disciplines, training, education, and ongoing improvement, 2 years later, we screen all of our primary care patients for a variety of behavioral and social conditions that affect their health, including housing insecurity. HealthBegins was our original inspiration to address social needs and is now a vital force in supporting us as we refine our processes to track patients and assure that they've reached the resources they need.

But something was missing from both clinical practice and public discourse: the social determinants of health. To those of us on the front lines, it seemed like few in the mainstream of US health care were discussing what we could plainly see in our clinics. Long-neglected "upstream" social ills and "pathologies of power,"[1] such as housing instability, food insecurity, and structural racism, were wreaking havoc on the lives of our patients, on the care we delivered, and on the communities we served. Meanwhile, organized medicine and health care payers were largely silent in the face of upstream policy prescriptions and calls to action, such as those in the 2008 report from the World Health Organization (WHO) Commission on Social Determinants of Health. Federal programs like the Community Transformation Grant, though notable, barely registered on the day-to-day radar of clinicians. Upstream imperatives and initiatives seemed like footnotes to domestic healthcare priorities.

We were not deterred. Like many who work on the frontlines of health care and social services in low-income communities, we persisted. Against the backdrop of health care reform, we experienced setbacks and successes and learned practical lessons about ways to help health care systems and their community partners to assess and address the upstream needs of patients with resourcefulness and rigor.

Thanks to increasing payer commitment to value-based care, the concept of moving upstream to address social determinants of health is now entering the mainstream in US health care. If the past 10 years were about health care's awakening to the realities of social determinants of health and *why* they matter, the next 10 years will focus on *how* to address them as clinicians, as organizations, and as partners to our civic, public health, and social-sector peers. As my colleagues at HealthBegins can attest, there is growing demand among health care systems for practical tools and methods to do this work well. For primary care—and health care writ large—moving upstream will bring its own setbacks and successes. Along the way, this will and should lead to hotly contested debates about our very notions of care models, capacity, and culture.

## CARE MODELS

As the shift from volume to value raises questions about the role of primary care vis-à-vis the social determinants of health, we must first acknowledge and then push past the limits of our current model of care. Our model of primary care today is itself a by-product of a long, ongoing debate. In the 1970s, global failures in the provision of basic health services and the promise of community-based solutions led world leaders to create the WHO Alma Ata declaration. Acknowledging the "social roots of illness," government officials articulated primary health care as an important component to advance broad, intersectoral, rights-based approaches to improve care and the social determinants of health.[2] This comprehensive vision and role of primary health care, however, was quickly challenged by more selective, technical definitions of primary care.[3] In 1979, early critics argued that "until primary health care can be made available to all, services targeted to the few most important diseases may be the most effective means of improving the health of the greatest number of people."[4]

In contrast to the sociological and communal underpinnings of Alma Ata, this narrower, selective definition of primary care reinforced a biomedical and individualistic paradigm that has come to dominate our attitudes and approaches to health care and health.[5] Ironically, the reductionist nature of this paradigm, wherein "cognitive" disease evaluation and management activities have lower perceived value than "technical" interventions, has made it even easier to undervalue primary health care and overvalue specialty care in the United States. We now spend only 5% or so of total health care spending on primary care.

The selective, biomedical paradigm is reflected in nearly every aspect of our current US model of primary care. Hamstrung by lopsided fee-for-service reimbursements, primary care physicians devote much of their time to a discrete set of clinic-based activities, such as sick visits, that are largely reactive in nature and narrow in scope.[6] This is true even in America's community health centers, which were founded on the principles of Community-Oriented Primary Care (COPC)[7] and serve as informal US embassies of the Alma Ata approach. Even in these settings, the bulk of day-to-day work of primary care is focused on providing individuals with a selective range of discrete biomedical clinic-based treatments, counseling and education, and limited clinical preventive services "targeted to the few most important diseases."[8] A direct result of this selective, biomedical approach to primary care is a lack of clinician or practice-level readiness to assess, let alone address, the social determinants of health. Only one out of every five physicians in the United States feels confident to address the health-related social needs of patients.[9] Only one in three primary care practices in the United States feels prepared to coordinate care with social service providers.[10]

Another consequence of the biomedical paradigm is reflected in what health care leaders mean when they refer to "social determinants." Transportation is a good example. Instead of investing in transportation as a resource for healthy engagement in work, family, or civic life, many leaders in the medical community only consider the utilitarian aspects of transportation as a means to improve patient adherence and facilitate reimbursable visits to the hospital or clinic.[11] Although these self-directed interests of clinical service providers are understandable, they can also be at odds with the broader social needs and interests of the communities they serve. Health care leaders who seek to move upstream to address the needs of the community must guard against the gravitational pull of the biomedical paradigm, which conflates and muddles the social determinants of "health care" with the social determinants of "health" and the social and political determinants of "health equity."[12] The underlying model of care that we have come to accept, after all, is still largely technical and selective, just as was recommended nearly 40 years ago by critics of Alma Ata.

For those interested in reimagining the paradigm of primary care to improve care *and* the social determinants of health, there is reason for hope. Transformation efforts, such as the PCMH, and best practices from "direct primary care" clinics have highlighted ways to improve care coordination, efficiency, and the quality of patient–provider relationships. New regulatory standards and data integration opportunities are beginning to push and pull primary care practices to collect and help address patients' health-related social needs.[13,14] Together, these models and standards form the paths that health care can traverse to move upstream. They provide opportunities to test and expand new care models that not only improve the technical integration of health care and social services but also shift toward a broader social paradigm for primary care itself.

Considering newer models of care that are already expanding our notions of *where* primary care can be provided can help us to understand these opportunities. The marked increase in the number of urgent care and "retail" clinics at pharmacies and large chain stores, the expansion of telemedicine, and the growth of "on-site" and "near-site" employer-sponsored clinics are all bellwethers of major changes in the location of primary care. From a social determinant of health perspective, these new settings for care delivery not only create opportunities for primary care practices to gather data and insights on health-related social risks, but also help address them in new ways.

During my time as Chief Medical Officer for a self-insured employer in California, for instance, my colleagues and I built and ran on-site primary care clinics for thousands of rural, agricultural employees who disproportion-ately suffered from diabetes and other chronic conditions. The location of our practices (e.g., at large agricultural processing plants) spurred clinical innova-tion. In addition to traditional office-based care, our clinicians, health coaches, and other staff helped reform the menu at the plant cafeterias where thousands ate every day. This led to improved food quality and employee satisfaction while dramatically reducing the exposure to processed, unhealthy carbohydrates and sugar-sweetened beverages. At one of our sites, clinic staff, including phys-ical therapists and physicians, worked with *promotoras* (lay Hispanic/Latino community members who are trained to dispense basic health education in the community) from Latino Health Access to design and lead worksite ed-ucation efforts for more than 1,300 employees on safety, nutrition, exercise, and mindfulness; this led to marked improvements in health knowledge and behavior. Clinicians introduced screening questions for insecurity related to food, finance, and housing into company-wide employee health surveys and routinely organized individual sessions at the onsite gym and diabetes peer-groups at a local community center. Locating primary care where people work certainly led to new forms of clinical engagement and new models of care de-livery and disease management. It also led to new opportunities to better assess and address health-related social needs. As the reach of primary care expands to nonmedical settings (i.e., where people live, work, eat, sleep, learn, and pray), we can and should expand our model of primary care to help address the full spectrum of the biopsychosocial needs of patients.

## CAPACITY

For many primary care clinicians, the promise of addressing the biopsychosocial needs of patients and communities is what drew them to the field in the first place. In addition to the built-in limitations of a fee-for-service, biomedical model of care, however, primary care clinicians face another barrier to realizing these upstream hopes: the lack of capacity. Recent critics of efforts to integrate social determinants of health into US primary care point to barriers such as competing demands on physician time and existing levels of burnout among primary care physicians.[15] From this perspective, physicians are overworked, and any demands to integrate social determinants in primary care may exacer-bate burnout. Although concerns about burnout are relevant and pressing, re-search suggests that an inverse phenomenon may be at play when it comes to our understanding of primary care capacity and social determinants of health. For instance, in a cross-sectional study of more than 500 primary care physicians, physician perception of *higher* clinic capacity to address patients' social needs was the strongest independent predictor of *lower* rates of burnout.[16] In other words, the lack of clinic capacity to address social determinants of health may be driving physician burnout. This research resonates with experiences of many frontline practitioners in primary care. When caring for patients who routinely present with physical and psychological sequelae of unmet social needs, such as hunger, substandard housing, or toxic workplaces, it can be professionally unsatisfying and frustrating to work in a clinic or system that lacks the capacity to understand and help address these upstream issues. It is not that primary care clinicians are too burned out to integrate social determinants of health interventions. Rather, primary care clinicians are burning out because, in large part, our clinics and systems don't have the capacity to address social determinants of health.

As clinical–community partnerships around the country are teaching us, the good news is that we can build the capacity of primary care to better assess and address social determinants of health. This starts with acknowledging that effective social determinants of health integration will not be achieved through the adoption of new software or scaling of novel programs alone. Integration of social determinants of health is a major business change and, as such, requires intentional collective behavior change on the part of clinical and community-based organizations. The only way to help organizations navigate successful changes such as these is through complex systems redesign, as we have found with other major changes to the day-to-day business of medical practice, such as the implementation of EMRs or PCMH transformation. Before we *build* the capacity of primary care practices to address social determinants of health, therefore, we must first *assess* their capacity for systems redesign and identify opportunities to build specific social determinants capabilities, including the capacity to effectively partner with social sector, public health, and community-based organizations (CBOs).

A growing number of tools are now available to assist in this process. HealthBegins, for instance, developed an organizational *Upstream Capability Assessment* based on its own experiences and feedback working with hundreds of clinical and CBO leaders and staff, as well as best practices from organizational development theory and practical implementation science.[17–19] The tool was designed to help health care systems and CBOs determine the maturity of their respective organizational competencies and processes to support clinical–community partnerships to advance social needs interventions for specific priority populations (Table 9.1).

As primary care systems assess their organizational capabilities to address social determinants, another dimension of capacity to be considered is *scope*. For many health care systems, issues such as food insecurity, homelessness, and structural racism can feel overwhelming and beyond the scope or reach of conventional clinical practice. To make the move upstream less daunting, primary care providers can use a taxonomy of clinical–community partnerships to categorize unmet social needs and identify opportunities to intervene on seemingly intractable social determinants of health in concrete, actionable ways. The *Upstream Strategy Matrix* (Table 9.2), for example, uses levels of prevention (i.e., primary, secondary, and tertiary) and levels of intervention

| **Table 9.1** ▼ Health care organizational competencies for effective social determinants of health integration | |
|---|---|
| **1. External environment:** *Assess the favorability of the external environment for your organization to address social determinants of health.* | **6. Project management of upstream interventions:** *Assess the maturity and style of project management for social determinants of health interventions.* |
| **2. Perceived value of moving upstream:** *Identify the perceived value of a change to assess and address social determinants of health.* | **7. Workflow integration:** *Assess the degree to which your social determinant of health intervention is integrated in care delivery workflows.* |
| **3. Executive sponsorship:** *Assess the quality and degree of executive sponsorship to advance social determinants of health interventions.* | **8. Quality improvement:** *Assess your organization's quality improvement culture and processes as they relate to social determinants of health interventions.* |
| **4. Staff and team roles:** *Identify if staff and team roles have been clearly defined and integrated into upstream work.* | **9. Organizational infrastructure:** *Consider the organizational infrastructure and supports for your social determinants of health intervention.* |
| **5. Scope of work of upstream interventions:** *Consider if the scope of the proposed or current upstream intervention has been defined.* | **10. Financial readiness:** *Identify the degree to which financial risks and rewards and payment models have been optimized for your intervention.* |

*From HealthBegins Upstream Capability Assessment. HealthBegins, 2018. Reproduced with permission.*

(i.e., individual, organizational, and population) to help health care systems and their community partners understand local needs and resources as well as the opportunities to improve specific social determinants of health for priority patient populations.[2]

Table 9.2 provides an illustrative example of how health care and community partners can map potential upstream "early win" opportunities across different levels of intervention and prevention to improve outcomes by addressing food insecurity for a priority population of adult diabetics. Using this strategic framework, primary care clinics can circumscribe their roles in potential clinical–community partnerships (i.e., where health care professionals can lead, partner, and/or support). In our experience, the majority of health care institutions that are currently working on social determinants of health are engaged in activities that fall in the bottom left (see Table 9.2) (i.e., individual-focused, tertiary prevention activities designed to mitigate and reduce the impact of disease and preventable utilization among high-need, high-cost patients). Health care "hotspotting" is an example of this type of tertiary-prevention activity.[20] If we hope to make substantial progress in improving the health of patients and communities over the next decade, however, health care's scope of engagement with the social determinants of health will need to move beyond what's shown at the bottom left of this matrix (see Table 9.2). Success in population health will depend on our collective ability to partner and influence other areas of impact. Over time, we will need to expand our scope of engagement and lead, partner, and/or support concrete social determinants of health initiatives in the communities we serve across many more levels of intervention and prevention.

Primary care practices can begin this process by leveraging existing data to build and strengthen partnerships with CBOs and public health agencies that are already engaged in addressing social determinants of health and health disparities. In addition to reviewing and sharing aggregate, de-identified data from patient registries with public health partners interested in disease surveillance and disparities, clinics have a variety of ways in which they can leverage their data to uncover unmet health-related social needs and engage in community health partnerships to address them. For instance, clinics can partner with public health departments to identify community-level "hot spots," where high-utilizers and disease are disproportionately concentrated. As clinical coding systems for social determinants of health become more sophisticated and increasingly more practices collect social risk data using EMRs, primary care clinicians will also have increased opportunities to support community coalitions that seek to identify and address "cold spots" (i.e., the places where the social determinants of health, support, and access to primary care have broken down).[21,22] Over the next decade, those who have dedicated themselves to the work of primary care will find ample and welcome opportunities to build capacity to address social determinants through partnerships with patients, public health, and community-based organizations.

| Table 9.2 ▼ Upstream strategy matrix for diabetes mellitus 3 × 3 | | | |
|---|---|---|---|
| | **Patient level of intervention** | **Organization level of intervention** | **General population level of intervention** |
| **Primary prevention** | Financial literacy, support, and nutrition programs for low-income families with strong family history of diabetes mellitus (DM) | Provide on-site farmers' market, gym, walking trails, or financial counseling for families at risk for DM | Advocate for local increase in minimum wage and supports for low-income families, particularly those at risk of DM |
| **Secondary prevention** | Poverty screening and financial assistance for DM patients at risk of end-of-month hypoglycemia | Subsidize vouchers to local farmer's market or hire a financial counselor for at-risk employees | Change timing and content of WIC and school food programs to avoid food insecurity among those with DM |
| **Tertiary prevention** | Reduce hospital use among high-utilizer severe diabetics using food and income support | Coordinate with local banks, collectors, lenders, to reduce debt burden for utilizer diabetics | Support legislation/ regulations to provide financial and "hot spotter" services to severe diabetics |

## CULTURE

Beyond implications for care models and capacity, the move upstream will likely create shifts for the culture of health care as well. As with all major organizational changes, primary care efforts to address social determinants of health through partnerships with the social sector will spur an evolution of conventional norms, values, and behaviors in health care. Although many of these cultural changes will not take place in a smooth, linear fashion, some of these changes are certainly desirable. For example, the inclusion of new staff, such as community health workers, is now recognized as a means to expand, if not reflect, sociocultural competence among primary care teams.[23,24] With increasing pressure from value-based payment models to bring in community health workers to help address social and contextual drivers of health and disease, the trend toward greater sociocultural competence among primary care teams will undoubtedly continue.

What remains to be seen is whether and how the integration of community partners and the addition of community health workers and other unconventional roles (e.g., health coaches, patient navigators, social workers, lawyers) to move upstream will transform deeper subjective cultural norms in primary care. This includes our most fundamental notions of power and how we, as primary care professionals, exercise power relative to new colleagues and community partners. Social psychologists have defined at least six sources of power used to achieve desired outcomes in workplaces and other settings: (1) coercive, (2) reward, (3) legitimate, (4) referent, (5) expert, and (6) informational power.[25] Community health workers (CHWs), much like staff and leaders from nonmedical CBOs and social service agencies, have high levels of referent, expert, and informational power within their neighborhoods and communities. As Dr. America Bracho and others have put it, CHWs possess *community* and *relational* expertise that is qualitatively distinct from the *technical* expertise that is often prized in clinical medicine.[26]

Traditionally, however, US physicians and other health care professionals have undervalued CHWs and CBO staff and have poorly understood their extensive sources of power and expertise. As a result, many US health care systems that currently engage in population health planning simply and narrowly relegate CHWs and CBO staff to "clinical extender" roles. They are seen, at best, as supporters rather than as leaders of primary care transformation. This perspective fails to recognize and learn from the deep, relational, and nuanced insights, as well as the technical expertise, that CHWs and CBOs bring to bear in the lives of patients and communities. As nascent cross-sector efforts to improve social determinants of health spread and scale over time, we may see a shift in cultural norms and attitudes of primary care practitioners toward a more ecological and biopsychosocial perspective. Rather than just seeing CBOs and CHWs as "clinical extenders" of care delivery, health care professionals might also come to see ourselves as "extenders" of community and public health initiatives. To achieve this more balanced, integrated vision, we will have to expand opportunities for professional, leadership, and faculty development, not only for primary care clinicians, but also for CHWs and CBO staff. In the near future, for example, we should all hope to see more instances in which community and social sector experts, such as CHWs, social workers, public health practitioners, and public interest lawyers, are presenting at hospital grand rounds, leading CME and CNE courses, and sharing platforms at health care conferences that have long been reserved for those with privilege and power in clinical medicine. We should also expect and support efforts to reduce historic levels of structural inequity within and across communities and sectors. For example, US health care institutions and payers, which have historically received the lion's share of societal resources compared to public health and social sectors, will be called on to transfer capability and resources to CBOs as they expand investments in social determinants of health interventions. To truly realize the potential of clinical–community partnerships, both sides will need to transform organizational cultures and learn to recognize, share, and exercise power in new ways.

## CONCLUSION

This is a time of extraordinary change and promise for primary care clinicians, public health practitioners, and social sector leaders. For the first time in a generation, underlying financial, cultural, and regulatory drivers in US health care are converging to create windows of opportunity to improve care, address the social determinants of health, *and* advance equity, especially for our most vulnerable patients and communities. The question before us all is this: Can we ensure that our collective efforts to move upstream are sufficiently rigorous, effective, transformative, and sustainable? In the coming years, we will certainly bear witness to increasingly more innovative experiments, needed investments, and policy changes vis-à-vis social determinants of health and primary care. As we journey upstream, we can leverage new care models, assess and build capacity, and navigate cultural norms to find answers to that fundamental question.

### REFERENCES

1. Farmer P. *Pathologies of Power: Health, Human Rights, and the New War on the Poor*. Berkeley: University of California Press; 2003.

2. Manchanda R. Practice and power: Community health workers and the promise of moving health care upstream. *J Ambul Care Manage*. 2015;38(3):219–24.

3. Baum FE, Legge DG, Freeman T, Lawless A, Labonté R, Jolley GM. The potential for multi-disciplinary primary health care services to take action on the social determinants of health: actions and constraints. *BMC Public Health*. 2013;13:460.

4. Walsh JA, Warren KS. Selective primary health care—an interim strategy for disease control in developing countries. *N Engl J Med*. 1979;301:967–74.

5. Robinson W, Navarro, V. The Political Economy of Social Inequalities: Consequences for Health and Quality of Life. *Contemporary Sociology*. 2002;31(6):685.

6. Breaking the fee-for-service addiction: Let's move to a comprehensive primary care payment model. Health Affairs Blog, August 17, 2015. https://www.healthaffairs.org/do/10.1377/hblog20150817.049985/full/

7. Mullan F, Epstein L. Community-oriented primary care: New relevance in a changing world. *Am Public Health* November 1, 2002;92(11):1748–55.

8. Walsh JA, Warren KS. Selective primary health care—an interim strategy for disease control in developing countries. *N Engl J Med*. 1979;301:967–74.

9. Fenton M. Health care's blind side: the overlooked connection between social needs and good health. The Robert Wood Johnson Foundation. Published Dec 2011. http://www.rwjf.org/en/library/research/2011/12/health-care-s-blind-side.html.

10. Osborn R, Moulds D, Schneider EC, Doty MM, Squires D, Sarnak DO. Primary care physicians in ten countries report challenges caring for patients with complex health needs. *Health Aff*. 2015;34(12):2104–2112.

11. Health Research & Educational Trust. *Social Determinants of Health Series: Transportation and the Role of Hospitals*. Chicago, IL: Health Research & Educational Trust; 2017. www.aha.org/transportation.Accessed March 15, 2018

12. Jones CP. Addressing the social determinants of children's health. *J Health Care Poor Underserved*. 2009;20:1–12.

13. Magnan, S. 2017. Social determinants of health 101 for health care: Five plus five. NAM Perspectives. Discussion Paper, National Academy of Medicine, Washington, DC. https://nam.edu/social-determinants-of-health-101-for-health-care-five-plus-five.

14. Garg A, Jack B, Zuckerman B. Addressing the social determinants of health within the patient centered medical home: lessons from pediatrics. *JAMA*. 2013;309(19):2001–2.

15. Solberg LI. Theory vs practice: Should primary care practice take on social determinants of health now? No. *Ann Fam Med*. 2016;14(2):102–3. doi:10.1370/afm.1918.

16. Olayiwola JN, Willard-Grace R, Dube K, et al. Higher perceived clinic capacity to address patients' social needs associated with lower burnout in primary care providers. *J Health Care Poor Underserved*. 2018;29(1):415–29.

17. Weiner BJ. A theory of organizational readiness to change. *Implementation Science*. 2009;4:67.

18. Scaccia JP, Cook BS, Lamont A, et al. A practical implementation science heuristic for organizational readiness: R = MC². *J Commun Psychol*. 2015;43(4):484–501.

19. Greenhalgh T, Robert G, MacFarlane F, Bate P, Kyriakidou O. (2004). Diffusion of innovations in service organizations: Systematic review and recommendations. *Milbank Q*. 2004;82(4):581–629.

20. Healthcare Hotspotting. A project of the Camden Coalition of Healthcare Providers https://hotspotting.camdenhealth.org/. Accessed April 18, 2018.

21. DeSilvey S, Ashbrook A, Sheward R, Hartline-Grafton H, Ettinger de Cuba S, Gottlieb L. *An Overview of Food Insecurity Coding in Health Care Settings: Existing and Emerging Opportunities*. Boston, MA: Hunger Vital Sign National Community of Practice; 2018. http://childrenshealthwatch.org/foodinsecuritycoding/.

22. Westfall J. Cold-spotting: Linking primary care and public health to create communities of solution. *J Am Board Fam Med*. 2013;26:239–40.

23. Rogers EA, Manser ST, Cleary J, Joseph AM, Harwood EM, Call KT. Integrating community health workers into medical homes. *Ann Fam Med*. 2018;16:14–20.

24. Mobula LM, Okoye MT, Boulware LE, Carson KA, Marsteller JA, Cooper LA. Cultural competence and perceptions of community health workers' effectiveness for reducing health care disparities. *J Prim Care Community Health*. 2015;6(1):10–5.

25. Raven BH. Social influence and power. In Steiner D, Fishbein M, eds. *Readings in Contemporary Social Psychology*. New York: Holt, Rinehart, & Winston; 1965:371–82.

26. Bracho A, Lee G, Giraldo G, de Prado RM. *Recruiting the Heart, Training the Brain: The Work of Latino Health Access*. Berkeley: Hesperian Health Guides; 2016.

# Collaboration: The Role of Multiple Sectors in Improving Health

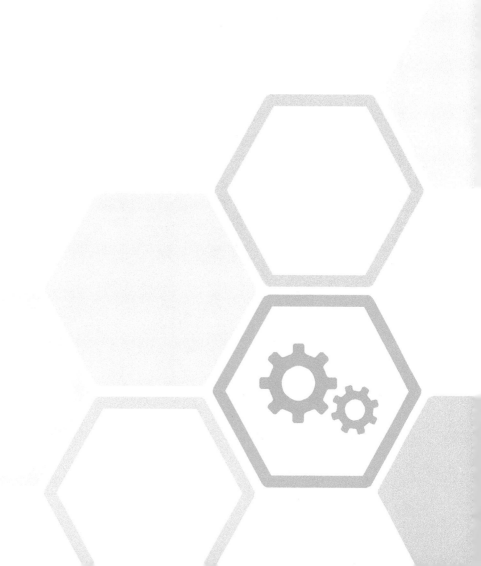

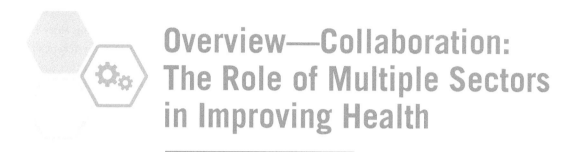

# Overview—Collaboration: The Role of Multiple Sectors in Improving Health

## DON W. BRADLEY AND BRIAN C. CASTRUCCI

The American culture of rugged individualism, a strong work ethic, and entrepreneurial competition has yielded one of the world's largest and most technologically advanced economies. At the same time, multiple stakeholders working hard and with good intent, but along parallel and disconnected paths, have yet to produce the health outcomes we might expect given the time, energy, and money this country has devoted to health care. If "The definition of insanity is doing the same thing over and over again, but expecting different results" according to the quote often attributed to Albert Einstein, then it is time to try another and anecdotally more successful model: collaboration.

The chapters in this section illustrate some of the critical components of a successful collaboration, identify how various community sectors can and do contribute to collaborations, and show how to scale up and sustain community health collaborations.

The secret sauce for a successful collaboration is community engagement, a method that has been studied and refined over the past several decades into a set of core principles, including the need to go to and learn from the community, begin with their community's strengths and concerns, build trust, and partner through long-term engagement.[1] "Engaging Residents for Health Transformation" (Chapter 11) presents a typology for engaging communities (residents) at three levels: (1) awareness and participation, (2) feedback and input, and (3) active resident leadership, and it offers lessons, tools, and practices to facilitate true engagement.

These engagement tools and principles, notably trust and relationship, have benefited from continuing research in and experience with collaboration since first edition of *The Practical Playbook: Public Health and Primary Care Together* was published.

In Chapter 15, Joyner and Treyz share a powerful story from Edgecombe, North Carolina, about parlaying the trust and relationship inherent in many faith communities into successful collaborations with the local school system and their Federally Qualified Health Center (FQHC). The keys to this story are the Rev. Joyner's holistic view of his congregation's spiritual and physical health and his recognition that the contribution of his congregation, in this case a bountiful garden and beehives, synergizes with the work of other community stakeholders to produce remarkable results.

Primary care has built on its historical roots of holistic family-centered care to embrace the broader concept of population health (Chapter 12), in which Grumbach and Woods note the evolution of care models from patient-/family-centered to panel management (the sum of patients being cared for by a primary care practice), to community health management. This broader concept of health necessitates collaboration with partners outside the clinical practice, including public health professionals, policymakers, and professionals from schools, housing, parks and recreation, law enforcement, transportation, and food systems.

In Chapter 17, Phillips shares a compelling and personal story of collaboration among primary care, mental health, schools, students, foundations, and government to reduce the risk of suicide in his community. He notes both positive and some negative experiences that the "community of solutions" faced in reducing substance abuse and building student resiliency.

Elected officials can facilitate collaborations at multiple levels, from implementation of operational regulations to passage of legislative statutes. Understanding officials' perspectives, motivations, and timelines is important, and Hunter (Chapter 14) details 10 practical tips for working with elected officials. The story of the Near Northside community in Houston (Garcia and Mendoza, Chapter 13) illustrates how using those tips helped form and sustain their Safe Walk Home initiative.

Multisector collaborations appear to produce superior results compared to well-intentioned but siloed initiatives. That said, collaborations are subject to the availability of resources and often remain relatively isolated in scope.

The California Endowment offers "Sustainability Through Accountability: The Accountable Community for Health Model" (Chapter 18) as one model for sustaining community collaborations. This chapter identifies seven key elements for success. The Wellness Fund is a unique component, though many of the success factors and lessons learned are in alignment with other models.

Beyond sustainability, Calvo (Chapter 16) discusses taking collaborations to scale, noting the importance of data and of the concept that "all teach, all learn," as well as the ever-present need for relationship and trust.

The original *Practical Playbook* appropriately emphasized collaboration between primary care and public health as an approach to population health. As the movement has matured, its scope, scale, and sustainability have grown tremendously, and it now encompasses a broader and more diverse set of partners.

Finding and forming a collaboration can be hard. Henry Ford once said, "Coming together is a beginning, staying together is progress, working together is success." Other sections of this book address the tools and resources necessary to power successful collaborations. Data and information are critical to drive decisions and evaluate progress. Innovation is a necessary spark plug to push progress (remember the earlier Einstein quote), training of the workforce is necessary to carry out collaborative initiatives, and policy helps sustain our progress.

## REFERENCE

1. NIH, CDC, and ATSDR. *Principles of Community Engagement* (2nd ed.). Washington, DC: Author; 2011(11-7872):xv. https://www.atsdr.cdc.gov/communityengagement/pdf/PCE_Report_508_FINAL.pdf. Accessed on 1/16/19.

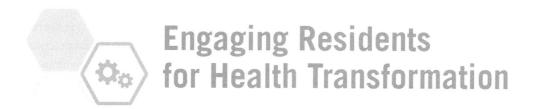

# Chapter 11

# Engaging Residents for Health Transformation

PEDJA STOJICIC

O ver the past two decades, the term "community engagement" (as well as resident, patient, and client engagement) has become such an important buzzword that rarely will a public health initiative neglect to explain, in detail, its plans for engaging the "community." Multisector partnership (MSP) members proudly report employing a variety of methods of engagement: surveys, focus groups, town hall meetings, design charrettes, and more. In fact, community engagement has become a catch-all phrase that is used to describe almost any activity that involves local residents. If a goal is to transform health systems to improve population health, then multisector partnerships and their individual stakeholders need to learn how to influence and create conditions for residents to act collectively, with the purpose of creating health. For many multisector partnerships, this will require a deep re-examination of how they approach their work with communities and residents.

*Residents are those who live and work in the community and are not professionally involved in a multisector partnership or organizations.*

This chapter provides clarity about what is actually meant by the word "engagement," unpacks the actual practices associated with the word "engagement," and learns more about the outcomes that partnerships can expect to achieve by implementing any one of those practices.

The findings are the result of the research project conducted by ReThink Health, an initiative of the Rippel Foundation in 2017. They interviewed a diverse group of more than 50 stakeholders to hear firsthand their goals, methodologies, challenges, and successes when engaging residents. These stakeholders included representatives from hospital systems, philanthropies, community-based organizations, public health departments, and insurers, as well as resident leaders themselves. In addition, researchers conducted an extensive review of the literature to examine the role of ordinary people in shaping big cultural shifts from the past. Topics included how resident engagement plays (or does not play) a role in anti-smoking, recycling, and other social movements.

The analysis of the interviews showed no single "best way to engage residents" and indicated that practices varied depending on the type of stakeholder and their capacity and leadership skills.

It's also worth noting that the stated goal (shared by participants at the beginning of every interview) was not always in sync with the actual practices performed. As an example, someone might say that their goal for community engagement is to build social cohesion or a sense of belonging, but if they are only doing occasional surveys or focus groups, it is highly unlikely that they will succeed in their goal. The practice and the goal are a mismatch.

The study analyzed the actual practices associated with the word "engagement" and learned more about the outcomes that partnerships can expect to achieve by choosing any one of those practices. The result was the creation of a Resident Engagement Practices Typology (Figure 11.1) that classifies the practices based on the three outcomes that partnerships or other organizations could actually achieve:

- Increase resident *awareness and participation* in the services provided by organizations
- *Secure feedback and input* from residents to improve services, processes, or policies
- Support *active resident leadership (community activation)* by creating conditions for large groups of residents to lead and be involved in transformational efforts

As a note, the following list is the end-all be-all of practices that engage residents, but from these interviews, literature review, and experience working in the field, these are what surfaced, and we will continue to add to this typology. While constructing the typology, two major lessons emerged that could enhance your partnership's work. They are:

1. *Partnerships could be much better at ensuring that their practices align with desired outcomes.* If your goal is to cultivate active resident leadership, for example, providing community services cooking classes or Zumba classes may not achieve this (that practice is associated with another outcome—resident awareness and participation).

2. *Partnerships should invest more effort in supporting active resident leadership (community activation) to create a balanced set of practices that could achieve health system transformation.* Transforming a region's system for health requires blending and balancing practices across all three outcomes.

If any one outcome is not pursued, there is an imbalance. One finding from ReThink's research is that the vast majority of partnerships and organizations involved are focused on increasing resident awareness and participation and/ or getting feedback and input from residents; rarely are they pursuing active resident leadership. This lack of balance in their resident engagement portfolio creates consequences, including diminishing trust of the MSP within the

# Figure 11.1 ▽

Resident engagement practices typology.

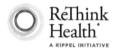

Resident Engagement Practices Typology

"Residents" are those who live and work in the community and are not professionally involved in a multisector partnership.

| Outcomes | Practices | Description |
|---|---|---|
| **Resident Awareness and Participation** | Provide services and programs in the community | Provide services and programs to residents in the community (e.g., cooking classes, farmers' markets, mobile vans, etc.) |
| | Incentivize behavior | Offer incentives to residents with the intention of changing their behavior (e.g., health care organization pays patients to show up for appointments) |
| | Share information | Share information about services, programs, and healthy behaviors with residents through flyers, blogs, reports, social media, and more |
| **Feedback and Input from Residents** | Conduct surveys, interviews, and focus groups | Gather feedback and input from residents on specific projects, services, or programs through in-person surveys, interviews, and focus groups |
| | Invite feedback via social media | Gather feedback and input from residents on specific projects, services, and programs through social media |
| | Invite representation on advisory committees and governing boards | Invite residents to serve on advisory committees and governing boards to gain their perspectives and input |
| | Host community meetings/town halls | Receive input from a broad group of residents through community meetings or town halls. |
| | Conduct listening campaigns | Organize a focused effort to build community and identify concerns and priorities in a specific region through one-on-one or house meetings |
| | Organize public deliberation processes | Organize public deliberation processes for the discussion and decision-making necessary to solve community problems |
| | Co-design of services and/or programs | Facilitate resident input in the design of community-related services and programs |
| **Active Resident Leadership** | Provide grants for resident-driven initiatives | Invest financially in resident-driven and -led initiatives (e.g., grants for programs or for hiring and training community organizers) |
| | Open opportunities for shared decision-making | Provide opportunities for a large number of residents to participate in decision-making on specific issues (e.g., participatory budgeting) |
| | Offer physical space for community gatherings | Provide free access to community spaces for residents to gather and self-organize |
| | Deploy a cadre of residents as community organizers | Recruit, hire, and train residents as community organizers to build community power |
| | Open opportunities for residents' to build their capacity for leadership | Offer training in leadership and other skills to residents seeking to build their capacity for leadership positions |

**Figure 11.1** ▽

Continued

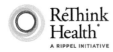

Resident Engagement Outcomes

This **Resident Engagement Practices Typology** classifies resident engagement practices based on the three outcomes that organizations or partnerships could actually achieve:

- Increasing **resident awareness and participation** in the services provided by organizations
- Getting **feedback and input from residents** to improve services, processes, or policies
- Supporting **active resident leadership** (community activation) by creating conditions for large groups of residents to lead and be involved in transformational efforts

Transforming a region's system for health requires the
balance between practices across all three outcomes.

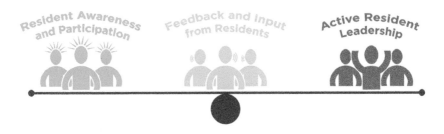

If any one outcome is not pursued, there is an imbalance.

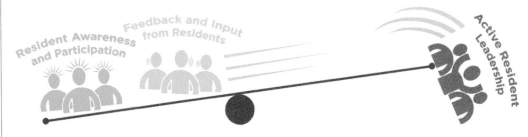

> **Box 11.1 | How Can Partnerships Use the Resident Engagement Practices Typology?**
>
> The Typology is not only a collection of practices, but it can also be used to initiate a conversation within your partnership to align your goals around resident engagement, to strategize a portfolio of activities appropriate for achieving those goals, or to identify the gaps in efforts or initiatives you are currently implementing. In your next partnership meeting, you could share the Typology and conduct a sharing exercise with two simple questions:
>
> • What needs to shift for your practices to balance your resident engagement portfolio?
> • Can your organization actually make that shift? What are the limitations (e.g., state regulations, resources)? How can you partner with someone else to overcome any limitations?
>
> Answering these questions will enable participants to identify gaps and needs in their current engagement practices.

community. Residents sense an inability to influence things, which creates a sense of being excluded and powerless (Box 11.1).

## POWER, TRUST, AND SENSE OF BELONGING

In our research, we observed that the partnerships and other organizations that are most effective at creating the conditions for residents to lead and get involved ensure that their practices are helping residents experience all of the following: (1) a sense of belonging, (2) a sense of trust, and (3) a sense of power (Figure 11.2).

### Sense of Belonging

For almost anyone, a sense of collective and cultural identity is a powerful source of motivation for active involvement and leadership. If residents feel as if they don't belong to a place or a region, it is difficult for them to invest time and energy to work on improving things around them. (And it doesn't hurt that sense of belonging contributes directly to health outcomes—since that's the ultimate goal.)

### Sense of Trust

Low levels of relational trust among residents, and between residents and local institutions, are an enormous barrier to engagement and transformation. Change happens at the speed of trust, so all resident engagement practices should create opportunities for cultivating trust and accountability.

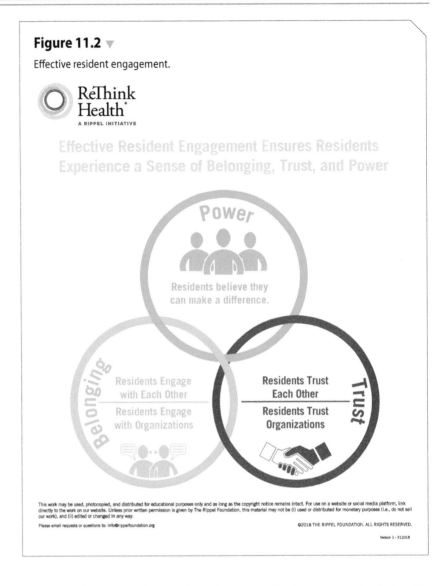

**Figure 11.2** ▼

Effective resident engagement.

ReThink Health®
A RIPPEL INITIATIVE

Effective Resident Engagement Ensures Residents
Experience a Sense of Belonging, Trust, and Power

Power

Residents believe they
can make a difference.

Belonging

Residents Engage
with Each Other

Residents Engage
with Organizations

Residents Trust
Each Other

Residents Trust
Organizations

Trust

For example, partnerships and residents can develop a mutual relationship in which both parties take risks—the organizations trust the decisions and behaviors of residents rather than dictating to them, and residents trust the intentions and support offered by the organizations and professionals (Figure 11.3).

## Sense of Power

The power, or sense of agency, to influence your community is essential for exercising leadership. Without a sense that their efforts and opinions really matter—which partially depends on feelings of belonging and trust—people rarely find the motivation to be actively involved in the initiatives or sustain the long-term efforts needed for community transformation.

**Figure 11.3** ▽

Resident engagement outcomes.

Resident Engagement Outcomes

Transforming a region's system for health requires the
balance between practices across all three outcomes.

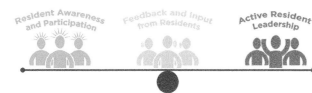

If any one outcome is not pursued, there is an imbalance.

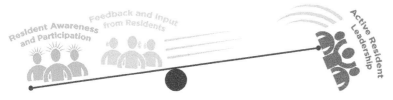

---

## Box 11.2 | Putting Belonging, Trust, and Power into Practice

Let's consider one of the most common resident engagement practices—a survey conducted across the community—to explore how partnerships working on health system transformation can approach resident engagement.

To conduct a survey, partnerships tend to set up an internal team, develop a set of survey questions to explore the health-related priorities of residents, transfer the questions to an online platform (e.g., SurveyMonkey), and distribute the survey through various communication channels. After the information is collected, someone in the partnership analyzes the results and develops the presentation of residents' priorities that will be used to, among other things, inform decisions about community investments or improving specific services.

If a partnership implements a survey with residents' sense of belonging, trust, and power in mind, the process looks quite different. Instead of designing the survey on its own, the partnership would ask itself three questions:

1. How is this practice creating a *sense of belonging* for residents in our region?
2. How is this practice fostering a *sense of trust* among residents in our region and trust in our organization or partnership?
3. How is this practice increasing residents' *sense of power* to change and influence the region where they live?

Answering these questions could lead the partnership to involve residents and community organizations (which often represent residents) to co-design the survey. Then, the partnership might distribute the survey in partnership with local residents, by intentionally working with people from the community to ensure that information is collected from everyone and not just from people who usually participate or have online access. The partnership might also provide resources to residents who are open to organizing outreach events that will nurture and celebrate local values and history.

When the survey is complete, the partnership might create a transparent process of sharing the results with the community. For example, it could coordinate a series of town hall meetings in partnership with local churches, civic centers, or active community organizations. Instead of just presenting the information, the partnership might invite people to join in a dialogue about how to implement some of the findings and invite residents to take action. The partnership could also ask residents to help create a process for holding the partnership accountable for implementing the decisions that impact the community and develop a long-term plan for regular "check-ins" with residents.

If performed well, this process will increase residents' sense of belonging, trust, and power as well as increase the likelihood of success for the partnership's health transformation efforts in the communities it serves.

Importantly, there is no particular order in which residents experience a sense of belonging, trust, and power, and the three are incredibly interconnected. For example, to develop power, you need to have trust. Furthermore, you can often gain a sense of power when you have a sense of belonging, and you can feel a sense of belonging even if you don't feel a sense of trust (Box 11.2).

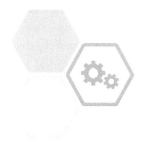

# Chapter 12

# The Role of Primary Care in Population and Community Health: Pragmatic Approaches to Integration

JULIE WOOD AND KEVIN GRUMBACH

It is well known that the United States has an ineffective health care system. It has the highest per capita investment in health care of any nation in the world,[1] yet it ranks consistently low in quality measures compared with other industrialized nations.[2] Efforts to improve the system have been focused on integrated, high-value health care that positions family medicine and primary care as an important solution to the health care crisis. It is "one of the first objectives for family physicians to understand the living conditions patients face when they leave our office or when they leave the hospital."[3] This is paralleled by a growing awareness of the social, environmental, and community determinants of health.[4-6] However, for successful broad system change, primary care physicians must align with the public health sector; they are two fields with a common interest, yet they have been functioning independently for the past century. In this chapter, we first briefly describe the population and community framework and its historical role in the development of primary care, and then we turn to the proposal of pragmatic approaches that busy primary care clinicians and care teams can use to integrate population health approaches into their practices.

## THE POPULATION AND COMMUNITY HEALTH FRAMEWORK

For many years, the training model for physicians has focused on the individual and solving the presenting clinical problem, with a reactive rather than proactive or preventive approach. Although individual care remains important, there is an evolution toward broader considerations of population and community with a long-range view of patient wellness to keep individuals healthy for as long as possible and promote healthy communities. There are many stakeholders doing so, with a variety of definitions, interests, and desired outcomes, leading to confusion about terms, concepts, and approaches.

"Population health" is a term frequently used in both health care and public health. It has been used to mean different things, depending on context and perspective. The American Academy of Family Physicians offers this definition of population health from the perspective of the family physician and primary care:

> Population health is "the health outcomes of a group of individuals, including the distribution of such outcomes, within the group." The population being considered may vary based on an individual's perspective and goals. For the family physician, the most obvious "group of individuals" is their patient panel. This is where most family physicians focus their energies and where they often have the greatest impact. Population health also includes the health status and outcomes of the larger communities to which the physician and patient belong. It is essential when caring for their patients that family physicians consider the factors beyond the walls of their practice that influence their patients' health. The family physician must consider the social and physical environments in which their patients live and work in order to effectively improve health outcomes."[7]

This definition captures the most salient features of a population health approach: (1) considering the health of groups and not just individuals, (2) specifying the relevant group that is of interest (e.g., all patients cared for by a primary care practice, all residents within a specified geographic community, or a particular demographic stratum, such as homeless individuals), and (3) attending to the social and environmental determinants of health and illness.

Although a population health approach has not been fully woven into most contemporary primary care practices in the United States, there are many prominent threads in the history of primary care. One bright strand is the Community-Oriented Primary Care (COPC) model, developed in the 1940s by physicians Sidney and Emily Kark in South Africa.[8] The COPC model became an organizing framework for the community health center movement in the United States in the 1960s, with leaders such as Jack Geiger pushing care beyond the clinic walls to engage with community members and address social determinants. The Folsom Report of this same era,[9] which was published in 1967 and helped catalyze the establishment of the specialty of family medicine in 1969, called for a strong link between primary care and community health service delivery to create "communities of solution."[10] Despite this impetus in the 1960s toward an integration of primary care and population and community health, models such as COPC remained largely confined to safety net practices, and, even in those settings, the models have receded in prominence as funding models drove clinics to focus on individual care and clinic visit productivity.

Recent trends are moving population health back into the mainstream of primary care practice. The national health "Triple Aim" calls for improving patient experience and the health of populations while reducing unnecessary costs.[11] The Affordable Care Act enacted in 2010[12] includes many elements focusing on population health management and has promoted the development of new care models, such as accountable care organizations (ACOs) and the patient-centered medical home (PCMH). Payment and quality improvement policies are increasingly using a population health framework. Ongoing efforts to integrate with the National Academy of Medicine's (formerly the Institute of Medicine) Primary Care: America's Health in a New Era[13] and The Future of the Public's Health in the 21st Century[14] initiatives developed the momentum that led to the 2012 release of the National Academy of Medicine's Primary Care and Public Health: Exploring Integration to Improve Population Health initiative,[15] demonstrating successful models of integration and accountability sought to ensure quality patient care. These reforms all recognize that individual health is inseparable from the health of the larger community, which ultimately determines the overall health of the nation.[16] To better align these individual and community forces, primary care and public health need to reconnect.

Many local, state, and national efforts and collaboratives have been developed to facilitate mechanisms for this integration to occur at all levels. Review of the changing landscape of health care delivery and payment structure, as well as interprofessional educational reforms, is needed to educate physicians in training, as well as those in established practices.[17]

## INTEGRATING PRIMARY CARE AND POPULATION AND COMMUNITY HEALTH: PRAGMATIC APPROACHES FOR PRIMARY CARE PRACTITIONERS

How can physicians, nurses, and others working in primary care clinical settings take pragmatic steps to integrate a population health approach into their practice? Are there ways to do this that do not overwhelm already busy clinicians and aggravate already high levels of burnout in primary care? We discuss several strategies, starting with the population of patients empaneled in a primary care practice and extending to broader community-based population health approaches.

### The Empaneled Patient Population

*Empanelment* refers to the process of attributing individual patients to a primary care physician or care team. Empanelment is a vital enabler of many elements of high-performing primary care.[18] Empanelment formalizes a relationship of continuity between patients and their primary care team and medical home. It also provides a population denominator for measuring and holding primary care teams accountable for quality of care, such as the percentage of patients who are up to date on breast cancer screening. These population-based metrics are increasingly being used by payers and regulators for primary care assessments. Empanelment most formally occurs when payment to primary care is by capitation and patients must register with a primary care physician, as occurs in capitation models in Canada, Britain, and other nations, and in the United States under "direct primary care" and some managed care payment models. In fee-for-service payment models that do not require formal registration, payers using "value-based payment" models, such as accountable care organization (ACO) arrangements, are attributing a population of patients to primary care practices and health care organizations based on patterns of care use and using this attributed population for measuring performance and determining risk-based contracting payments.

These payment and related reforms are moving many primary care practices into a population health framework, emphasizing accountability for the entire group of patients under their care. Practices are adopting approaches such as "panel management," in which clinicians and care team members review data on which patients in the panel are up to date on preventive and chronic care services and then proactively reach out to patients needing to have care gaps closed (e.g., to have colon cancer screening performed) or to have chronic conditions better managed (e.g., diabetic patients with elevated glycosylated hemoglobin levels).[19]

Appreciation of the powerful influence of social determinants on health is also prompting some primary care practices to begin to more systematically assess the social vulnerabilities of the group of patients empaneled in their practice. Although obtaining a thorough social history is a core task of traditional primary care practice, there is evidence that primary care clinicians do not consistently ask patients about many important social factors, such as food insecurity, and that using more structured screening tools may elicit more complete, clinically relevant information. Screening tools also allow for data on social needs to be entered more easily as structured data in electronic health records. In Chapter 26 of this book, Gottlieb and Fichtenberg describe how primary care practices can systematically collect data on patient social needs to guide "socially informed care" (e.g., identifying patients with limited English proficiency who need interpreter services) and "socially targeted care" (e.g., referring patients with food insecurity to a neighborhood food bank). The chapter also highlights methods for socially targeted care that do not place a major onus on the primary care clinician to personally manage these types of referrals. The AAFP EveryONE project, described in Box 12.1, is another example.

One recent study found that enhancing the capacity of primary care practices to address the social needs of their patients may not only be beneficial for the health of the patient population served, but also for the well-being of the clinicians working at the practice.[20] The study found that clinicians who reported that their practices had more resources available to address patients' social needs were less likely to have high burnout on standard burnout assessment

## Box 12.1 | EveryONE Project Provider Toolkit

The American Academy of Family Physicians (AAFP) defines social determinants of health (SDOH) as the conditions under which people are born, grow, live, work, and age. Prominent factors of SDOH include socioeconomic status, racism and discrimination, poverty and income inequality, and lack of community resources. One study suggests that social and economic factors account for as much as 55% of health outcomes. Other studies have shown that a substantial proportion of all deaths are attributable to poverty (2–6%), income inequality (9–25%), and lower socioeconomic status (18–25%). Primary care physicians provide the majority of health care in the United States. Specialists in primary care are a natural point of integration among clinical care, public health, behavioral health, and community-based services. In addition, family medicine was developed as a medical specialty, in part due to the recognition of the role that social factors have on health. This makes primary care, especially family medicine, a critical component of the nation's health system for addressing patients' SDOH. In their patient-centered practices, family physicians and their staff identify and address the SDOH for individuals and families, incorporating this information into the biopsychosocial model to promote continuous healing relationships, whole-person orientation, family and community context, and comprehensive care. This implementation guide provides suggested changes that family physicians and their practices can make to address their patients' SDOH as a means for advancing health equity. As you address SDOH in your practice setting, bring together your health care team to provide the services efficiently and establish a process that works well for the team. This requires clear instructions on roles and responsibilities.

### Team-Based Primary Care

Team-based primary care addressing your patients' SDOH) requires a team-based approach and is not intended to be implemented by the physician alone. The procedures outlined within this implementation guide are intended to support team-based care and recognize the unique skills of different types of health care workers and how they can contribute to addressing SDOH in primary care.

*From: American Academy for Family Physicians. Addressing Social Determinants of Health in Primary Care, Team-Based Approach for Advancing Health Equity. Published online by AAFP. 2018. https://www.aafp.org/dam/AAFP/documents/patient_care/everyone_project/team-based-approach.pdf*

measures. Serving the health needs of primary care patients requires team work inside the office and, increasingly, outside as well.

## Moving from Empaneled Patients to the Broader Community

Public health agencies define populations based on geographical location, stratified by demographic factors such as race, ethnicity, gender, age, language, disability, or disease status.[7] For primary care clinicians, embracing this broader geographic community framework requires a large professional cultural shift from the prevailing medical definition of population as an empaneled aggregate of individual patients whom a single healthcare organization has cared for over a period of time to a geographically defined population that includes many individuals who are not under the care of that particular health care organization. Is it feasible for primary care clinicians to include this broader framework in their practice?

We believe that there are a number of pragmatic ways to integrate this broader framework into primary care practice under what has been described as a *clinical population medicine model*.[21] This model includes three elements: (1) health assessment, (2) policy development, and (3) assurance. An example of health assessment well-known to many primary care practitioners is surveillance for public health outbreaks and disease clusters. Traditional disease surveillance has involved sentinel practice reporting systems for seasonal influenza incidence. Screening children for elevated blood lead levels has allowed primary care clinicians to collaborate with public health department environmental control divisions to identify housing that needs lead abatement treatment. The advent of electronic health records now provides a much more powerful means of using "Big Data" from clinical records to identify population health patterns, such as census tracts in which residents have high rates of preventable hospitalizations, which may in turn inform public health efforts to target "upstream" interventions—in partnership with practices—to address social and environmental factors driving the poor health outcomes in these census tracts.

At the level of policy development, simple steps can promote more integration between primary care practices and public health departments to address community-wide health issues. An example is involving primary care clinicians in public education campaigns addressing local community health priorities. For example, many public health departments have sponsored campaigns to reduce the consumption of sugary beverages, which may include billboard and public service announcement messaging, "Drink Water Said the Otter" coloring books for children, and related outreach efforts. These campaigns can be amplified by distributing these materials to primary care practices and engaging primary care clinicians as powerful reinforcers of these public health messages.

An additional role for primary care clinicians in addressing community health is the role of advocate. Surveys indicate that physicians and other health professionals, particularly those working in primary care, remain highly respected and trusted by the public. Health professionals have an influential voice, whether exercised through professional societies or individual actions. Primary care clinicians have a role to play in public health assurance by speaking out about the profound public health implications of issues such as housing insecurity, gun violence, climate change, and inadequate investment in early childhood education.

## CONCLUSION

A congruence of factors, from payment reform to growing recognition of the importance of social determinants of health, is returning primary care to a population health model. As primary care moves in the direction of population health, it need not stop at the concept of population as defined simply by the patients empaneled in a practice, but should also continue to find ways to embrace a broader view of community-wide population health and integration with public health. There are practical and feasible steps that primary care practices can take to make steady progress on the road to population and community health integration.

### REFERENCES

1. World Health Organization. *The World Health Report 2000—Health Systems: Improving Performance*. Geneva, Switzerland: World Health Organization; 2000. http://www.who.int/whr/2000/en/(www.who.int). Accessed on 1/16/2019.

2. Davis K, Stremikis K, Schoen C, Squires D. *Mirror, Mirror on the Wall, 2014 Update: How the US Health Care System Compares Internationally*. Washington, DC: The Commonwealth Fund; 2014. Accessed on 1/16/2019.

3. Woolf S. 2011 AAFP National Conference. Family physician urges residents, students to consider "social determinants" of health. 2011. http://www.aafp.org/news/health-of-the-public/20110803ntlconfwoolf.html. Accessed on 1/16/2019.

4. World Health Organization. *Commission on Social Determinants of Health—Final Report*. Geneva, Switzerland: World Health Organization, 2008. http://www.who.int/social_determinants/final_report/en/index.html(www.who.int). Accessed on 1/16/2019.

5. Christiani DC. Combating environmental causes of cancer. *N Engl J Med.* 2011;364(9):791–3.

6. Schensul JJ. Community, culture and sustainability in multilevel dynamic systems intervention science. *Am J Commun Psychol.* 2009;43(3-4):241–56.

7. Kindig DA, Stoddart G. What is population health? *Am J Public Health.* 2003;93:366–9.

8. Mullan F, Epstein L. Community-oriented primary care: New relevance in a changing world. *Am J Public Health.* 2002;92:1748–55.

9. National Commission on Community Health Services. *Health Is a Community Affair: Report of the National Commission on Community Health Services (NCCHS)*. Cambridge, MA: Harvard University Press; 1967.

10. The Folsom Group. Communities of Solution: The Folsom Report revisited. *Ann Fam Med.* 2012;10:250–60.

11. Berwick DM, Nolan TW, Whittington J. The triple aim: Care, health and cost. *Health Affairs* (Milwood). 2008;27(3):759–69.

12. Patient Protection and Affordable Care Act of 2010. 42 U.S.C. §§ 298d, x5313.

13. Institute of Medicine. *Primary Care: America's Health in a New Era*. Washington DC: The National Academies Press, 1996.

14. Institute of Medicine. *The Future of the Public's Health in the 21st Century*. Washington DC: The National Academies Press, 2002.

15. Institute of Medicine. *Primary Care and Public Health: Exploring Integration to Improve Population Health*. Washington, DC: The National Academies Press.

16. Koh HK, Piotrowski JJ, Kumanyika S, Fielding JE. Healthy people: a 2020 vision for the social determinants approach. *Health Ed Behav*. 2011;38(6):551–7.

17. Centers for Disease Control and Prevention. *Advancing Integration of Population Health into Graduate Medical Education: The CDC Milestones Project*. Atlanta, GA: Centers for Disease Control and Prevention; 2013. http://www.cdc.gov/primarycare/docs/milestonemeeting-report082013.pdf(www.cdc.gov).

18. Bodenheimer T, Ghorob A, Willard-Grace R, Grumbach K. The 10 building blocks of high-performing primary care. *Ann Fam Med*. 2014;12(2):166–71.

19. Grumbach K, Olayiwola JN. Patient empanelment: the importance of understanding who is at home in the medical home. *J Am Board Fam Med*. 2015;28(2):170–2.

20. Olayiwola JN, Willard-Grace R, Dubé K, Hessler D, Shunk R, Grumbach K, Gottlieb L. Higher Perceived Clinic Capacity to Address Patients' Social Needs Associated with Lower Burnout in Primary Care Providers. *J Health Care Poor Underserved*. 2018;29(1):415–29.

21. Orkin AM, Bharmal A, Cram J, Kouyoumdjian FG, Pinto AD, Upshur R. Clinical Population Medicine: Integrating Clinical Medicine and Population Health in Practice. *Ann Fam Med*. 2017;15(5):405–9.

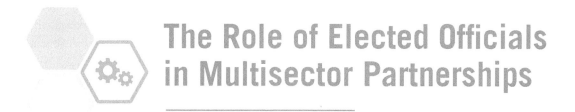

# Chapter 13

# The Role of Elected Officials in Multisector Partnerships

SYLVIA GARCIA AND ELSA MENDOZA

## CASE STUDY: NEAR NORTHSIDE COMMUNITY, HOUSTON

I am an avid believer in cross-sectional partnerships being necessary to sustain meaningful progress in communities. The role of an elected official is to listen to and understand the needs of the population of the district being represented and to create and/or effect policy that in turn addresses those needs. I am committed to understanding the priorities of my constituents in order for them to live affordable, healthy lives.

### Collaboration with the Community

For the Near Northside community in Houston, dealing with crime, homelessness, and drug activity is for many, unfortunately, an everyday occurrence. After a senseless stabbing of an 11-year-old boy as he walked home from school, I dedicated resources with the intention to find solutions for safety concerns in the Near Northside and in communities with similar problems.

It was through a community needs assessment conducted by my office that I learned of the various situations contributing to the neighborhood's dangerous environment, in which this murder was possible. The community assessment gathered information from already existing neighborhood assessments, small business owners, school leadership personnel, long-time residents, and local nonprofit organizations. At the same time, a grassroots effort that focused on making routes safer for walking students was gaining traction. The program, known as Safe Walk Home, became the immediate response that the community needed to regain any sense of security.

Safe Walk Home is composed of Near Northside residents who commit their time to monitor students during peak walking hours. Behind the scenes, the members educate themselves on how to properly report crime and how to administer basic first aid, and they are involved in safety initiatives across the community to continuously improve their practices.

Throughout my time as an elected official, and also due to my social work education, I have come to value understanding the interconnectedness of circumstances that produce social injustices. Some solutions may not initially make sense to constituents, but in understanding the connections that problems have to one another, it is important to communicate to constituents the link between the solutions to many or all of their issues.

In recognizing that much constituent frustration against lawmakers stems from misunderstanding the legislative process and its long-term benefits, I saw the opportunity to work with the Near Northside's Safe Walk Home group to alleviate some of the frustration the neighborhood was experiencing. For that reason, through my time in the legislative session of 2017, my office worked on maintaining the Safe Walk Home program, and some residents of the Near Northside engaged during the process. With their support, and trusting that they know best what their community struggles with, I successfully passed legislation that aims to improve transportation for walking students living in high crime areas.

Having the group be part of the legislative process, from advocating on the Hill to testifying at Senate hearings, was the perfect opportunity for me and my legislative team to teach a mourning community how to advocate for themselves by becoming civically engaged. The group asked questions and we answered them. It simply took us working together and taking the time to break down a complex process into simple language, with action plans of advocacy. To sustain support of constituents, they have to comprehend what my role is and how we are useful to one another. In the end, we succeeded in a victory that was needed for a community used to obituaries and not winning.

Currently, I continue to work with the Safe Walk Home group as they have become an integral leader in safety advocacy for the Near Northside neighborhood. We discuss ways to improve the neighborhood's quality of life, from simple fixes to legislative possibilities. The empowerment of a group such as this one, or of a neighborhood creates trust, compassion, and sincere dialogue among community and elected officials.

The following are key points for ensuring effective collaboration between constituents and elected officials:

- *Empower constituents with resources*, do not just give them resources. Meaning, discuss contextually how resources can be used.
- *Motivate constituents to ask questions*, and have honest and simple answers to legislative processes. Keeping in mind to always to talk to them, rather than talk down at them. It helps to break information down without using legal bureaucratic language and acronyms.
- *Do not miss the chance to discuss the interconnectedness of issues beyond the neighborhood's scope* that may be contributing to the neighborhood's immediate problems.

- *Make constituents aware that legislative solutions come from detailed logical explanations of the community's concerns*, as gaps in services or problems in procedures are distinguished more easily.

The following are key points for ensuring effective communication between elected officials and health care providers, both clinicians and public health care officials:

- *It is useful for elected officials to be aware of any issues in communication* between government agencies and health care providers that may affect the eligibility, accessibility, and understanding of resources. Being aware of these issues will allow officials to identify if there may be any legislative solutions.
- *Invite elected officials to events that showcase the work being done in the community on behalf of your group*. It is essential for elected officials to understand what resources are available in their districts as constituents normally need referrals and are unaware of what may be available to them.
- *Inviting elected officials to tour facilities* in order for them to personally observe what constituents have to go through to receive services. This helps officials understand how policy is translated into real-life implications.
- *If collaborations and partnerships are occurring, invite elected officials to partake*. It is helpful for an elected official to be aware of relationships between stakeholders so that he or she can strengthen the mission if it aligns with the agenda of the elected official.

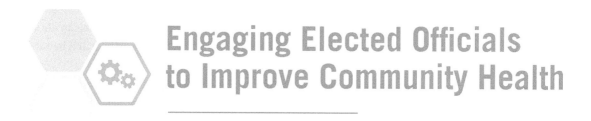

# Chapter 14

# Engaging Elected Officials to Improve Community Health

EDWARD L. HUNTER

I mproving the health of populations and communities requires an "all hands on deck" approach. Elected officials can be important allies in efforts to achieve health goals at all levels of government, but they are often overlooked as potential collaborators. Public health and health care partners can enhance the impact of cross-sector collaborations with greater awareness and preparation for working with elected officials.

Engaging with the political process is important for advancing community health goals,[1] yet engaging with elected officials isn't always about partisan politics or even about enacting legislation. Because determinants of health span many sectors, many decision-makers important to advancing health are elected: legislators, county executives, mayors, councils, school boards, sheriffs, and commissioners in a diverse range of subject areas. Particularly at the local level, many who make administrative decisions are elected officials, and many are nonpartisan. Regardless of their specific job and connection to partisan politics, it's important to understand their roles, drivers, and influences.

## IMPORTANT ROLES FOR ELECTED OFFICIALS

Clearly, the most important role for elected officials is the establishment of public policies and providing for the administration of public agencies. Section VI of this book, "Policy: Achieving Sustained Impact," addresses the critical role of policy as a tool for improving health; it provides examples of policy interventions at all levels of government.

Policy can include the use of law, regulation, and administrative action, most often by political leaders empowered by voters. Through the legislative process, broad and sustainable changes in communities can be achieved; similarly, authority for public programs is established and funding is provided to executive agencies. These actions often take successful pilots or geographically limited programs to a broader scale or provide sustainability for programs that start with private funding.

The importance of using policy as a tool is increasingly highlighted by efforts to move health "upstream" and by attention to the role of public health officials as health strategists for their communities.[2,3] Cross-sector collaborations can play a critical role in Influencing elected officials to adopt these tools, particularly as upstream interventions often require action beyond the health sector.

Beyond these roles in making or enacting public policies, elected officials can be effective collaborators for other reasons. A few examples follow:

- An important part of the job of political leaders is to engage in problem-solving for constituents, intervening when agencies take action that affects constituents, or engaging on issues where advocates seek action. For advocates, this provides an opening to approach elected officials with health problems they want prioritized for action. For public agencies, this provides opportunities to help elected officials solve problems, an important way to develop constructive relationships that can advance goals.
- In a health crisis or controversy, elected leaders with whom health officials have positive relationships can be key allies in crisis communications, calming the public or other elected officials. Conversely, those same leaders can amplify controversies if they are uninformed.
- Leaders can help make connections across communities and to non-health sectors. Particularly at the local level, elected officials may also be important in business or other circles. For example, state legislator is often a part-time position, so a majority of time is spent in private pursuits (including as business leaders, members of trade associations, or with other pathways to influence in the community). An elected official convinced of the need for a public policy action can become an effective ambassador and help build needed support elsewhere.
- Because of their connections across diverse elements of communities, elected officials can often provide a reality test for what is possible to achieve in a community as well as help strategize about ways to work with other political leaders. The essay in Chapter 13, by Texas State Senator Garcia and her staff person, Elsa Mendoza, is a great example of an elected official serving this supportive, facilitating role.

## UNDERSTANDING WHAT MOTIVATES ELECTED OFFICIALS

Elected officials are subject to drivers and influences that are often different from those of health care or public health officials, and it is important to understand the experience and perspective of an individual elected official before engaging with him or her. A few examples follow:

- Health officials are driven by evidence-based science, whereas elected officials are unlikely to be skilled consumers of science and have multiple real-world influences.

- Many advocates for health policies presume a positive role for government, whereas many elected officials favor private or market solutions to problems. Others differ about which level of government (federal, state, or local) is the appropriate locus for action.
- Health interventions, particularly for chronic diseases, may have a long time frame before an outcome can be measured, whereas elected officials often need results keyed to an election cycle.
- Distributional impacts may be viewed differently. Health officials may evaluate approaches through a health equity lens, in which aiding populations in greatest need is a pre-eminent value. Officials standing for election not only need a positive record to point to (and therefore "wins" from a policy choice, including health equity), but also are concerned with the distribution of losers and will need to understand the implications of a policy choice for their constituents, supporters, and contributors.

Despite differences, there are many commonalities that provide the basis for constructive engagement: elected officials are motivated to improve the community, respond to residents' interest in their own health, understand that economic development requires healthy communities, and they are motivated by budget considerations to achieve more value from health spending.

## TEN TIPS FOR WORKING WITH ELECTED OFFICIALS

1. *Seek engagement with political leaders*. Don't be afraid: advocacy is just another word for telling a story and showing the value of approaches to improving health of communities. There are likely many more ways you can work with the political system than you may think.
2. *Understand the difference between advocacy, lobbying, and political activity*. Some activities are likely off limits for many health advocates and officials (e.g., fundraising or campaigning for an individual). Others are more subtle, and the particular rules that govern you because of your tax status or funding source are key. Federal funding, for example, is subject to specific appropriations language that prohibits *lobbying* but enables many forms of education and advocacy.[4] Nonprofit organizations have restrictions on lobbying that are governed by the Internal Revenue Service.[5] A few of the more clear distinctions are presented in Table 14.1).
3. *Understand your own organization's approach to engagement* and the rules or clearances you may need in taking positions on policies. In private organizations, this may be your general counsel; in public agencies it may be the legislative affairs office. Beyond legal considerations, avoid conflicts by understanding the policy positions of your organization and any strategies they may be pursuing with the same officials on related issues, or make appropriate disclaimers.

| Table 14.1 ▼ Lobbying versus education and advocacy | |
|---|---|
| **Lobbying** | **Education and advocacy** |
| Direct contact with an elected official in support (or in opposition) to a specific piece of legislation. | Holding briefings and meetings to present evidence on the importance of a health problem or issue, and the need for solutions. |
| Encouraging the public to contact their elected officials in support of a specific measure. | Convening public forums to discuss the importance of an issue or problem, and presenting objective evidence. |
| Directly approaching an executive branch official to argue for the adoption of a specific regulation or administrative action. | Presenting elected officials with evidence on the effectiveness of policy approaches, including stories from other jurisdictions where a policy has been implemented. |
| | Describing the implications of a policy approach in an elected official's own jurisdiction, or a specific population. |
| | Describing the impact of increases or decreases in funding levels of a health program, or policy change. |

4. *Understand the elected official you want to engage with.* Don't make assumptions about motivations, influences, and predispositions; do the research you need in order to find a way to connect. There's almost always some common interest or personal contact to build on. For example, the further away from "home" elected officials may be, the more they will value your specific knowledge of what is happening "on the ground" in their community and how they can use your connections to be current with their constituents.

5. *Use language that resonates.* Find ways to communicate on *their* terms and in their language. Don't assume they understand science/evidence or that it is the dominant factor in their decision-making process. There are existing and emerging resources for facilitating communication that are helpful,[6] but it starts with thinking through how you would have a conversation with a neighbor or family member who is unfamiliar with health issues.

6. *Invest in relationships.* It takes time to develop credibility and trust and to demonstrate that your evidence and solutions are consistent with the interests of the elected official. This means continuity of contact with the elected official and his office, and sometimes connections with the networks of organizations and individuals that elected officials belong to. It's important to invest for the long term: politicians aspire to upward mobility and have long memories. Find good prospects with a health interest and cultivate relationships with them before they are important and in demand. Finally, a good rule of thumb is that you never want to have to go to an elected official for the first time in the middle of a crisis.

7. *Rely on government affairs professionals* in your organization or find ways to access expertise if your organization doesn't have them. This can be helpful

in opening doors, identifying interests, and crafting messages. Many national associations have skilled people who can offer advice, relationships, and materials that have already been developed to help convey key messages.

8. *Have an offer, not just an "ask."* Health is a critical issue to voters, and professionals in health care and public health have useful information to provide to elected officials. Information about their community and constituents is often as valuable as a campaign contribution as it can help them look good and connect to voters. Find ways to routinely share information about events in the community, new initiatives being launched, and successful programs/interventions. Use your knowledge to advantage: be their go-to source for information about the constituents and communities they serve. And, within appropriate limits, give them preferential access to information, as you would do for the press or advocates, and work with them to make them part of announcements. Finally, consider building a relationship through your "offers" before you advance to your "ask."

## Figure 14.1 ▼

Ground rules for political engagement.

From Hunter EL. Politics and public health: Engaging the third rail. *J Pub Health Manag Pract.* 2016:22(5):436–41.

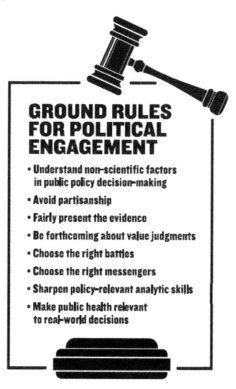

**GROUND RULES FOR POLITICAL ENGAGEMENT**

- Understand non-scientific factors in public policy decision-making
- Avoid partisanship
- Fairly present the evidence
- Be forthcoming about value judgments
- Choose the right battles
- Choose the right messengers
- Sharpen policy-relevant analytic skills
- Make public health relevant to real-world decisions

9. *Make any "ask" realistic and relevant* to the official you are appealing to. Most elected officials are approached by a wide range of advocates and constituents and need to decide where to invest their time and political capital. You can make this decision easier by providing practical solutions that are actionable and align with other interests the official may have. And as noted earlier, elected officials and their staffs may be great resources on how to make your "ask" more appealing to their counterparts as you grow a supportive coalition.

10. *Follow some simple ground rules for political engagement* This has already been verified, all set?>. Figure 14.1 is drawn from a longer commentary on engagement with the political system.[7] It is directed at public health officials but is generalizable to others in health advocacy.

## REFERENCES

1. Hunter EL. Politics and public health—Engaging the third rail. *J Public Health Mgmt Pract.* 2016;22(5):436–41.

2. http://www.resolv.org/site-healthleadershipforum/files/2014/05/The-High-Achieving-Governmental-Health-Department-as-the-Chief-Health-Strategist-by-2020-Final1.pdf. Accesed on 1/16/2019.

3. https://www.healthypeople.gov/sites/default/files/Public-Health-3.0-White-Paper.pdf. Accessed on 2/5/2019.

4. https://www.cdc.gov/grants/documents/Anti-Lobbying-Restrictions.pdf. Accesed on 1/16/2019.

5. https://www.irs.gov/charities-non-profits/charitable-organizations/political-and-lobbying-activities. Accesed on 1/16/2019.

6. PHRASES.org. https://www.ncbi.nlm.nih.gov/pmc/articles/PMC1449221/, https://journals.lww.com/jphmp/Fulltext/2017/07000/Crafting_Richer_Public_Health_Messages_for_A.15.aspx. Accesed on 1/16/2019.

7. https://www.healthypeople.gov/sites/default/files/Public-Health-3.0-White-Paper.pdf. Accesed on 1/16/2019.

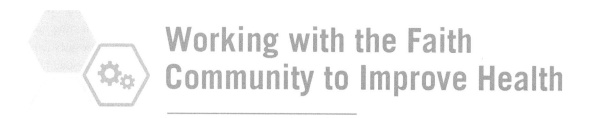

# Chapter 15

# Working with the Faith Community to Improve Health

### RICHARD JOYNER AND ALEXANDRA TREYZ

A faith community experiences the greatest joys and sorrows of its people: birth, marriage, death, a new job, a school graduation. As members of a faith community gather to worship, mourn, and celebrate, they bring not only their beliefs, but their physical bodies, both broken and healed. Although a faith community is not a hospital for the physical healing of bodies, it is a hospital for the healing of souls. And it also can be a hospital for preventative care, for paying attention to and addressing the health of the body. Therefore, a faith community should exist not solely for the practice of religion, but also for the healing of hearts, minds, *and* bodies.

When a faith community pays attention to and addresses the well-being of the whole person—body and soul—transformative healing is possible. Therefore, the faith community has a critical and powerful role in community health and upstream health intervention efforts. Additionally, a faith community is made up of human beings with human development potential, not only on Sunday mornings, but throughout the week. Human development in and through the faith community should therefore encompass all areas of an individual's well-being: social, emotional, physical, and spiritual.

## ACKNOWLEDGING THE WHY

When it comes to the health of its people, as the church, we must acknowledge the trauma and health challenges of the congregation as a result of the social contexts in which our parishioners live. As a pastor, I visit my congregants in the hospital and preside at graveside burials. If I don't ask myself *why* my people are sick from preventable diseases or *why* they have died young, I'm failing not only the sick and the dead, but also the living in my congregation, in the community, and our future generations.

In my church, Conetoe Missionary Baptist located in Conetoe, North Carolina, I first started the process of acknowledging the true causes of preventable disease more than a decade ago, when, in 1 year I presided over 30 funerals for people younger than 40. I had to ask myself: Is what we are offering at church just preparing us for another funeral? Why are we not being honest with ourselves about why so many people are dying so young in our congregation? What is that doing to our community? As I started to ask these questions, I started to unwind some critical truths about poor health, its causes, and the role of the church to address those issues.

Without this first level of acknowledgment, forward progress is never possible. Speaking the truth wakes up that which has been sleeping: our consciousness and our will power to bring about change. We must raise our consciousness concerning not just the habits and behaviors that might be making us and our communities sick, but also about the experience of the trauma of racism, poverty, and abuse that has devastated the social fabric in our communities, making chronic disease a symptom of our interpersonal dysfunction.

## SOCIAL DETERMINANTS, THE BUILT ENVIRONMENT, AND HEALING

Initially, when I began to name what was making us sick, I was preaching health messages from the pulpit, urging healthy eating at church gatherings and pointing out the poor eating habits within my congregation. And the congregation's initial response was anger. I was confused at the response. With time, I realized that they weren't angry at me, personally. Instead, I saw how their anger was unexpressed grief and rage at the unjust status quo of poverty, racism, unemployment, and lack of access to quality education, healthy and nutritious food, and affordable health care, all of which they felt powerless to address. This pain was driving the chronic illness. I had been trying to address social determinants with programs; what I needed was a place for human connection.

In addition to poor social determinants of health, the built environment in Conetoe did not support the health of my congregants. There were no sidewalks or common green spaces for physical activity or play. Apart from the church sanctuary and fellowship hall on Sunday, there was no common space for nurturing human connection. As the son of a sharecropping family in Eastern North Carolina who watched his parents work the land with little return, the last thing I wanted to do was start a garden and work this earth here in Coneteo. But, in the year after I presided over all of those funerals, I felt a call as clear as day: work this land, grow food, heal the community.

The garden that I started, and the garden for which my community has been known, is not about the garden. Yes, Conetoe is a food desert, despite its acres of arable and fertile farmland; yes, the built environment previously didn't support healthy activity; and yes, we urgently needed a source of healthy food. But even more so, we needed a place to be honest, a place to connect, a place to stand side by side with one another and open real conversations, to promote real community. We returned to the land to find healing, very hesitantly at first, given the history of slavery and sharecropping. We returned to the land and reclaimed it for the purpose of justice and human development.

## GARDENS, BEEHIVES, AND HUMAN DEVELOPMENT

To grow food, we called upon our greatest assets: human beings and the land. From the pulpit and in conversations with the community throughout the week, the church recruited youth to plant the first 2-acre garden. Over time, we began to farm more land and to harvest honey from more than 100 beehives dotting the landscape in Edgecombe County. The affiliate of Conetoe Chapel Missionary Baptist Church—the Conetoe Family Life Center—now sells produce from our gardens, honey from our hives, and seedlings from our hoophouses to farmers markets in Edgecombe County and as far away as Raleigh, the nearest Piggly Wiggly, and a local Ace Hardware.

The gardens and beehives have become the conscience and healthy heart-beat of the community. There we empower our youth and teach them leadership, social and emotional management, science, financial planning, and entrepreneurial know-how. There we grow food to nourish the bodies of our congregants and members of the greater community. The gardens tell the story of who we are as a faith community—a community that cares about the *whole* person, body and soul. A community that actively promotes long, healthy life for its members.

## PARTNERSHIPS TO PROMOTE HUMAN FLOURISHING

The church, however, is only one aspect of our congregants' lives. To achieve holistic health outcomes, we must partner with other key community partners. True partnership comes in recognition of our unique strengths, coming together under the goal of producing human gain, not as separate entities fighting for grant dollars. In Edgecombe County, the Conetoe Family Life Center has an ongoing relationship with the school system, where the Family Life Center provides wraparound social and emotional support for students struggling with behavior issues in the classroom. More often than not, children want to learn, but their home or community is producing an environment that makes learning impossible. There may be drug and alcohol abuse, there may be domestic violence, there may be no food, light, or heat.

In Conetoe, we increased our high school graduation rate from 40% to 98% over the course of 4 years by being honest about what was stopping our children from learning: incest, rape, and sexual abuse. We were honest with a hard conversation, especially a hard conversation within the context of the church, but our school system is not designed to address the issues in our children's homes.

We, the church, are. So we did, through counseling, family visits, and therapeutic time in the garden in a supportive, intergenerational framework that allowed children to talk, express their pain, and heal with the support of adults.

The school system refers its potential out-of-school suspension students to the Conetoe Family Life Center, and we in turn work with the children to increase the likelihood of their academic success. Our partnership with the school system expands also to the garden, where, with recent our Good Agricultural Practices (GAP) certification, we are able to sell our produce directly into the school system, allowing the children working in the garden to literally see the fruits of their labor during the school day.

Beyond the school system, it is important to help our children see the world beyond their own neighborhoods. To learn that their community has assets that others need, but also shares common challenges with other communities, we partnered with a secondary school on Hatteras Island and participated in a food equity exchange program. In the exchange, Conetoe Youth traveled to Hatteras Island to learn about the local thriving commercial fishing economy that co-exists with an acute shortage of healthy and nutritious produce. In turn, Hatteras youth traveled to Conetoe to learn about our gardens and bee operation. This partnership encourages our youth to grow in curiosity and knowledge regarding pathways to healthy food and community building.

Partnerships with health organizations have been most successful when, once again, we have been honest about the needs and strengths of each organization involved. the Opportunities Industrialization Center (OIC) in Rocky Mount, North Carolina, has been an ongoing health partner, as they run the Federally Qualified Health Center (FQHC) in our area. We have partnered with OIC to provide fresh produce to their patients based on their dietary needs and specific disease states, and we have been working on growing specific produce designed to impact chronic disease, such as high blood pressure, diabetes, and certain types of cancer. This partnership has proved to help reduce weight, reduce hemoglobin A1C levels, and bring down the medical costs for patients by helping them reduce their number of prescription medications.

Our partnerships with hospitals have focused on reducing 30-day hospital readmissions, with a robust community health worker program. This project has been most successful when it has remained in community, as opposed to institutionalized within a broader system. When community members, who know their fellow congregants and neighbors, are involved in the discharge plans and support of their fellow community members, hospital readmissions go down. Over the course of a 4-year period, we saw that number decline as a result of this process. A similar process, based on our model but using hospital staff instead of the community, ended up costing more than 10 times as much, with none of the same results.

The church is not the solution to solving community health issues, but it can be a strong partner in understanding and addressing the point at which these issues are arising. The church can bring people together, the church can create a space for honest conversation, and the church can be part of healing the community—as long as the community is ready to be honest about what needs healing and how to heal.

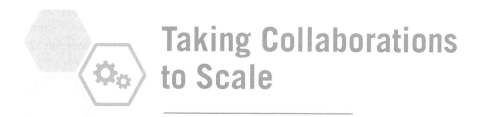

# Chapter 16

# Taking Collaborations to Scale

AHMED CALVO

T his chapter discusses taking collaborations to scale: that is, aiming at enlarging the number of partners on a scale that requires collaboration over larger distances that encompass perhaps a region, a whole state, a nation, or international dimensions as opposed to only having a partnership at the local community level.

This is not to say that partnerships at the local level are not important. Local partnerships need to be diligently and carefully cultivated because that is exactly where individuals live and interact every day and where most human collaboration begins as people start to work out solutions to issues of importance to them and to their communities. Collaboration at the local level is important for beginning any of the scale-up aspects of collaboration discussed in this chapter*.

From the start, local collaborators must include various simultaneous considerations to optimize the success of the scale-up. As one reads this chapter for the first time, these components initially can appear to be unrelated, but, in the examples discussed, they were critical to the success of scale-up and especially valuable when leveraged together proactively by strategic planning. To understand the different components technically, this chapter first discusses these different dimensions individually. Some of the important dimensions are addressed as intertwining components later in the chapter, to show how they might fit together to help with scale-up to help improve population health multisector collaboration.

## THE IMPORTANCE OF DATA

A practical key consideration is to *start on a small scale for demonstrating or implementing the collaboration as a proof-of-concept.* For going to scale, this

---

* This writing was conducted by the author and is not to be construed as representing the opinions of the federal government or any of its agencies. The opinions are solely those of the author

proof-of-concept needs to meet a built-in assumption regarding data. From the very beginning, the local collaboration must be careful to develop as much robust data as reasonably possible, perhaps with the co-evolution of appropriate analytics processes factored into the collaboration. This is necessary to create some objective information for sharing with others to describe concretely the subsequent insights gained by the collaboration. Data are needed for evaluation. Data are also critical for assessment of attribution and impact of the intervention. Subsequently, they are valuable for gauging the level of fidelity in the scale-up of the intervention. One widely used and practical method for organizing the data to be gathered and used is the *small tests of change approach* utilized in many quality-improvement efforts in primary care and in public health, as well as in multisector collaborations.[1]

Doing good collaboration without generating data about its impact hinders its future scale-up potential because funders need the data to justify investment, and possible future collaborators will need the data to understand what was done. Gaining other partners will be easier if the story can be told well, with insightful perspectives built from accurate real-time data.

## THE IMPORTANCE OF EVERYONE HAVING RESPONSIBILITY FOR TEACHING

For scale-up, it is useful for staff be clear up front that there is value in being able to explain the collaboration to others who also may want to try it. With this approach, it will not be enough to merely learn the work of the collaboration. Being able to teach the activity to others and describe what is being done with data are necessary for successful scale-up. The approach enables individuals to learn the content more thoroughly since participants feel the responsibility to teach it to others, which helps the individuals become more proactively engaged.

Knowing that there is an expectation for everyone to teach the activity to others helps create a sense of perspective that is less subjective, which in itself can help local collaboration to be more successful precisely because the idea of explaining the effort to others in the future creates a separate aspiration.

Local partnerships that have this type of "chemistry" are able to share well in a small room with a few partners or in conference facilities with many people and via webinars involving a large number of organizations. Practicing teaching to others can be taught, learned, and used repeatedly as the scale-up efforts progress, allowing many to get proficient at the teaching, which also helps to better propagate insights.

Framing this expectation can be done by emphasis on having a "conversation of the whole." For this, I have often used the "all teach—all learn" approach to frame the start of the conversation in the room, which helps open the conversation to all participants. Resource materials on this method are available in a variety of places, many currently using the new phrase *collaborative improvement and innovation networks* (CoIIN).[2] The method helps engender the learning needed to achieve the collaboration process and to carry out the work.

This additional dimension can help get through what might otherwise become a more difficult issue of local power struggle. All collaboration runs the risk of power struggles arising, as partners' levels of engagement may ebb and flow over time. The tendency can be anticipated of one or more of the partners trying to exert control over others due to enthusiasm for the project or due to characteristics of the organization. It is naïve to expect a perfect balance to always be in play throughout the continuum of a long-term collaboration effort.

An example of a practical approach to the issue of framing the importance of "teaching others" is having an up-front discussion with clinicians involved in the collaboration to emphasize that activity meetings are not intended to be continuing medical education for any one individual. Instead, for collaborations that are intended to be taken to scale, the following notions need to be clearly disseminated: (1) that teams are involved, (2) that people who are traveling to a given meeting are part of a "travel team," and (3) that the travel team has responsibility to teach what they've learned when they get back to the "home team."

This means that the material being learned by any one individual participant is not meant to be "secret knowledge," to be hoarded by that individual and kept from members of the home team who did not get to attend the meeting. Information and insights need to be shared widely with the home team, which then can lead to new insights being added at the local level. And since the group is typically smarter than any one of its individual members, the open discussion of ideas and brainstorming about the issues that need to be solved can yield valuable perspectives about what is to be done together, leading to a better chance of success in the process of scale-up.

## THE IMPORTANCE OF TRUST BUILDING

To optimize teaching and learning, constant attention to the relationship of the collaborating parties is required, regardless of the specific tactical activity of the effort. The most critical insight that needs to be understood in any collaboration is very similar to what is needed for successful relationships, marriages, and partnerships: the importance of trust.[3]

*Going to scale happens at the speed of trust.* Trust is the key ingredient in any collaboration being taken to scale, regardless of any other technical components, such as the fidelity of the model or intervention.

*Local collaboration also happens at the speed of trust.* This is also true for spreading the scale-up to other communities or other partnerships. This aspect can often be forgotten in the process of teaching the technical considerations of the collaborative effort. Although technical components are important when devising a strategy to take a cross-sector collaboration to scale or when working in a cross-sector local collaboration, in my experience, establishing a solid foundation for collaboration based on relationship and trust is crucial. Failure to attend to this principle can lead to failure in the scale-up of an effort, unrelated to whether or not the components of the intervention have undergone rigorous evidence-based development and assessment.

So, a key practical consideration to address when taking collaboration to scale is the need *not* to focus on the technical aspects only. Factoring in trust and the related aspects of building and maintaining trust are needed throughout the process for the collaboration's success and for the success of any scaling-up that is attempted. Collaboration is a process that involves people: a social process by definition. An effort that relies mainly on a "computer programming algorithm" mentality runs a significant risk of failing because the individuals involved in the collaboration are not computers or robots. People doing the collaborative work need to be treated with respect and attention to how they are feeling about doing the work. These are aspects of trust building that are required for successful outcomes of collaboration, and they apply not only to individuals as people, but also to the organizations that are involved in the collaboration. Regardless of the actual intervention's details, developing, establishing, and nourishing the trust of partners is the most important aspect of successful collaboration and scale-up of an intervention (Box 16.1).

---

**Box 16.1 | Scale-Up Resources**

The hyperlink https://www.healthcarecommunities.org/aboutus.aspx will direct the reader to a web portal that contains a library of resources for primary care practices interested in the scale-up work described in this chapter.

The web portal is run by CSI Solutions, a company that originally developed the web portal in 2005 to support the Health Resources and Services Administration's (HRSA) Health Disparities Collaboratives working with the Federally Qualified Health Centers (FQHCs) and their infrastructure. The portal has grown from more than 3,000 users to more than 30,000 users, and it is currently funded by the Center for Medicare and Medicaid Innovation (CMMI) at the Centers for Medicare and Medicaid (CMS) for national efforts at quality improvement to generate value for the nation.

The portal supports more than 70 virtual communities, including CMS's Transforming Clinical Practice Initiative (TCPI), Partnership for Patients (PfP), and the QIO 11th Scope of Work. This library of resources is being used in every single state and territory as the entities work on quality, safety, and affordability. The web portal also provides opportunities for third-party sponsorship of communities seeking to collaborate but who do not have the resources to support the effort.

---

# THE HRSA HEALTH DISPARITIES COLLABORATIVES: A SCALE-UP EXAMPLE

The US Department of Health and Human Services (HHS), via the partnership of two of its agencies, the Health Resources and Services Administration (HRSA) and the Centers for Disease Control and Prevention (CDC), supported the initial national effort at quality improvement collaboration that came to be known as the HRSA Health Disparities Collaboratives (HDC).[4] Managed by the health center program operated by the Bureau of Primary Health Care within HRSA, the HDC engaged more than 80% of all of the primary health care corporations that operated facilities that delivered care to underserved communities throughout the nation in 2006. These clinical delivery facilities are known as Federally Qualified Health Centers (FQHCs). The HDC multiyear effort meets the straightforward test of an effort that was taken to scale as it started with the participation of only five FQHCs, via a 1998 effort with the Institute for Healthcare Improvement (IHI).

Opinions have been published to the effect that proper evaluation of quality improvement collaboratives, such as the HDC, need external evaluations outside of the so-called *black box framework*.[5] Many descriptive publications of the HDC scale-up historically have focused on the models that were taught: the Wagner Chronic Care Model, the plan-do-study-act (PDSA), the small tests of change method for quality improvement science, and the IHI Breakthrough Series Collaborative learning model.[6] Most of the assessments of both process and health outcomes of the HDC have used standard methodologies; many developed as federal evaluations by the Agency for Healthcare Research and Quality (AHRQ), the National Institutes of Health (NIH), and other agencies. For purposes of this discussion on scale-up, however, I believe that people who have looked at the HDC to understand what the intervention was and how it was done may have missed a key ingredient that led to the success of the scale-up. The HDC success did not merely involve the use of evidence-based interventions.

The antecedent fact of the establishment of the Clinician's National Forum (CNF) in 1997 was critical. This interdisciplinary group of clinicians from FQHCs committed to (1) "be a creative and innovative force in reducing health disparities in care to the underserved by accelerating beneficial improvements in the delivery of care" and (2) to "furnish front-line clinicians with the tools, systems, and resources they need to carry out meaningful work and provide quality care."[4] This commitment of the CNF seems to me to be very similar to the approach and aim of this edition of the *Practical Playbook*.

From my perspective for understanding what was done so that others can benefit from the HDC in planning for scale-up, it is particularly important to realize that the CNF had a built-in element of trust which was inherent in the group's formation and a clear commitment to mission that was ingrained in the group's "front-line vision and commitment to action."

CNF brought to bear the associated infrastructure of the safety net, which evolved a collaborative network of partners that spread at the speed of trust. This network included the Migrant Clinicians Network, Health Care for the Homeless, the Primary Care Associations, and the National Association of Community Health Centers.

Of particular interest to this edition of the *Practical Playbook*, the HDC also enabled partnerships between primary care and public health at both national and local levels, for example, by linking local activity of the CDC-funded state health department diabetes control program coordinators and the HRSA-supported FQHCs so that the entire integrated national and state network of primary care and public health departments learned together to improve diabetes care. The same was true regarding screening for cancer, for example, involving (1) primary care done at FQHCs supported by HRSA, (2) CDC-funded cancer screening expertise at public health departments, and (3) the teaching by NIH cancer screening experts of recommendations from the US Preventive Services Task Force.

In retrospect, to take their effort to scale, CNF was able to gain support from the HRSA and the CDC, as well as from multiple other federal agencies over time (e.g., the Substance Abuse and Mental Health Services Administration, the Environmental Protection Agency, and the National Institute of Diabetes and Digestive and Kidney Diseases [NIDDKD], National Heart, Lung, and Blood Institute [NHLBI], and the National Cancer Institute [NCI]). The effort also gained funding from the HHS Office of Women's Health, the Office of Minority Health, and a large variety of other federal, state, and local government programs. The CNF was able to leverage its deep commitment; and engagement with private foundations and other nonprofit and for-profit organizations created many private–public partnerships important for sustaining the quality improvement activity (Box 16.2).

## THE POLITICAL WILL OF THE CNF INTEGRATED THE DIFFERENT COMPONENTS

The HDC improvement network scale-up was focused on the safety net of the nation. It leveraged the mission-driven commitment of staff already working in the safety net. At the true center of this effort were the clinicians of the CNF, which was a community of trust that continued to work together in the HDC activity as it was being scaled up. They enabled others from the surrounding clinical community of interest of the safety net infrastructure to become involved and helped to evolve the entire effort into a national community of practice for better care of chronic diseases and prevention. Overall, therefore, the relatively small cornerstone community of trust of the CNF created a community of solution. This was an act of political will by the CNF that deftly integrated the different types of components described in this chapter, and it did so with strategic sophistication.

> **Box 16.2 | Community of Interest, Community of Practice, Community of Solution**
>
> A *community of interest* is a group of people who share a common interest or passion.[1] There is no geographic implication in the sense of a "local community"—people could be on the other side of the planet.
>
> A *community of practice* is similar to a community of interest, but individuals in the community need to be in action professionally or in a craft.[2] Communities of practice are trying to solve some issue, although may not yet have a solution yet.
>
> A *community of solution* is a community of practice that actually has shown results in some area, and they are interested in disseminating that solution more widely and effectively.[3–5]
>
> For this to work in a modern sense, and for wide dissemination with efficiency, there is need for support infrastructure in the form of *information and communication technology* (ICT). This means of dissemination includes webinars, the Internet, conference calls, data analytics, and new metrics (including person-centered metrics, population health metrics, team-based care metrics, etc.).
>
> **References**
>
> 1. Wikipedia. Community of interest. https://en.wikipedia.org/wiki/Community_of_interest. Accessed April 1, 2018.
> 2. Wikipedia. Community of practice. https://en.wikipedia.org/wiki/Community_of_practice. Accessed April 1, 2018
> 3. Grishwold KS, Lesko, SE, Westfall JM. Communities of solution: Partnerships for population health. *J Am Board Fam Med*. 2013;26(3):232–38. doi:10.3122/jabfm.2013.03.130102.
> 4. National Commission on Community Health Services (NCCHS). *Health Is a Community Affair: Report of the National Commission on Community Health Services (NCCHS)*. Cambridge, MA: Harvard University Press; 1967.
> 5. The Folsom Group. *Communities of solution: The Folsom Report revisited. Ann Fam Med*. 2012;10:250–60.

Over time, the experience leveraged the national infrastructure of the FQHCs and state-based and nationally based support systems and generated new insights for dissemination of scale-up into what became a much larger community of trust. This was the true success of the HDC effort, and it continues to instill its effect locally in many places, as well as nationally within the safety net.

In addition, the development of the apparatus within the safety net enabled maturation of a larger national community of interest on quality improvement—the broader quality improvement activity connected to IHI and later to the Centers for Medicare and Medicaid (CMS) Center for Medicare and Medicaid Innovation (CMMI) of mainstream medicine. This can be seen in the variety of models being tested by CMMI that leverage insights and even staff that came from the HDC. By linking to studies from AHRQ and other research networks, such as those funded by the new Patient-Centered Outcomes Research Institute, the staff of CMMI helped to scale up the evidence-based interventions while continuing to work out the rigorous attribution aspects needed to gain an additional level of confidence. This is an ongoing effort.

The key point to understand from this sequence is that the scale-up occurred due to political will prior to the development of many traditional evidence-based, peer-reviewed publications. The implication is that trust was a key ingredient that enabled the scale-up of the work. At the speed of trust, the HDC grew much more quickly than the typical 15- to 17-year lag seen in the deployment of something that has been well-documented and well-published in the peer-reviewed literature.

And, in the process of the scale-up, the HDC managed to get many others to participate via new strategic partnerships that brought together the expertise of different sectors to work in a synergistic manner that helped speed the scale-up. "All teach—all learn" was explicitly used and linked to the adage of "steal shamelessly and share senselessly."

The practical focus became the use of a variety of data and analytic methods to track intervention outcomes, or the tests-of-change known as the *PDSA cycle data*. The interventions used were delivered via interdisciplinary team–based activities that were organized via the Chronic Care Model. The data were tracked using new population-based electronic registry systems developed for the specific topic of each collaborative. Policy levers also were used, such as the formal decision by HRSA to fund part of the activity, with contributions of time and energy from the existing state and national health center infrastructure.

The entire effort of the HDC was always a population-based approach to delivery of teams-based care. The HDC built on the FQHC history of Community-Oriented Primary Care, which was the genesis of the health centers developed by Jack Geiger using the perspective that he had learned from Sidney and Emily Kark.[7] For the scale-up, all of these different components were interlaced via the individuals dedicated to doing the work of the CNF. In other words, ultimately, the CNF leveraged use of political will to help the implementation and dissemination of its tools and insights to frontline providers and teams. The CNF members were unified in their mission, and their commitment was long term. And it took a long-term and patient effort. But many others became involved in the process.

## THE IMPORTANCE OF STARTING WITH THE END IN MIND

It must be understood concretely that, from the very beginning of this effort, the CNF was interested in both local- and national-level innovation and improvement, and the clinicians worked hard at linking them. The effort was never only about helping one or a few local communities or FQHCs. From the start, there was a need to think at the national scale and its implications. This can be described as "starting with the end in mind."[8]

Starting with the end in mind in this context means beginning a particular local collaboration with the strategic grand plan of enlarging the partnerships to a much greater number of partners or, minimally, being willing to share the gained insights with a larger national or international community of interest. This consideration changes the approach of many of the initial local partners; it helps partners to not be parochial about activities; and it helps to create an objectively different point of consideration, which can be missed if only the local preexisting collaboration history is taken for granted. Experience with the scale-up of the HDC showed the value of starting local collaborations with the aim of taking the collaboration to scale in the future; that is, to think up front about the idea of spreading the insights to others, whether on a state/regional level or a national/international level. Serious effort has been used to institutionalize the experience within the health center program. This is still a work in progress.

In translating these insights of the safety net to primary care settings or public health entities for this edition of the *Practical Playbook*, careful attention needs to be paid by the participating organizations in a given collaboration to development, nurturing, and sustaining the trust needed by participating organizations. This is the critical aspect that will get the effort through difficulties that might be encountered along the way. For primary care practices, it may be valuable to network with other primary care private practices interested in the same type of collaboration. For public health departments, there is a natural and powerful network of public health departments that can help keep perspective as the going gets tough.

Local primary care practices have state- and national-level networks that can be brought to bear, such as primary care academic and residency training groups as well as professional networks for each specialty (e.g., family medicine, internal medicine, and pediatrics). Close collaboration with these entities probably will help any given primary care medical practice that is contemplating participating in a collaboration that they hope can be taken to scale.

Even if a practice or local public health department wants to focus only on the local environment, there is much to be gained from being in touch with what is happening at the state and nation levels that can be helpful in collaborative work. Staying aware of such developments, such as those contained in the this edition of the *Practical Playbook,* is a place to start.

## PATIENT-CENTERED MEDICAL HOMES: ANOTHER EXAMPLE

An example of scaled-up development in the primary care community is the effort regarding the *patient-centered medical home* (PCMH). The PCMH model originally was developed via HRSA-funded activity from the Maternal and Child Health Bureau and was focused on children with special needs. PCMH first was reported in the literature by the American Academy of Pediatrics in 1967. Scaling the PCMH idea also took an act of political will, with superior timing leading to powerful branding success, which functionally was an embodiment of practice redesign principles.[9]

This political will, in theory, took the form of professional organizations of primary care coming together in 2007 to issue their "Joint Principles of the Patient Centered Medical Home." The key organizations involved were the American College of Physicians, the American Academy of Family Physicians, the American Academy of Pediatrics, and the American Osteopathic Association.

In practice, the real engagement of the primary care medical practices and clinicians, health care delivery systems, and self-insured corporations whose internal data enabled them to see the value of organizing primary care delivery into PCMH activity (e.g., IBM) occurred with the launch of the Patient-Centered Primary Care Collaborative (PCPCC). This led to the accumulation of concrete examples and sharing of resources, tools, studies, and reviews of the evidence and results.[10] The true strategic success of the PCMH scale-up is not yet clear; it is also a work in progress.

## MAXIMIZE THE CULTURAL SIMILARITY OF ANCHOR ORGANIZATIONS

In retrospect, some nuance regarding what type of political activity to push and who to engage therein for successful scale-up needs to be carefully considered. A key consideration in building a successful multisector collaboration for population health at scale may be to consider how to *maximize the cultural similarity of anchor organizations*. This aspect may enable the subsequent spread of the particular intervention to other similar entities in other communities and other partnerships.

For the HDC, participating entities were similar in mission, although they were dispersed throughout all states and territories. The staff of the FQHCs, the leadership of the FQHCs, and the local boards of directors of the FQHCs were structurally very similar. Ultimately, this helped tremendously in the subsequent scale-up of insights and activity in support of the clinicians' effort. Although the local partnerships were diverse in the mix of partners from different sectors, there was an FQHC anchor organization that was similar enough in each of the efforts to help spread the models, insights, and dedication to scale up the activity. This may have been taken for granted at first, but, looking back, it was a key consideration; it is an advisable pathway for others attempting new population health scale-up efforts.

A similar analysis applies to the PCMH activity of the PCPCC, which employed the enthusiasm of anchor primary care medical practices coupled with the support of professional organizations of primary care as well as the academic and residency training networks. Like the HDC, there have been many policy levels triggered within federal agencies, such as at the CMMI and others.

To address population health via multisector collaboration, which can be more difficult due to the mix of organizational cultures, the strategic solution will involve building trust, both as a consideration of the anchor organizations of any given collaboration and of the larger scale-up multisector activity required.

A few caveats should be factored in. One cannot assume that the models that work for large multispecialty practices can translate easily (or at all) to small primary care practices. The size of the organizations may be different enough to present a significant challenge. Further study is necessary to sort this out. I suspect that trust is also a factor herein. Small primary care practices many not trust the insights from a large multispecialty group practice. With multisector activity, the difficulty of trust-building among the partners will be key to the success of the scale-up effort, and it may continue as a struggle due to the natural waxing and waning of all long-term collaboration.

## IMPORTANCE OF POLITICAL WILL HARNESSED APPROPRIATELY FOR SCALE-UP

The experiences of the CNF and the PCPCC demonstrate that successful scale-up involves political will power and not just use of evidence-based interventions.

If enough audacious will is applied diligently over time, it is possible to scale up an effort. This is true even if the specific activity has not yet met some traditional evidence-based criteria or has accumulated enough of an evaluative basis for others to think that this threshold has been met.

This political will power needs to be timed to a situational awareness of the context. This combination can achieve grand strategy, but it needs attention to details related to the different types of components discussed in this chapter. The critical components include the following:

1. The importance of starting small, but with a grand plan.
2. The importance of data (and the related analytics capacity).
3. The importance of a teaching framework that requires all to teach.
4. The importance of trust building as the key glue for the participants.

The combination of these components, leveraged together synergistically, is needed for successful scale-up. However, it is not for the faint of heart. Scale-up requires dedication and long-term political will to continue the struggle of trying to change things for the better.

## REFERENCES

1. The National Institute for Children's Health Quality. Quality improvement 101—The fundamentals of changes that lead to improvement. Boston. 2018. www.nichq.org/resource/quality-improvement-101. Accessed on 1/16/2019.

2. The National Institute for Children's Health Quality. Infant Mortality CoIIN Prevention Toolkit. Boston. 2018. www.nichq.org/resource/infant-mortality-coiin-prevention-toolkit. Accessed on 1/16/2019.

3. Covey SMR. *The Speed of Trust*. New York: Simon and Schuster; 2008.

4. Stevens DM. Health centers after fifty years: Lessons from the health disparities collaboratives. *J Health Care Poor Underserved*. 2016;27:4:1621–31.

5. Mittman, BS. Creating the Evidence Base for Quality Improvement Collaboratives. *Ann Intern Med*. 2004;140(11):897-901.

6. Kilo, CM. A Framework for Collaborative Improvement: Lessons from the Institute for Healthcare Improvement's breakthrough series. *Qual Manag Health Care*. 1998;6(4):1–13. https://www.ncbi.nlm.nih.gov/pubmed/10339040. Accessed 1/16/2019

7. Gofin J. On "A Practice of Social Medicine" by Sidney and Emily Kark. *Soc Med*.2006;1: 107–15. www.socialmedicine.info. Accessed on 1/16/2019.

8. Covey SR. *The 7 Habits of Highly Effective People: Powerful Lessons* In *Personal Change*. New York: Simon and Schuster; 1989.

9. Kilo CM, Wasson JH. Practice redesign and the patient-centered medical home: history, promises, and challenges. *Health Aff*. May 29, 2010;5:773–8. doi:10.1377/hlthaff.2010.0012 7.5.w328

10. Patient-Centered Primary Care Collaborative. http://www.pcpcc.org/about.

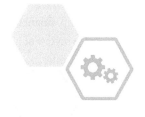

# Chapter 17

# Case Study—Addressing Behavioral Health with a Multisector Approach: Why We Started Community of Solutions

ROBERT L. PHILLIPS, JR, CAROL V. DAVIS, ETHAN J. PHILLIPS, HEATHER DAVIES, VALERIE FLOWE, MARY BETH QUICK, AND LAUREN TERRY

We often think of the boys who died by suicide at our local high school even though it's been a few years. We're not even their moms or dads. We are moms, dads, and siblings of their classmates. We are some of the many people in our Fairfax, Virginia, community who still think about the boys who left us much too early in 2012, 2013, 2014, and 2016, and what we might have done to help.

We think of their moms and dads, too. We wanted to prevent other parents from having to endure what they've had to go through—and continue to go through—by helping provide education and awareness about the problems teenagers face and the solutions we can find to address those issues with our children, our students, and our neighbors. They are one of the reasons we felt compelled to help organize the Community of Solutions. We hope what happened here never occurs in another community. Three boys at W. T. Woodson High School took their lives within 6 months, a total of eight over 5 years.

The name Community of Solutions (CoS) is derived from the 1967 Folsom Report, *Health Is a Community Affair*, a national report co-sponsored by the American Public Health Association and the National Health Council, and led by Marion Folsom, former Chair of Eastman Kodak and the second Secretary of Health, Education, and Welfare.[1] The first recommendation of that report states that "the planning, organization, and delivery of community health services by both official and voluntary agencies must be based on the concept of a *community of solution.*" The second to last recommendation said of the role of "voluntary citizen participation" that "[a] central factor in the growth and development of . . . personal and community health has been the participation of individuals and voluntary associations through dedicated leadership, financial support, and personal service."[2] A review of that landmark report, a review of its impact, and a translation for modern times was published in 2012, offering an important context for the Woodson High School suicide cluster.[2,3]

Carol, an instructional designer and adult educator, knew some of the boys through her son and her volunteer work at the high school. Bob, a physician who works on behalf of an association for family medicine, knew some of the boys through Boy Scouts, coaching basketball, and through his own sons. Bob and Carol's boys were friends, and the two started discussing how they could help.

"These were our neighbors, our kids. I could not stand by," Bob recalls. He was giving a lecture at the Centers for Disease Control and Prevention (CDC) to the very group that performs Epi-Aids—field investigations of epidemics and disease outbreaks—when he learned about the fourth suicide at the high school. He knew the boy, whose name was Ethan. Ethan had coached his younger brother's elementary school basketball team while Bob coached another team. Bob set about finding out who at the CDC could authorize an investigation into the rash of suicides in Fairfax.

While working on getting a CDC Epi-Aid authorized, CoS began focusing on local efforts. "Bob and I quickly pooled our resources to facilitate a meeting at our community center that was attended by 20 parents, two representatives from Fairfax County Public Schools (FCPS), and six teens," Carol recalls. The meeting agenda intentionally kept the focus away from suicide because we wanted to learn about what our teens were experiencing and help them cope. It was important that we hear it from their perspective instead of putting our own parental spin on what might be happening. We also agreed we would not blame our particular high school or the FCPS system. Our approach would be one of building bridges and strengthening relationships. Living up to our name, finding solutions as a community, and moving forward would be much more productive than passing judgment on what was wrong with the system.

During the meeting, people shared fears about the pressure to succeed in academics and extracurricular activities. They talked about drugs and alcohol and mentioned depression. A school psychologist opened our eyes to the reasons why students don't seek out help for depression: (1) they believe they can solve the problem themselves, (2) they think the problem will go away, (3) they don't think their parents will understand or support them, (4) they are concerned they will be hospitalized, and (5) they don't know where to go for help.

That evening, we also learned that there was hunger for progress on all of these issues.

We left the meeting agreeing to find answers to our questions and to help share the information, and we left that meeting with the hope that our community could prevent further suicides. We knew we were trying to tackle a huge, tragic problem facing our world. We agreed to do something, anything, for our community. That's when the organization we called CoS was born (Box 17.1).

Participation in the CoS swelled as concern swept the community. A group of volunteers—parents, students, teachers, school counselors, psychologists, administrators, and public health behavioral specialists—began to meet regularly to console, to listen, and to take stock of our collective skills and will to work on this crisis. CoS members would break out into self-organizing groups to take on specific tasks and create timelines to accomplish them. We conducted a survey of attendees and, based on this, held a formal strengths, weaknesses, opportunities, threats (SWOT) analysis that produced our work plan. This was important for getting specific about participants' concerns, prioritizing them, and organizing them into specific tasks (Box 17.2). We offer these here as they may be generally useful to other communities experiencing teen suicide, but also as a process for focusing effort (Box 17.2).

We purposefully moved our meetings between neighborhood community centers and the school, inviting the school system and county government to give us updates, slowly pulling them into the solutions. The leadership group recognized the need for steady work on priorities, growing trust, and building relationships to accomplish meaningful change. Nearly all of the boys who died

---

**Box 17.1 | Community of Solutions Charter**

Our organization facilitates action to raise the profile of mental health and substance use and abuse and to balance daily pressures of adolescence by fostering resilience. We identify resources and create community collaboration which begins with hearing different perspectives and working toward positive action that supports our teens.

*Mission*: Help teens deal with adversity and build resilience through idea and resource sharing between teens, parents, and professionals.

*Vision*: Teens who are comfortable with seeking help from parents, friends, and professionals; teens who are mentally healthy and who realize that suicide is not the answer.

*Values*: Listening; fostering resilience/practicing mindfulness; collaboration; building trust; positivity; connecting ideas, people, and resources; taking risks in a safe environment

For additional information, visit https://www.facebook.com/groups/CommunityofSolutions/

and https://communityofsolutions.org/.

**Box 17.2 | Top Four Survey Action Foci from Community of Solutions Members**

1. Offer students who are feeling acute and overwhelming stress (due to homework that is piling up or due to overlapping large assignments) an opportunity to create a work plan with teachers.
2. Promote an accepting environment for discussing mental illness and encourage help-seeking behavior, both for themselves and their peers.
3. Enforce county school system policy limiting the amount of homework that can be assigned per night.
4. Educate teens on how to differentiate between normal teen ups and downs and more serious mental health issues; provide teens more information about how to assist their friends in distress.

Other items rated very important by 75% or more of respondents:

1. Train teachers regularly about warning signs of mental illness and ways to approach teens, as well as provide more in-depth training about mental diagnoses.
2. Remove coaches, teachers, and staff who regularly bully and demoralize students.
3. Provide more mental health awareness education and training for parents.
4. Ensure that teens know what mental health treatment entails and that treatment is effective for a high percentage of people.
5. Promote an accepting environment for discussing mental illness and encourage help-seeking behavior, both for themselves and their peers.
6. Offer students who are feeling acute and overwhelming stress (due to homework that is piling up or due to overlapping large assignments) an opportunity to create a work plan with teachers to stretch out deadlines in a reasonable way so they can get all their work done.
7. Survey teens and ask them to identify what is causing them the most stress.

by suicide were athletes, so we specifically sought out the county director of student activities to pursue Mental Health First Aid training for all athletic trainers, screening students for depression during the formal health screenings for student athletes, and doing a trial of a collegiate mindfulness training for sports performance enhancement. Research shows that adolescents are more likely to reveal risky behavior electronically than to verbalize it, which led us to support moving the traditional crisis phone line to a text-based process. This produced a tripling of reports. Learning from parents that the mobile crisis unit of the community services board (CSB) was overtaxed, we testified to the county government for an additional $1 million in funding that supported a second unit, among other services. The successes and failures each represent handfuls of people committedly working a shared goal. They mostly organized organically, and this grew to be a leadership team of six people creating a framework of support in which to work.

Students also played a key role in the actionable solutions that came out of the CoS work. When CoS was created, the goal of responding to student needs necessitated teen involvement and input. A few of the sons and daughters of parent leadership created a teacher-student forum at W. T. Woodson High School to foster collaborative conversation around the issues that needed to be addressed. Although the topics discussed did not always pertain directly to student mental health, the fact that discussion had a place to occur opened the possibility of a school culture between the faculty and the student body that would create changes based on student need. More recently, the same model has been taken to Thomas Jefferson High School for Science and Technology (TJ), another community school that has long struggled with adequately responding to student mental health and had experienced a teen suicide in March 2018. By bringing together students, parents, teachers, administrators, and counselors, these forums allow the school community to create holistic and collaborative answers to the mental health problems faced every day by those same stakeholder groups. The goal is consistent: to create a *community of solutions*. Ethan Phillips, a student member of CoS who brought the forum model to TJ in the fall of 2017 recalls, "I saw the same issues that CoS sought to address in the Woodson community being ignored at TJ. We had the resources to do better for students and the desire to solve the problems that we faced, all we needed was a platform to make it all happen." These forum models have already shown their effectiveness in bringing together leaders from all involved stakeholder groups, creating discussion, and initiating changes. However, only so much can be done at the individual school level. For this reason, the future of the forum model calls for expansion to more high schools and to the county as a whole. As the reach of the discussion regarding student mental health is broadened, greater change can be made to prevent what occurred at Woodson from ever happening again.

## HIGH-LEVEL ACCOMPLISHMENTS

- Secured resources from the Fairfax County government for behavioral health
- Facilitated a change of the crisis phone line to a text-based system, more than tripling the number of concerns reported
- Introduced Mental Health First Aid training into several schools, for students and for staff, and rapidly expanded trainings with the considerable help of the CSB (a Fairfax County Government Agency)
- Hosted mindfulness courses for students and faculty
- Developed teacher-student forums, initiated by student members, about shared concerns in one school, and another school may adopt the model

- Partnered with a sister-city, Palo Alto, California, which also experienced a devastating suicide cluster
- Worked with the public health department to bring the CDC and the Substance Abuse and Mental Health Services Administration (SAMHSA) to Fairfax for the first joint Epi-Aid evaluation of a suicide cluster; they recently completed the second in Palo Alto
- Organized a parent information session with National Institute of Mental Health expert[3]
- Formed local National Alliance on Mental Illness support groups in affected schools

Box 17.3 lists specific successes to inform other communities seeking to change their own suicide risk.

## CHALLENGES

CoS faced many challenges along the way. The first was general reticence to discuss suicide and the related problem of how to discuss it when parents are very fearful. An early community listening session held at the affected high school brought out more than 1,000 parents and students, and emotions ran high. CoS parental participation peaked at 30 to 40, and regular attendance numbered fewer than 25 (parents, FCPS staff, students, CSB staff). Each suicide fanned discussion and fear for short bursts of time, but, despite a high level of sustained fear, open discussion was difficult to maintain.

The second challenge was engaging the school system. Initially, FCPS circled its wagons out of fear of blame, even counseling the Parent Teacher Student Organization to avoid involvement. CoS leaders worked hard to build trust and a place to avoid blame and seek shared solutions. We became a resource and advocate to try new efforts that might reduce what we came to call a "slow-burn cluster."[4] It was not typical of other contagion clusters in that it occurred over several years. There was some evidence of contagion effect in that a pair of Woodson suicides were associated, temporally, with suicides in other local high schools. We were also told that student reports of suicidal ideation in area schools surged after they experienced suicides, but also after students at other schools died by suicide (anecdotal). What is clear is that the CDC/SAMHSA Epi-Aid revealed a more than doubling of local emergency department visits by adolescents for suicidal ideation or attempts over the same period. The CoS leadership became concerned that we might be dealing with a long-term problem of cultural suicide acceptance rather than the more typical copy-cat contagion effect. Furthermore, this coexisted with a culture of avoidance around discussion and change. To their great credit, FCPS became an informal partner to CoS in communicating to the group about its efforts to improve screening and services and reduce risk. They also allowed CoS to hold meetings in the schools and to organize educational sessions, and they

**Box 17.3 | Community of Solutions Successes: Collaboration with Fairfax County Public Schools**

1. Mental health first aid (MHFA):
   - Training 50 students in six schools in MHFA, which is only the second implementation of student training in the United States of this international curriculum. The goal was to create peer resources in schools. This was a partnership between the Parent Teacher Student Organization, the Josh Anderson Foundation, and the Fairfax-Falls Church community services board (CSB).
   - Securing resources to train teachers, coaches, and athletic trainers in MHFA in all schools Fairfax County Public Schools (FCPS) and CSB. This will expand the number of MHFA trainers in the county.
2. Listening:
   - Student input into clarifying FCPS "consequences" for seeking mental health help or reporting concerns about friends.
   - Students request for a counseling process when they seek help for friends; provided feedback to FCPS administration that changed policy.
   - Introduction of depression (PHQ2) screening into school sports physicals.
3. Fostering resilience/practicing mindfulness:
   - Exploration of introduction of Mindfulness for Sports Performance Enhancement (Catholic University research focus) into athletic programs in FCPS. Pilot in planning stages while exploring funding of a randomized trial. (All suicide victims were athletes.) Athletics is also looking for ways to emphasize mentoring, modeling, monitoring, and mindfulness.
   - Development of mental health, suicide, and resiliency components for concussion training course required of all parents of athletes.
   - Introduction of mindfulness exercises as routine part of classroom and after-school programs.
   - Implementation of Virginia Tech program Actively Caring (www.ac4p.org) to give students a way to recognize healthy, supportive behavior.
4. Student-teacher forum:
   W. T. Woodson student group worked with school administration and teachers to organize a series in which students and teachers could identify and talk about shared concerns. These fora effectively changed the school tardy policy and resulted in repairs to several bathrooms. The forum did not survive student leadership transition but is being adopted by another high school (TJ).

**Collaboration with Boy Scouts**

- Mental Health First Aid training of leaders of the Boy Scouts of America (BSA) incorporated into local University of Scouting.
- National Capital Area Council of BSA created formal training for troop leaders that we're now trying to spread across the country.
- Formation of a 501c3 to fund training.

**Collaboration with the Community**

- Advocacy efforts for county Systems of Care program funding for mental health services ($1 million additional dollars secured in 2014).
- Grand Rounds hosted by pediatrics and including family medicine to make county depression and suicide statistics more apparent, to discuss screening, to identify ways to help health care providers access mental health services, and to challenge clinicians to consider community leadership roles.
- Lectures to family medicine residency about Community of Solutions (CoS) and community leadership.
- Networking and presentations to the community.
- Active Facebook feed and resource website.
- Provided physician alerts through the Medical Society of Northern Virginia.
- Collaborated with local drug-free community coalition.

allowed us to initiate student and teacher services (mindfulness training, yoga, stress-less days, and a Mindfulness for Sports Performance trial with sports teams). Mary Beth Quick, a CoS leader, conducted mindfulness training and yoga sessions to which students and alumni still point as being valuable for their ability to deal with stress.[5] Thanks to Heather Davies and Valerie Flowe, CoS sponsored parenting workshops, organized National Alliance on Mental Health (NAMI) groups, and held several student-parent depression panels at neighboring schools. We also conducted a trial of a formal curriculum of Mindfulness for Sports Performance Enhancement, which demonstrated both significant reduction in depression/anxiety symptoms and improved performance.[6] The relationship continues to be helpful when other school crises or concerns occur.

The third challenge was the Fairfax County Public Health Department (FCPHD). At the previously mentioned community listening session (attended by more than 1,000 people) held after the fourth student died by suicide, health department staff—seemingly trying to calm the crowd—announced that the county adolescent suicide background rate was lower than that in the rest of the state. This message, although well intended, was not received well. We struggled with the health department's resistance to embracing the cluster as a public health crisis and invested considerable time in trying to understand their perspective. We attempted to reframe it, suggesting that while syphilis rates in the county are low, multiple cases in a single school would be investigated directly. CoS members met many times with health department leaders in person and on calls to maintain good-faith communications. The CDC/SAMHSA Epi-Aid that eventually investigated risks for youth suicide took more than a year to organize. The CDC had undertaken Epi-Aids for prior suicides, most notably in Delaware[7] and Maine,[8] and early conversations with Dr. Phillips led to conversations with SAMHSA to develop one jointly. Epi-Aids are traditionally called for by local health authorities, but it took calls from CoS and others to the state health department to dislodge resistance to a local request.[9,10] Once that occurred, a conference call with CoS leaders, Fairfax County Health Department staff, Virginia Department of Health staff, and CDC staff produced the shared aims. Call participants were copied on the email to the CDC leadership that laid out these aims:

- Review all relevant information sources that might shed light on potential associations between the Woodson suicides to see if there are patterns that may suggest an existing unusual risk.
- Look at suicide attempts by Woodson students in the same period that the seven suicides have occurred to see if those add additional information about potential patterns.
- Review data about suicides in students who live in the Woodson community but are home-schooled or in private school.

The email further clarified, "Our goal is not necessarily to identify causal links, but rather to gain information that could help us enhance and tailor ongoing postvention activities and plans, as well as guide local investigations of future suicides."

When the Epi-Aid was conducted, however, the protocol did not look like what was agreed on, nor did it look like Epi-Aids done in Maine or Delaware. None of its work centered on Woodson High School, and none of the related community meetings was held at Woodson—in fact, the community meetings were held very distal to the Woodson Community. The FCPHD website explains the deviance from the plan and from precedence thusly:

> In the early planning stages, some community members were concerned about youth suicides at one high school and its unique risk factors, including the potential role of social media (e.g., youth using social media to share information about a suicide at one high school being a risk for suicide at another high school). Preliminary data analyses showed that youth suicides were occurring at multiple high schools, and in October 2014 there were three youth suicides at three separate high schools. Based on this information and community goals to prevent all youth suicides, the Epi-Aid partners selected a county-wide approach to identify risk and protective factors for the county as well as unique to any particular school. A community and multi-school approach to the Epi-Aid in Fairfax County has many advantages that can inform suicide prevention community-wide as well as at any particular school. It allows for a comparison of risk and protective factors across schools so that schools can more reliably understand their strengths and challenges in context. It also better informs community-wide prevention approaches.[11]

There was real value in the resulting Epi-Aid report, but the capacity to investigate the Woodson cluster was lost. It remains unclear to CoS leadership why the Epi-Aid could not accomplish both goals—a study of Woodson-specific and county-wide risks. Despite its valuable components, the study echoed the early FCHD statement, "Suicide rates for all age groups in Fairfax

County, Virginia are lower than the overall national suicide rate for 2003–2012." The follow-on travesty of the Epi-Aid refocus is that the same approach was repeated when Palo Alto called for CDC and SAMHSA to repeat the study for their community.[12] Palo Alto school leadership acknowledged that the 10-year suicide rate for their two high schools was four to five times higher than the national average.[13] CoS calculated that the Woodson rate from 2011 to 2014 was 7/3,600 (denominator calculated to avoid double counting same students in multiple years), or nearly 60-fold higher than the county rate for 10- to 19-year-olds. We addressed these concerns in a formal letter to FCHD, but it remains unwilling to call adolescent suicide a public health crisis. The health department also declined requests for developing clinician notifications about student deaths by suicide, similar to notifications that occur regularly about infectious disease cases. Thankfully, the Medical Society of Northern Virginia collaborated with CoS in communicating to its membership about a suicide cluster occurrence. The Epi-Aid identified the significant rise in emergency department visits for adolescent suicidal ideation and attempts, and CoS continues to believe that local clinicians need to be aware when their adolescent patients might be affected.

The fourth challenge is sustainability. CoS leadership began with concerned parents and students, but those students have graduated and most of the parents no longer have children attending W. T. Woodson High School. Unlike Palo Alto, which partnered very effectively with Stanford University, none of our local universities or hospitals offered similar community engagement or support to local health practitioners. Lauren Terry developed a wonderful CoS website linked to a Facebook page managed by Heather Davies, which continues to be a resource to more than 400 registered users, many of whom continue to post information about relevant meetings and resources. In Palo Alto, sustainability of focus and effort is maintained by a Project Safety Net Task Force made up of school leadership, community leaders, students/teens, parents, foundations, and the Santa Clara Health Department, to name a few. FCHD did form a temporary, internal Youth Behavioral Health Task Force (which no longer appears on their website), but there was no sustaining focus on long-term reduction in adolescent suicide that included community members or students. While the Fairfax County Government has continued to put more resources into the CSB, it is unclear if there is any organized, sustained effort to study whether the past suicide cluster in Fairfax County has lasting, cultural risk in our schools or if we've appropriately addressed the need to reduce risk of teen suicide.

For now, the CoS remains a small, focused group that continues to work at improving student awareness and resilience, building resources for mental health and substance use, and reducing suicide risk. We hope that our story will help galvanize other parents, educators, medical professionals, and community members to take action to prevent tragedies like the ones in our community by working together to find solutions. Our community offers lessons—some positive, some not—that we hope might be instructive. We have a lasting hope that the CDC and SAMHSA might rethink their approach to suicide clusters that more closely approximates what they do for other disease outbreaks—namely, studying the cluster itself, as well as its proximate environment, to understand potential sources and any ongoing risk of spread.

## REFERENCES

1. Roberts DW. Health is a community affair: Preview of the final report of the national commission on community health services. *JAMA.* 1966;196(4):332–33.

2. Group TF. Communities of Solution: The Folsom Report Revisited. *Ann Fam Med.* 2012;10(3):250–60.

3. Woolsey A. Youth Suicide forum coincides with death of Woodson student. *Fairfax County Times.* May 11, 2017. http://www.fairfaxtimes.com/articles/youth-suicide-forum-coincides-with-death-of-woodson-student/article_b1faf6e0-368e-11e7-8d1b-67520d424ecb.html. Accessed on 1/16/2019.

4. Scutti S. Woodson High School suicides: Some question whether suicide is contagious after cluster of teen deaths in Virginia. Medical Daily. http://www.medicaldaily.com/woodson-high-school-suicides-some-question-whether-suicide-contagious-after-cluster-teen-deaths. 2014. Accessed on 1/16/2019.

5. Pannoni A. Teachers: Use mindfulness to help students' academics. *US News World Report.* 2018. https://www.usnews.com/high-schools/blogs/high-school-notes/articles/2018-01-01/teachers-use-mindfulness-to-help-students-academics. Accessed on 1/16/2019.

6. Kaufman K, Glass C, Pineau T. *Mindful Sport Performance Enhancement: Mental Training for Athletes and Coaches.* Washington, DC: American Psychological Association; 2017.

7. Fowler KA, Crosby AE, Parks SE, Ivey AZ, Silverman PR. Epidemiological investigation of a youth suicide cluster: Delaware 2012. *Delaware Med J.* 2013;85(1):15–19.

8. Askland KD, Sonnenfeld N, Crosby A. A public health response to a cluster of suicidal behaviors: Clinical psychiatry, prevention, and community health. *J Psychiatric Pract.* 2003;9(3):219–27.

9. Spies E, Ivey-Stephenson, A, VanderEnde K, Lynch, S, Dean Jr. D, Gleason B. Epi-Aid 2015-003: Undetermined risk factors for suicide among youth, ages 10–24 Fairfax County, VA 2014. Centers for Disease Control and Prevention; Substance Abuse and Mental Health Services Administration. 2015. https://www.fairfaxcounty.gov/health/sites/health/files/assets/images/suicide-epi-aid-final-report.pdf.

10. Associated Press. Feds look into possible Fairfax County suicide clusters. 2014. WJLA. http://wjla.com/news/health/feds-fairfax-county-look-into-northern-virginia-suicides-following-3-deaths-since-september-109169.

11. Fairfax County Health Department. Epi-Aid 2015-003: Undetermined risk factors for suicide among youth, ages 10–24 Fairfax County, VA 2014: Questions and Answers. 2015. https://www.fairfaxcounty.gov/health/sites/health/files/assets/images/suicide-epi-aid-questions-answers.pdf.

12. Chawla I. CDC releases preliminary findings on Palo Alto suicide clusters. *The Stanford Daily News.* July 21, 2016. https://www.stanforddaily.com/2016/07/21/cdc-releases-preliminary-findings-on-palo-alto-suicide-clusters/. Accessed 1/16/2019.

13. Rosin H. The Silicon Valley Suicides: Why are so many kids with bright prospects killing themselves in Palo Alto? *The Atlantic* 2015. https://www.theatlantic.com/magazine/archive/2015/12/the-silicon-valley-suicides/413140/. Accessed 1/16/2019.

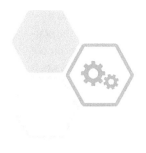

# Chapter 18

# Sustainability Through Accountability: The Accountable Community for Health Model

MARION STANDISH, BONNIE MIDURA, BARBARA MASTERS,
PATRICIA POWERS, AND LAURA HOGAN

Public and private funders have long supported community collaboratives to address a wide range of health issues. Although these collaboratives accomplish important goals, they rarely continue beyond the funding or yield lasting systems change. The accountable community for health (ACH) is a multisector collaborative with an embedded sustainability capacity—a Wellness Fund—built into it from the start. A Wellness Fund is an expression of the ACH's shared responsibility for the health of the community. Operationalizing shared responsibility or collective accountability through the Wellness Fund and other aspects of the ACH, such as achieving agreed-upon outcomes, is central to the success and sustainability of an ACH.

Collective accountability (Box 18.1) has been identified as a key indicator of systems change, recognizing that it is very difficult to achieve and sustain.[1] It demands a shift from "business as usual" to an innovative, dynamic, and iterative process of "we are in this together"—an important goal of the ACH.

## THE ACCOUNTABLE COMMUNITY FOR HEALTH MODEL

The ACH model is gaining traction across the country. A recent review of this trend found that "[a]ccountable health initiatives fundamentally embrace the concept that there is a shared responsibility for the health of a community or patient population across sectors. By focusing on the alignment of clinical and community-based organizations, they offer an integrated approach to health, health care, and social needs of individuals and communities to achieve equity, better population health outcomes, reach a higher quality of health care, and reduce costs."[2]

## Box 18.1 | Collective Accountability

Collective accountability assumes a much deeper commitment to the change process within and across organizations and between the practice and policy levels, building on previously established buy-in and a comprehensive understanding of the problem. Collective accountability occurs when organizations develop the capacity to balance internal interests with interests across other organizations and systems to support a common goal or address a shared community need.[1]

An ACH represents the next generation of health system transformation by extending the boundaries of the current health care delivery system to include community organizations and social services; other sectors, such as education and public safety; and the broader community environment.[3] There are variations in the specific components of an ACH, and the California Accountable Communities for Health Initiative (CACHI), has its own. (CACHI has its origins in the state's Let's Get Healthy California [LGHC] Task Force, which was launched in 2012 by California Governor Jerry Brown. Funders participating in LGHC [The California Endowment, Blue Shield of California Foundation, Kaiser Permanente, and Sierra Health Foundation] subsequently decided that the opportunity was ripe to implement the ACH model in California (Box 18.2). They pooled nearly $10 million over a 4-year period to test this new model of health system transformation in partnership with the California Health and Human Services Agency.) CACHI launched in 2016, and identified the following seven key elements of an ACH—all of which are infused with an equity lens.

## Box 18.2 | California Accountable Communities for Health Initiative (CACHI)

CACHI (CACHI.org) includes 15 communities participating through two cohorts: six Catalyst communities and nine Accelerator communities. A program management team housed at Community Partners, a fiscal intermediary based in Los Angeles, manages the six Catalyst communities, while the Public Health Institute oversees the nine Accelerator communities. The initiative is grounded by strong relationships between the funding partners, an explicit intent for communities to co-design the initiative alongside funders (a "build as we fly" approach), and a focus on sustainability from the start. The evaluation reinforces this learning-by-doing approach and links to a broader ACH evaluation framework developed by the Health and Human Services Agency.

1. *Shared vision and goals*, based on a common understanding of the problem.
2. *Explicit governance arrangement*, including identified leaders and champions and meaningful partnerships across different organizations and sectors.
3. *Resident engagement at all levels of the ACH*, from governance to workgroups, as well as the design and implementation of the portfolio of interventions.
4. *Backbone entity* that serves as the ACH's convener and facilitator.
5. *Data analytics and sharing capacity*, which will enable the ACH to effectively implement the portfolio of interventions, track progress, and communicate impact.
6. *Portfolio of mutually reinforcing interventions across five domains*: (1) clinical care, (2) community programs and social services, (3) community-clinical linkages, (4) environment, and (5) public policy and systems.
7. *Wellness Fund and sustainability plan* that can attract, braid, and blend resources to support the goals of the ACH.

It is important to distinguish the ACH model, which is relatively new, from the accountable care organization (ACO)—a prescriptive health care delivery system model (e.g., https://khn.org/news/aco-accountable-care-organization-faq/) that has been around for more than a decade. An ACO is a formal organization focused on *care,* whereas the ACH is a *community collaborative* aimed at *health and wellness.* Accountability is a common thread between the ACO and the ACH. However, while the ACO achieves accountability principally through financing agreements and, ultimately, shared savings, in an ACH, accountability operates at multiple levels, including, but not limited to, financing and the Wellness Fund.

## ACCOUNTABILITY: THE CRITICAL INGREDIENT FOR BUILDING COLLABORATIONS THAT LAST

The central operating principle of an ACH is that collective accountability is both a driver and an indicator of permanent systems change. It recognizes that for accountability to be meaningful across sectors, it must extend beyond financial arrangements. It is essential that all partners be explicit and continually revisit the questions of *to whom is* the ACH accountable and *for what.*

### To Whom Is the ACH Accountable?

Accountability requires participating individuals and organizations to agree to the mutual and shared responsibility for the ACH's activities, outcomes, successes, and failures. This applies to an ACH leadership team as well as to the wider circle of partners. Equally important for CACHI sites is accountability to the residents of the community.

Accountability can be assessed as the ACH balances the needs of its stakeholders with their commitment to principles and practices (Figure 18.1). Shared accountability not only means ensuring that the right stakeholders are at the table and that they are heard, but it also requires an ACH to do the following: (1) garner *commitment* from and foster *trust* among leadership team members, other partners, and the organizations they represent, which ideally deepens over time; (2) create a *distributed leadership* model where many people assume responsibility for various agreed-upon activities and participate in decision-making; (3) periodically evaluate whether any appropriate interest group/leader is not represented and, if so, how to best ensure *inclusion and diverse, equitable representation*; (4) continuously generate support and "buy-in" through transparent *feedback loops* leveraging data and information[1]; and (5) implement *authentic community engagement with an equity lens*. A brief description of each of these is provided in the following list:

*Mutual trust is the result of accountability.*
—*Pedja Stojicic,*
*ReThink Health*

- *Commitment and trust*: Building leadership team and partner organizations' commitment to the ACH and to each other takes time. As an ACH creates a vision and transparent governance structure and develops a portfolio of interventions that cuts across multiple sectors and organizations, participants begin to appreciate the scale and impact of the ACH. It becomes increasingly clear how their own organizational interests fit. The give and take of this process inspires a shared sense of mission and its collective benefits. They combine to strengthen trust. A more formal governance structure with organizational leadership team commitments further strengthens accountability.
- *Distributed leadership*: Although an ACH relies on a backbone organization for overall management, leadership team members assume

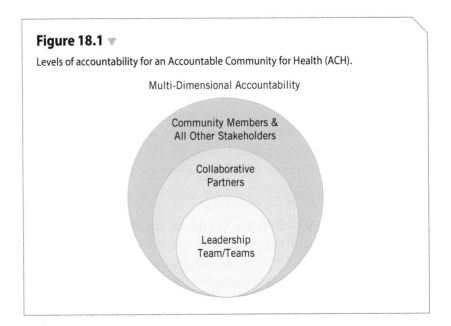

**Figure 18.1** ▼

Levels of accountability for an Accountable Community for Health (ACH).

Multi-Dimensional Accountability

Community Members & All Other Stakeholders

Collaborative Partners

Leadership Team/Teams

responsibility for specific activities. Given the diverse needs/expertise of the ACH, spreading these roles throughout the collaborative adds to trust building and mutual accountability. Just as obtaining organizational rather than individual commitments is important for governance stability and overall accountability, a distributed leadership model creates greater cohesion for the ACH, embedding it more broadly within the community. Figure 18.2 depicts a distributed leadership model developed by Merced County, where the backbone organization resides with the Department of Public Health, United Way serves as the Wellness Fund administrator, a local health information exchange and its vendor are taking the lead on data sharing, and clinics and community organizations are managing other key ACH activities.

- *Inclusion*: As the ACH develops, regular check-ins are needed to ensure that the governance structure and participants reflect the composition of the community. Leadership teams receive training in equity, diversity, and inclusion and are mindful of the risk of reinforcing accountability that skews toward stakeholders with power at the expense of those less powerful, but who are directly affected by the ACH's work.[4]

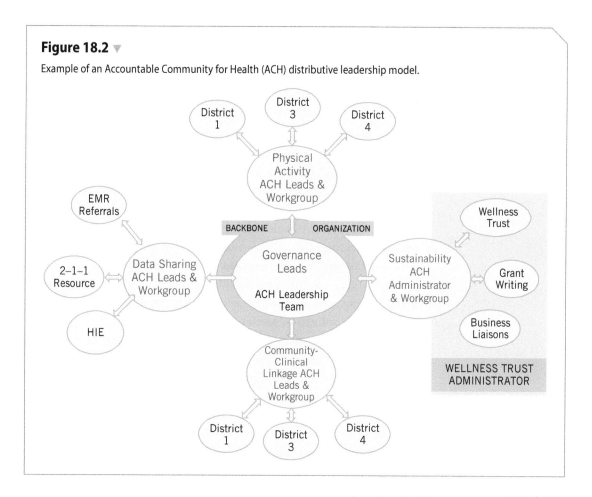

**Figure 18.2** ▼

Example of an Accountable Community for Health (ACH) distributive leadership model.

- *Transparent feedback loops*: The ACH uses a logic model to identify short-, intermediate-, and long-term outcomes. Because ACHs are breaking new ground where evidence and data may be thin, creative workarounds to consolidate data and gather "best available" information for monitoring and decision-making are necessary while working on longer term data-sharing strategies. In addition, each logic model includes metrics to gauge progress of the ACH infrastructure by which all involved can hold one another accountable.
- *Authentic community engagement with an equity lens*: Authentic community engagement requires that the ACH provide vehicles through which the community expresses its preferences, opinions, and views and can receive updates on progress and results. Moreover, the ACH should possess the agility to respond to the community and reflect a willingness to change its governance structure, policies, and programs as appropriate.

Accountability to the community ensures that the ACH addresses issues and interventions that matter to people. For example, residents participating in a San Diego community engagement meeting raised issues related to trauma and its contribution to cardiovascular disease, the focus of the ACH. This community priority was subsequently incorporated into the ACH portfolio of interventions. In Stockton, after knocking on residents' doors to gather their priorities, leaders recognized that their long-term focus on economic development and the prevention and treatment of trauma had to include attention to improving parks and eliminating local drug dealers.

## For What Is the ACH Accountable?

Improving population health requires a multifaceted and coordinated strategy at multiple levels, from individual provider practices to community-wide efforts. Creation of a portfolio of interventions is predicated on the idea that, to achieve change at scale, a coordinated set of interventions is required that consistently reinforce each other to strengthen and amplify the impact of individual activities. Ideally, the portfolio should encompass a full range of upstream and downstream activities to address all stages and aspects of an identified health issue, and it should be strategically assembled so that the interventions are aligned, reinforcing, and connected. A portfolio is not simply a collection of siloed activities operating in parallel, but rather a coherent set of interlocking activities that, when combined, can achieve a common set of outcomes.

Implementing a portfolio is a developmental process, and each iteration of the process results in an improved strategy and deeper acceptance among community residents and organizational partners. Portfolio development also affords opportunities to strengthen program alignment and to better articulate the communities' overall approach to a selected health issue. The process of developing a portfolio *and* the choice of its metrics and outcomes depends on and deepens collaboration and accountability. Figure 18.3 reflects the portfolio development process that CACHI is employing.

**Figure 18.3** ▼

The process of developing a portfolio of interventions.

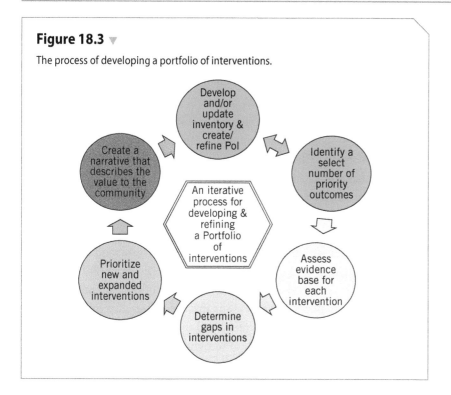

- Facilitated by the trusted backbone, communities inventory existing interventions mapped to portfolio domains (e.g., clinical care, community programs and social services, community–clinical linkages, environment, and public policy and systems).
- Simultaneously, communities establish portfolio outcomes that cut across all of the interventions, rather than individual program outcomes. This is critical for collective accountability, as multiple stakeholders will contribute to each outcome and its ultimate success.
- With the inventory and a common set of outcomes at hand, communities can then continue through the process to assess evidence, identify gaps, refine the portfolio, and develop a narrative of how the portfolio will improve health.

Using the process, CACHI sites have revised and prioritized portfolios so that they reflect local needs, assets, and aspirations. Outcomes have been developed to meet criteria such as producing measurable, feasible for data collection that is compelling to multiple audiences and increasing equity. Developing this aligned set of interventions and outcomes raised several issues relevant to building a sense of collective accountability:

- Ensuring that *equity* goals are elevated and articulated throughout the portfolio
- Using consistent and straightforward *language* that is understandable by all participants, including residents

- Learning about best practices and agreeing on what constitutes *evidence* for portfolio programs
- Agreeing about *outcomes* that are achievable and important
- Connecting the portfolio to *sustainability* planning and the Wellness Fund

More than any other element of the ACH, the Wellness Fund requires—and is an expression of—collective accountability. The Wellness Fund is the vehicle for an ACH's sustainability and is governed by the ACH itself. In this way, the ACH governance links strategy (the portfolio) to sustainability (the Wellness Fund) and formalizes accountability to the community. Embedding sustainability and accountability is a critical goal of CACHI, so that attracting and prioritizing resources to sustain and expand the portfolio and ACH infrastructure are contained within the same governance structure, and its accountability is squarely with the community. In one CACHI community, the county host agency has developed a formal memorandum of understanding (MOU) for approval by the Board of Supervisors that formalizes governance between the ACH (not an organizational entity) and the Wellness Fund. This governance structure allows communities to recognize and prioritize needs, such as scaling interventions and addressing gaps in the portfolio, alongside decisions for infrastructure sustainability, like backbone support, data, and community engagement.

## EARLY LESSONS

With just under 2 years of CACHI implementation, lessons are already emerging regarding the essential role of accountability in the development and implementation of an ACH.

- *Development of an accountable health system is an iterative effort.* Grantees are working on all seven elements of the ACH simultaneously, necessitating continual review and updates. The iterative process itself strengthens understanding and accountability for the ACH among all partners.
- *ACHs develop faster and with greater likelihood of sustainability when they build on and incorporate past efforts that include community capacity and leadership development.* Many of the ACHs are utilizing existing platforms and tables, and many of the leaders have experience with previous initiatives. Preexisting and trusting relationships provide a solid foundation for the ACH.
- *Sound governance means that there is broad and deep ownership of the ACH.* Although strong individual leaders are important to catalyze action, sustainability requires multiple leaders, broad ownership, and

organizational buy-in of the ACH. Four of the six CACHI communities are undergoing leadership transitions, underscoring this need.

- *Community engagement—and ultimately activation—ensures that the ACH is accountable to the community in a meaningful way.* The ACHs are implementing robust community engagement efforts to train residents and develop community leaders on health. This requires overcoming past failed promises of action and widespread "input" fatigue. Relatedly, ACHs are developing concrete mechanisms of accountability to the community, such as dashboards and other means of communication, to ensure that community residents are kept apprised of progress and meaningfully involved in the effort.
- *Strong accountability mechanisms enable the ACH to shift from project orientation to systems change.* The goal of CACHI is for each community to establish an enduring platform to tackle a range of community health priorities. Accountability mechanisms enable stakeholders to shift their mindset from a project to a sustainable community-wide effort.
- *Trust and clear accountability mechanisms are critical for selecting a Wellness Fund and ensuring sound governance.* The Wellness Fund and implementation of the sustainability plan should not be viewed as separate or distinct from other elements of the ACH. Accountability to the ACH, built on a platform of trust, will help investors and other stakeholders see the value of investing in the Fund.

## CONCLUSION

Improving the health of populations requires mutual and shared responsibility for outcomes. No single system, organization, or individual can achieve results on their own. With its focus on accountability across multiple stakeholders, especially community residents, the ACH is an emerging model that holds much promise for success. However, as noted, accountability cannot be limited to financial returns but must become meaningful and actionable across multiple dimensions and all stakeholders. This is the meaning of transformation, and it is an important mechanism for driving improved and sustainable positive health outcomes.

## REFERENCES

1. Linkins KW, Frost LE, Boober BH, Brya JJ. Moving from partnership to collective accountability and sustainable change: Applying a systems-change model to foundations' evolving roles. *Foundation Rev.* 2013;5(2):52–66.

2. Siegel B, Erickson J, Milstein B, Pritchard KE. Multi-sector partnerships need further development to fulfill aspirations for transforming health and well-being. *Health Affairs.* 2018 Jan; 37(1): 30-37

3. Mongeon M, Levi J, Heinrich J. Elements of accountable communities for health: A review of the literature. *Natl Acad Med*. November 2017. http://cachi.org/uploads/resources/Elements-of-Accountable-Communities-for-Health_updatedFINAL.pdf. Accessed March 15, 2017.

4. Stojicic P. *Restoring Trust and Building Power—Resident Engagement Practices*. ReThink Health. CACHI, December 2017. https://www.rethinkhealth.org/wp-content/uploads/2018/12/RTH-ResEngageToolkit_12172018.pdf. Accessed 1/23/2019.

# Data: Finding and Using Information

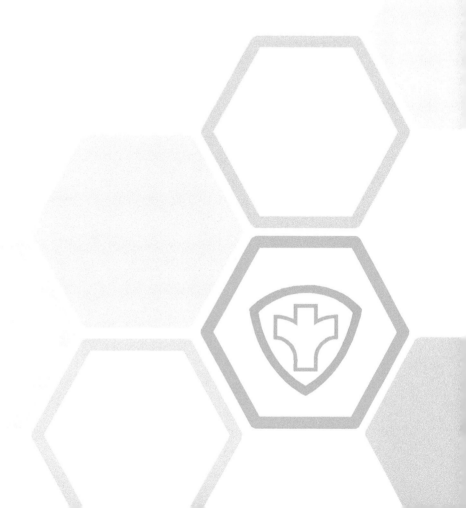

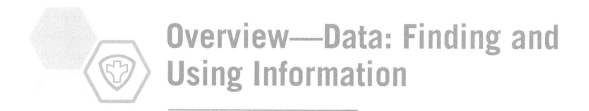

# Chapter 19

# Overview—Data: Finding and Using Information

BRIAN C. CASTRUCCI AND DON W. BRADLEY

Data on the causes of death and disease are necessary to drive well-informed, impactful resource allocation and policy decisions. As maintaining health has become more complex, so has the need for more complete data that extend beyond health metrics. Electronic health records have digitized patient encounters, creating an unprecedented volume of data on disease. But these data alone do not provide the information needed to improve health. Administrative data, including public park locations and safety, alcohol and tobacco sales outlet locations, housing foreclosures, and student test scores, along with data captured through, for example, sensors in bridges and roads, highway transponders, and grocery store loyalty cards, provide a nearly continuous stream of data that can, in unprecedented ways, describe our interactions with the communities in which we live. Technology promises to expand our ability to capture data even further. However, our ability to collect data far exceeds our ability to create usable information that can be applied to improve health.

The amount of data collected increases almost daily, but significant barriers exist to sharing data across sectors. When these data remain isolated, so do strategies informed by them. Simultaneous visualization of social and health information can provide a complete understanding of the factors influencing community health and design and can contribute to the implementation of effective and impactful clinical interventions, urban planning and land use, community development planning, and policy agendas. Data systems must be created that integrate data across various systems—health, health care, education, transportation, criminal justice, and utility payments—to create the information necessary to inform the creation of the best strategies and interventions to improve health. Although technical barriers are surmountable, the organizational barriers can prove to be an equal, if not a greater, challenge. While no blueprint currently exists to build these needed data systems, it is imperative to identify successful collaborations, strategies, and experiences to build the knowledge necessary to progress toward this goal.

## WHAT'S IN THIS SECTION

This section explores what is happening to build the trust and accountability necessary for partnerships in which data sharing is at the center. Highlights include use cases that guide health professions through and around Health Insurance Portability and Accountability Act (HIPAA) regulations when accessing the data they need (Chapters 20–23), tips on crafting data-sharing agreements (Chapter 22), lessons on managing data exchange between health care and public health (Chapter 21), instructions on how to find the data you need (Chapter 23), advice from the All In Data Collaborative for community health improvement (Chapter 20), and a case study from the Baltimore City Health Department (Chapter 24), just to name a few. Practitioners and analysts alike can find the angle they need to improve the way they use data and build data-sharing partnerships in these chapters. This section is truly meant as a resource guide and toolkit for all health professionals to improve the way they use and share data.

## WHAT'S NOT IN THIS SECTION

One of the most compelling and concrete reasons to build partnerships among health professions, as well as among different sectors, is that partnerships can increase access to new and better data. Nevertheless, many data-sharing projects and collaborations are still in their infancy. Future data partnerships should focus on the social determinants of health and combining data from different sectors outside health care. This combined data on social determinants can move interventions continuously upstream so that expensive clinical solutions to community health problems become the exception and not the norm. Data collection and use also have serious implications for health equity, especially when considering from whom we collect data and what we do with it. Using the lens of health equity, data can help us dive deeper into the roots of health disparities and find solutions that address those root causes. Data also have an important role to play in the creation of an evidence base that informs policy solutions. Combining strong evidence with powerful stories can motivate and inform policymakers to implement policy solutions with powerful implications for improving community health on local, state, and national scales. Finally, data are a resource in making our case for health solutions to other sectors, such as businesses. Health professionals can use data to translate our messages about health into messages about workforce, security, prosperity, or social good. In this way, public health and health professions can create an impact that reaches much farther than the walls of a health department or hospital. This is where the field needs to move with data, and partnership is how we will get there.

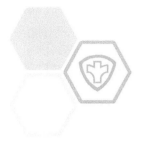

# Chapter 20

# All In: How and Why Communities Are Using Data to Drive Community Health Improvement

CLARE TANNER AND PETER ECKART

A s this edition of *Practical Playbook* makes clear, health is best under-stood as one of a number of important drivers of community well-being, combining with multiple social, political, and economic forces that influence residents' quality of life. Actors in multiple sectors—including clinical care, public health, housing, education, private industry, and all levels of government—see health goals as interdependent with safe communities, child-hood learning and development, economic prosperity, a clean environment, a socially engaged citizenry, and productive businesses.

Developing a shared data system is a natural extension of multisector work, though it is both an accelerator and a pain point for many initiatives. As these multisector initiatives proliferate, they are spinning off lessons of what works and what doesn't, and those lessons have much to offer to communities in the earlier stages of sharing data. This is why several national initiatives and funders have joined together to form All In: Data for Community Health, a learning network of communities across the country that are testing and evaluating new ways to transform health through multisector partnerships to share data (Figure 20.1).[1]

## TWO BROAD CATEGORIES OF MULTISECTOR DATA PROJECTS

Among the All In network, multisector data sharing initiatives focused on re-ducing health disparities fall into two broad categories: (1) those with a focus on sharing individual patient or client data to enhance whole-person systems of care and (2) those that use individual and aggregate data to improve population and community health and well-being. Figure 20.2 shows typical data sharing

### Figure 20.1 ▼

The All In community.

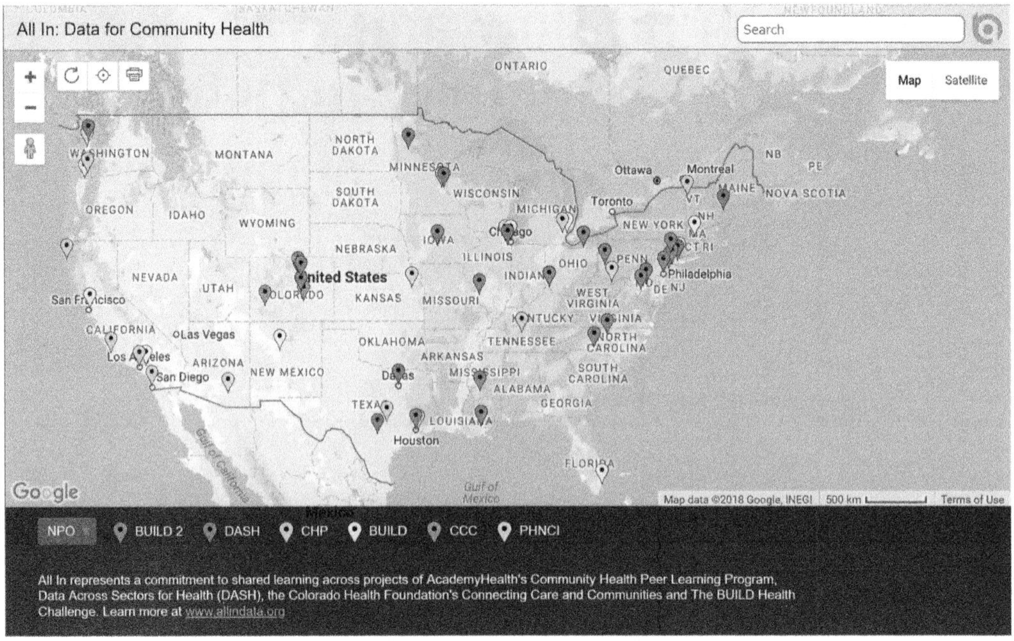

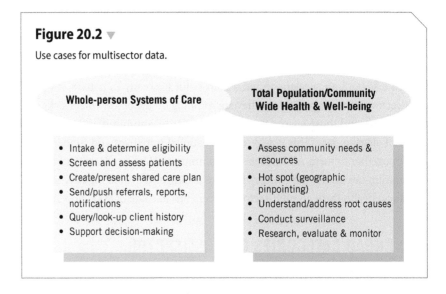

All In: Data for Community Health

NPO | BUILD 2 | DASH | CHP | BUILD | CCC | PHNCI

All In represents a commitment to shared learning across projects of AcademyHealth's Community Health Peer Learning Program, Data Across Sectors for Health (DASH), the Colorado Health Foundation's Connecting Care and Communities and The BUILD Health Challenge. Learn more at www.allindata.org

### Figure 20.2 ▼

Use cases for multisector data.

**Whole-person Systems of Care**

- Intake & determine eligibility
- Screen and assess patients
- Create/present shared care plan
- Send/push referrals, reports, notifications
- Query/look-up client history
- Support decision-making

**Total Population/Community Wide Health & Well-being**

- Assess community needs & resources
- Hot spot (geographic pinpointing)
- Understand/address root causes
- Conduct surveillance
- Research, evaluate & monitor

"use cases" in these two categories (a "use case" typically describes a typical way that organizations and individuals work within a system to achieve a particular desired outcome, like a reduction in youth homelessness or diverting individuals from the criminal justice system into behavior health care).

## Whole-Person Systems of Care

Hospitals, health systems, and their clinical partners are facing increasing pressures to expand their networks to embrace new kinds of expertise. "Pay for success" and "pay for value" strategies reflect the understanding that clinical care alone won't achieve desired outcomes for health, and person-centered care is driving a more holistic and relational understanding of health. Electronic health records (EHR) are increasingly being connected to data from behavioral and mental health providers and even from community-based social service organizations. Comprehensive individual assessment tools, shared care plans, and resource and referral systems are all examples of these new systems of whole-person care (Box 20.1).

## Population and Community Health and Well-Being

Public health has long sought population health solutions where the goal is to change the environment in which we live, eat, work, play, and pray. The use cases for these "place-based" strategies rely on the integration of governmental public health data and data from sectors shaping the social determinants of health, such as transportation, community safety, economic stability, education, and other social forces that are typically geographically focused. Common use cases include community assessment and planning, public health surveillance

---

**Box 20.1 | Altair Accountable Care for People with Disabilities**[1]

*Emily Yu and Clare Tanner*

Utilizing a partnership of multisector providers, Altair accountable care organization (ACO) has built a data platform to assist adults with intellectual or developmental disabilities in meeting their life goals, which include stable health, safe and secure housing, and employment. Altair ACO worked with a local health information exchange (HIE) to create an e-health infrastructure that improves coordination between primary care, behavioral health, and social services providers. The system notifies care teams about the behavioral health needs of people with disabilities in real time to ensure that they are providing the right services at the right time. For more examples of whole person systems of care, read the DASH issue brief.[2]

**References**

1. DASH Connect. Integrated care for people with disabilities: Lessons from an accountable care organization. http://dashconnect.org/2016/09/01/integrated-care-for-people-with-disabilities-lessons-from-an-accountable-care-organization/. Accessed May 2, 2018.
2. DASH Connect. Coordinated whole-person care that addresses social determinants of health. http://dashconnect.org/wp-content/uploads/2017/09/DASH-care-coordination-brief.pdf. Accessed May 2, 2018.

and reporting, hotspotting of adverse community and health conditions, and root cause analysis (Box 20.2).

## THE ENVIRONMENT FOR MULTISECTOR DATA-SHARING COLLABORATIONS

Data Across Sectors for Health (DASH) continuously monitors the environment for examples of multisector data sharing to support community health use cases. We have observed that successful data-sharing initiatives depend on the presence of strong interorganizational relationships, the existence of an official decision-making mechanism across the partner organizations, a foundational technical "infrastructure" or the capacity to develop it, and dedicated staff and funding for the multisector work.

With those foundational elements in place, community collaborations are ready to design and build the interconnected systems that enable data sharing. As they do so, they will need to address data governance (which specifies the contributions and obligations of the data owners and data users), security, privacy, and consent. They also attend to technical design, the interaction between users and technology, and how technology changes work processes.

## INSIGHTS AND RECOMMENDATIONS

Inevitably, combining and using data from multiple sectors to advance individual and community health is fraught with challenges. Frequently reported barriers include insufficient buy-in or trust across community partners, concerns or misunderstanding about privacy laws, difficulty in connecting specific data sets, and other technical challenges. Experience from across the country demonstrates that these barriers can be addressed, but it does take time, resources, and commitment to persist and iterate.

## 1. Successful Data-Sharing Collaborations Are Built on Honest and Mutually Beneficial Relationships

Multisector partners must be intentional about building trusting relationships. Getting to know prospective partners (e.g., what is important to them, the incentives that they are operating under, the level of infrastructure, constraints) helps a collaborative to craft a successful and productive outreach strategy, strengthen the coalition, and contribute toward sustainability by clearly articulating and defining the value that is being created by sharing data across sectors. When doing this, partners must be alert to differences in terminology that may get in the way.

A successful example comes from the statewide health information exchange (HIE), HealthInfoNet, in Maine. The HealthInfoNet staff conduct outreach to community action agencies (CAAs) so that the HIE can best understand their pain points, data system capacity, and workflows in order to facilitate their participation in the HIE. A representative from a CAA partner explained, " 'Social determinants of health' and 'enabling services' refers to what we do, but it is language from health care, not ours." Even so, this coalition overcame the barriers of language and data silos. "Our economic opportunity program aims to help families gain economic self-sufficiency. Health care costs and health care crises limit families' ability to achieve their goals of economic self-sufficiency. Education, life expectancy, and zip code predict health, and they also predict economic well-being. It goes hand in hand. It's all connected."

## 2. Legal Issues, Including Privacy and Consent, Require Significant Time to Discover and Address; Involve the Legal Teams Early on and Focus on Finding a "Path to Yes"

Most All In members are surprised at the time and resources it takes to get legal agreements in place for data sharing. The Health Insurance Portability and Accountability Act (HIPAA), the Family Educational Rights Privacy Act (FERPA), and the Substance Abuse and Mental Health Services Administration (SAMHSA) 42 CFR part 2 regulation all cover various aspects of data sharing and, depending on context, must be addressed. All In has witnessed a tendency to use or misuse these laws as justification to withhold data when the costs or risks seem to outweigh the benefits. Nevertheless, data-sharing partners have found a way to say "yes" to data sharing while protecting privacy and complying with applicable law. "Getting to yes" starts with trusted relationships and depends on a commitment to understand deeply what is and is not allowed by law in order to push back against assumptions or fears that are not supported by facts. Developing a successful data-sharing agreement ultimately involves organizational leadership, legal staff, IT, frontline staff, and, increasingly, the residents, participants, clients, and patients of the partner agencies.

In Chicago, the Department of Public Health and Chicago Public Schools developed a broad legal agreement—compliant with both HIPAA and FERPA—that would allow the school district and health department to share relevant data on an ongoing basis and avoid repeatedly creating one-off data-sharing agreements for specific use cases. Data elements that would be transferred between the two entities include demographics, immunizations, physical exams, chronic disease, academic performance, birth, vision and hearing, oral health, and other related social determinant metrics. Having a shared-values proposition was one key factor driving success, as both entities specifically identified what data and expertise they could bring to the table and how the partnership could be leveraged to further support their institutional missions.

### 3. Interoperability and Standards for Social Determinant Data Are Unlikely in the Near Term; Focus on Data Integration, Use the data that Partners Already Have, and Consider Proxies for Hard-to-Get Data

In its 2015 Environmental Scan, DASH found that stakeholders believed interoperability in the sharing of multisector data to be unlikely in the near future.[1] Since then, investment in new models of care, such as the common assessment form used by all ACHs, are driving discussion about harmonization of the ways that nonclinical health data are collected and documented. However, the federal government has been unwilling or unable to press for social services data interoperability in the way that standards for clinical data were developed as a part of health care reform, and there is no other value proposition for wide-scale data standards that reflect our broad understanding of how health is generated.

All In communities have learned not to make any assumptions about the quality and standardization of data in sectors outside of health care, which have not been the focus of investment and payment reform. For instance, the CAA, quoted earlier, reported having 150 different programs and funding streams, each with varying levels of accountability and requirements for data collection and reporting, to the extent that they were unable to track individual participants across their programs, much less share data with health care providers.

Without national standards to add stability to the health information technology market, many All In communities developing multisector care coordination systems have been able to collaboratively achieve a local understanding of the data they want to share and develop a common approach to connecting records to achieve their aims. To understand their problems and opportunities, communities can map desired data elements and potential sources of that data. Developing a common understanding of the data to be shared and the sources to be integrated can be solved locally, although these local solutions are often not generalizable to standards outside of the specific setting and use case being addressed.

## 4. Data Without a Practical Use Is a Waste of Resources; Choose Meaningful Data for Strategic Interventions and Action and Consider How These Data Will Be Incorporated into Programmatic Operations as Systems Are Designed

Some practitioners are attracted to data projects because of the potential insights and clarity that data provide. However, to ensure that multisector data has value, think through the organizational processes that will best leverage the data infrastructure being built. Adopting a technology and/or data-sharing system that enhances, rather than detracts from, effective workflow[2] is frequently a challenge (witness the debates about the impact of EHRs on physician workload to the detriment of patient interactions).

The challenge is that much greater when the changes in one organization's workflow reverberate across their partner organizations from other sectors with potentially conflicting operational priorities. (The term *workflow* is used to refer to a designed and repeatable pattern of activities to accomplish specific outcomes of an organization, such as the flow of clients through a system of care.)

As an example, a number of All In collaborations are trying to improve crisis or emergency services by supplying information about clients to the responding service providers (such as emergency medical services, police, or emergency department physicians). Several collaborations have found it challenging to deliver such information in a way that is acceptable to the provider in these fast-paced settings. However, North Coast Health Improvement and Information Network (NCHIIN) has found a way to connect busy emergency room physicians with housing case managers so that they can get information on patients' housing status at the point of care. NCHIIN maintains a multisector patient registry connecting clinical, housing, and incarceration data. As the regional HIE, NCHIIN also passes admit discharge transfer (ADT) notifications between health care providers. With each ADT transmission, the registry is queried to determine whether the patient admitted to the emergency department is also part of the registry. In those instances of a positive match, a notification is generated in real time back to the emergency department with the housing case manager's name and contact information.

## 5. Sustainability Must Be Addressed at the Community Level, as Well as Through Local, State, and National Policy

Multisector data-sharing projects, such as those in All In, are part of a major social experiment: Can individual and community health be improved by broadening and deepening the information used to create, operate, and evaluate our collaborative actions? And, if so, can that value be captured to support continued investment and innovation? At present, there is a proliferation of local examples, but the path toward scalability and replicability is still unclear. Early results suggest that multisector data projects can result in improved health, more equitable community outcomes, and financial savings. Yet because the resulting interventions are so local and diverse, it's difficult to measure outcomes and draw conclusions across multiple sites.

Conditions, however, are changing rapidly as leaders and practitioners in the field begin to apply greater rigor and new analytical approaches to assessing the financial impact of these interventions. Some approaches are federally funded, such as the State Innovation Models initiative, which seeks to build large-scale community approaches to whole-person health. Payers, health systems, and providers are building managed care networks under pay-for-success or pay-for-value approaches, where partners take responsibility and risk for the health of a designated pool of patients. New financing methods using social impact bonds are being tested, and many local initiatives are designed to save money by providing customized social services to high utilizers of expensive health care services. The ultimate answer to the question of sustainability will likely include a combination of these new approaches, as well as policy changes to the overall market incentives that are transforming systems of health (Boxes 20.3 through 20.5).

## CONCLUSION

It is a favorite aphorism of the All In community that "if you want to go fast, go alone, and if you want to go far, go together." Communities engaged in

---

**Box 20.3 | All In: Data for Community Health**

All In: Data for Community Health was established in 2015 and is maintained by state and national program offices that have combined forces to help communities connect and navigate the complex issues of multisector data sharing. Visit allindata.org to learn more about All In and its past and current partners.

*BUILD Health Challenge:* buildhealthchallenge.org
*Colorado Health Foundation, Connecting Communities and*
   *Care:* coloradohealth.org
*Community Health Peer Learning Program (CHP):* academyhealth.org/
   CHPHealthIT
*Data Across Sectors for Health (DASH):* dashconnect.org
*Public Health National Center for Innovations (PHNCI):* phnci.org
*Population Health Innovation Lab at the Public Health Institute:* http://www.
   phi.org/focus-areas/?program=population-health-innovation-lab
*New Jersey Health Initiatives:* https://www.njhi.org/

## Box 20.4 | Use Case 1: Is Childhood Asthma Rising or Falling?

*Joshua Sharfstein*

*Purpose.* The county health department is interested in reducing the burden of childhood asthma in the county. A core component of this effort is the regular assessment of the state of asthma. This is core public health surveillance—understanding the burden of disease to guide allocation of funds, inform program designs, and determine whether efforts are having the intended effect. Data reflecting time trends of asthma morbidity might allow the health department to strategically time the implementation of interventions to maximize impact. Time-series data pertaining to asthmatic episodes might also be used to inform health messages to the public about environmental conditions that are likely to trigger asthma attacks.

*Data request.* The health department requests a weekly data file from each area hospital with information about county residents younger than 21 years diagnosed with asthma during an emergency department (ED) visit or hospital admission. For each ED visit or hospital admission for asthma, the data file should include the following fields: date, age in years, gender, and race/ethnicity. The data file should not include name, social security number, address, or other demographic information. The health department asks that hospitals provide this data file at least weekly, with a lag of 2 weeks or less.

*Plan for data use.* The health department will combine and analyze the hospital data on a weekly basis for internal use. Analysis of these data will involve looking for trends by date, age, race/ethnicity, and gender. These reports will inform program development and facilitate monitoring of the burden of disease.

In addition, the health department intends to release a public report on childhood asthma every 6 months, with key findings from surveillance. The data will be reported in aggregate, without disclosure of identifiable patient information. The health department separately established a policy on patient privacy, based on a policy from the Centers for Medicare and Medicaid Services,[1] that requires the suppression of cell sizes of less than 10 in publicly released reports. This asthma report will be issued in accordance with this policy.

*Health Insurance Portability and Accountability Act (HIPAA) analysis.* As explained later, the health department's plan to use electronic health records (EHR) data to assess trends in asthma is permissible under the Health Insurance Portability and Accountability Act (HIPAA). It would be legal for hospitals to share the requested data for this purpose.

In this use case, the health department has clearly articulated a need for health information related to a public health activity—surveillance of pediatric asthma-related ED visits and hospitalizations by county residents. This clear articulation gives the health department the legal authority to request and receive protected health information from local hospitals and health care providers under HIPAA.

The health department has carefully described the data elements that are necessary for fulfilling the public health activity. This careful inventory of data elements meets the HIPAA minimum necessary requirement (described in greater detail in the report's HIPAA section) and allows hospitals or health providers to voluntarily share the requested information with the health department.

The health department may maintain and use the health data collected from hospitals and health care providers for its internal surveillance program. When the health department wants to release this data to inform the public, the information must be de-identified in accordance with HIPAA. The health department has a policy, based on the Centers for Medicare and Medicaid Services' policy regarding cell size suppression, which meets HIPAA standards for de-identification. This allows the health department to comply with patient privacy requirements while also providing valuable public health information regarding asthma to the public.

*Additional applications.* Real-time surveillance for other preventable conditions and manageable chronic illnesses using electronic health data can also facilitate health improvement. For example, health departments can monitor opioid overdoses via data on ED visits, complementing the reports of fatal overdoses from coroners or the office of the medical examiner. Health departments can also use electronic health data to conduct surveillance on preventable causes of injury resulting from medical treatment. For example, adverse drug events are a highly cited and preventable cause of hospital admission.[1] In two different studies, investigators utilized ED visits to monitor adverse drug events and develop prevention strategies.[2,3]

### References

1. CMS (Medicare) Data. CHS-NHLBI. https://chs-nhlbi.org/CHS_CMSData. Accessed March 26, 2017.
2. Budnitz DS, Pollock DA, Weidenbach KN, Mendelsohn AB, Schroeder TJ, Annest JL. National surveillance of emergency department visits for outpatient adverse drug events. *JAMA*. 2006;296(15):1858–66.
3. See I, Shehab N, Kegler SR, Laskar SR, Budnitz DS. Emergency department visits and hospitalizations for digoxin toxicity: United States, 2005 to 2010. *Circ Heart Fail*. 2014;7(1):28–34.

## Box 20.5 | Bronx Healthy Buildings Initiative

Sandra Lobo and Katherine Mella

The Bronx Healthy Buildings program (Healthy Buildings) is a collaborative, multisector approach to developing and implementing a community health initiative. This data-driven program aims to reduce morbidity among asthma patients living in the Bronx by holistically addressing several of the upstream causes—health behaviors, social and economic insecurity, and housing conditions—that exacerbate asthma symptoms. Healthy Buildings leverages the expertise of its strategic partnerships of community-based organizations, public agencies, and private-sector organizations, including the Montefiore Medical System, the MIT Community Innovators Lab, the New York City Department of Health and Mental Hygiene, and a.i.r. NYC, to implement asthma self-management support, community organizing, green and healthy building improvements, and development financing.

The Healthy Buildings program utilizes a variety of data sets to target distressed multifamily buildings that have the highest rates of asthma-related emergency room visits and hospitalizations, and which can greatly benefit from the range of program interventions. The program overlays electronic health records (EHR) data, data on rent-stabilized buildings, the NYC Clean Heat list,[1] and the Building Indicators Project's data (including housing violations, energy and water department benchmarking data), as well as estimated date of boiler retirement per Local Law 84[3,4] and the deadline for auditing and retro-commissioning buildings per Local Law 87.[5] This type of "hot-spotting" method allows for a comprehensive and holistic approach that not only addresses asthma, but also improves other health outcomes, addresses poor housing conditions, and contributes to environmental sustainability. Additional components of the program develop grassroots leadership within buildings by establishing tenant associations, and the program provides training in the social determinants of health as well as strengthens the local economy by contracting with local vendors. This comprehensive approach would not be possible without deep cross-sector, nontraditional partnerships which put the community as the lead and leverages resources and expertise across a range of organizations. This approach allows for collective problem-solving, decision-making, and iterative program development that contributes to the program's ongoing success.

**Notes**

1. This ensures a mechanism for affordability as landlords are prohibited from sharply increasing rent unless they undertake a Major Capital Improvement (MCI). Landlords will be prohibited from filing for an MCI as a result of the work funded or financed through the Healthy Buildings program.
2. A list that identifies those buildings still burning #4 heating oil, which was outlawed by the City of New York in 2011 and which owners will have to phase out over the coming years.
3. An index created by University Neighborhood Housing Program to identify multifamily buildings in physical and/or financial distress. Each building is assigned a composite score based on housing and building code violations, liens, and other building information to indicate overall level of distress.
4. Passed in 2009, as part of the Greener, Greater Buildings Plan, Local Law 84 (LL84), requires owners of buildings with greater than 50,000 gross square feet to annually measure their energy and water consumption in a process called *benchmarking*.
5. Also part of the Greener, Greater Buildings Plan, Local Law 87 (LL87) mandates that buildings of greater than 50,000 gross square feet undergo periodic analyses of their energy use and ensure correct equipment installation and performance.

multisector collaboration across the country are embracing and operationalizing this ideal in formal governance models, integrated data systems, and new ways of working together with powerful new information. A growing number of those communities are members of All In, where we add to the saying, "And if you want a better roadmap, go with us."

## HOW TO JOIN THE ALL IN COMMUNITY

All In is a learning community that shares experience, methods, advice, and tools. Community practitioners across the country contribute to and benefit from sharing their challenges and solutions.

The first step is to get in touch: http://www.allindata.org/get-involved/. There you can learn about the following resources:

> *Connect directly with other All In members on our online community*: https://allin.healthdoers.org/. The richest benefit of All In membership is the opportunity to connect with other members. Although each community is unique, there are people across the country who have faced similar challenges and have ideas, solutions, or support to offer. Joining the community is a great way to receive announcements about other financial and informational opportunities.

> *Webinars*: Recent webinars have showcased member accomplishments in the areas of Big Data, human-centered design, and data analytics and have featured subject matter experts in the areas of using electronic health data for public health, master person indexes, sustainability, and training and workflows for end users.

> *Affinity groups*: When there is sufficient demand, All In supports knowledge sharing through conference calls and online discussion forums. Previous affinity groups have addressed the challenges of accessing and analyzing health payer claims and encounter data, master person indexes, data visualization, and using housing data. Become a member and nominate a topic of importance to you!

> *Technical assistance*: All In hosts national and regional meetings at which members can connect with each other and with experts in the field. DASH and other partners may announce opportunities to access funding for comprehensive technical assistance for community-based multisector projects. Visit www.Allindata.org.

## ACKNOWLEDGMENTS

The authors wish to acknowledge the contributions to this chapter of Emily Yu, Executive Director of the Build Health Challenge; Jessica Solomon Fisher, Chief Innovations Officer of the Public Health National Center for Innovations at the Public Health Accreditation Board; Anna Barnes, Program Manager II at DASH; Jenna Frkovich, Communications Manager at DASH; and Melissa Moorehead, Project Manager at DASH.

## REFERENCES

1. DASH National Program Office. Early learnings from an emerging field: DASH Environmental Scan. For the Robert Wood Johnson Foundation. September 2015. http://dashconnect.org/an-emerging-field/. Accessed May 2, 2018.

2. Build Health Challenge. Build Health Mobility: Build 2.0 Awardee. http://buildhealthchallenge.org/communities/2-build-health-mobility/. Accessed May 2, 2018.

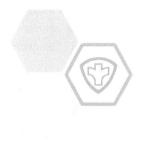

# Chapter 21

# Digital Data Exchange Between Health Care and Public Health: Lessening the Burden

JEFFREY P. ENGEL AND W. EDWARD HAMMOND

## SURVEILLANCE FOR A COMMUNITY OUTBREAK MET BY AUTOMATION

It's mid-summer in this fictional Midwestern city with a population of 250,000. The local health department environmental health unit has detected the presence of West Nile Virus (WNV) in mosquitoes collected as part of the vector-borne disease management program. Three years ago, the city experienced 25 human illnesses of WNV neuroinvasive disease with two deaths. The local health director has alerted the community and providers, and mosquito control efforts are under way.

The city is served by a single not-for-profit health care corporation that owns and operates the 150-bed acute care hospital, laboratory, and several out-patient clinics; all providers use an enterprise-wide electronic medical record (EMR) system. Electronic case and laboratory reporting from the medical record to the public health surveillance system was instituted several months ago. Since WNV neuroinvasive disease is a reportable condition, providers are confident that their reporting obligation will be met by automation. Reciprocally, the local health department will send an automated notification to providers when a WNV report is received.

## THE INFORMATION AGE HAS ARRIVED

The Information Age, also known as the Digital Age or Computer Age, was a shift in the industrialization enabled by the Industrial Age to an economy based on information technology. This transition occurred in the second half of the

20th century as a result of the advent of faster and smaller computers and the sophistication of the software that instructs them. The health industry, which accounts for more than 10% of the gross domestic product (GDP) of most developed countries, was a main driver of the Information Age, placing enormous demands on economies with its massive production of data and subsequent processing, storage, and analytic needs.

By the late 20th century, despite the data demand, not to mention the disproportionate impact on GDP in the United States, transition from the Industrial Age to the Information Age in the health industry was slow, iterative, and unorganized. Hospitals tended to lead the way with large mainframe computer systems for administrative data and for alphanumeric laboratory results, but most health records remained paper-based. In the government sector, public health agencies relied on telephonic information exchange and stand-alone data systems for vital records and population health monitoring. The expanding computer-based record keeping in both the health care and public health sectors had no data standard, hence machines could not communicate, even though the technology existed for this capability (known as *interoperability*). Many years passed in this siloed world of health information technology, the political will for change finally coming because of rising costs and quality concerns, as well as national health security.

In his January 2004 State of the Union Address, President George W. Bush outlined the President's Health Information Technology Plan to address health care quality and cost.[1] This plan had two notable initiatives: the creation of the sub-cabinet Office of the National Coordinator for Health Information Technology (ONC) and a mandate to move all health records from paper to an electronic format by 2015. The funding for the mandate came in 2009, when the US Congress passed the Health Information Technology for Economic and Clinical Health (HITECH) Act to promote and expand the use of health information technology nationwide, containing a $19.2 billion appropriation from the American Recovery and Reinvestment (Recovery) Act.[2]

While health care quality and cost were the main drivers for the health care sector, public health received its boost for modernization from the terrorist attacks of 2001. Although the September 11 attacks resulted in horrific death and destruction, it was really the anthrax attack through the US postal system in October that awakened the public health sector to its aging and obsolete information systems. Relying on paper, faxes, and telephonic exchanges, the public health surveillance enterprise encompassing local, state, and federal governments was inefficient, fragmented, and slow. The federal government response, led by the Centers for Disease Control and Prevention (CDC), lacked timely, complete, and accurate health reporting from the health care sector. Because of the threat to national health security, in 2002, Congress enacted the Public Health Security and Bioterrorism Preparedness and Response Act, and they appropriated nearly $1 billion annually to support state and local emergency preparedness and response to address bioterrorism threats.[3] A significant proportion of this funding was invested in data systems for improved public health surveillance.

Hence, facilitated by early 21st-century political exigencies and technological readiness, the US health data industry was poised by 2010 for real implementation of the Information Age. This chapter focuses on the developments that have enabled information exchange between public health and health care to advance to the level of automation. It focuses on how the computer can *lessen* the burden of the daily workflow for both sectors, resulting in efficiencies that promise to lower cost, improve quality, and strengthen health security through real-time information exchange (Box 21.1).

---

**Box 21.1 | Data Models**

Data models represent what data are required and what format is to be used. Data models include important attributes for the data element, such as name, data type, and units. Compound and complex models are represented with their relationships. An example of a data component is blood pressure that includes both systolic and diastolic pressures. Additionally, the model may include such related data elements as patient position, cuff size, arm used, and amplifying data, such as noting if readings were taken after exercise.

Data models are represented by data-modeling notation, which is often presented in the graphical format. Their focus is to support and aid information systems by showing the format and definition of the different data involved. There are three basic styles of data model, and, in most cases, all three are used for a project. The three styles are:

- Conceptual data models
- Physical data models
- Logical data models

Data models provide a framework for data to be used within information systems by providing explicit definitions and format. If a data model is used consistently across systems, then compatibility of data can be achieved. If the same data structures are used to store and access data, then different applications can share data seamlessly. Systems and interfaces are expensive to build, operate, and maintain. They may also constrain the business rather than support it. This may occur when the quality of the data models implemented is poor.

A *common data model* (CDM) permits the exchange of data among heterogeneous sites with unambiguous understanding. The problem is that there are many CDMs from which to choose. The Common Information Modeling Initiative (CIMI) is a Health Level 7 International (HL7) activity that has ties to another important HL7 standard, the Fast Healthcare Interoperability Resource (FHIR) that is discussed in Box 21.2. Other popular models include i2b2, the

---

Observational Health Data Sciences and Informatics (OHDSI), the OMOP CDM, Sentinel, PCORnet CDM, ONC US Core Meaningful Use CDM, and many others.

The Clinical Data Interchange Standards Consortium (CDISC) has a group of standards that support a CDM and data exchange for clinical research.

- *Study Data Tabulation Model (SDTM)*: A standard for organizing and formatting data for collection, management, analysis, and reporting for clinical research. SDTM is one of the required standards for data submission to the US Food and Drug Administration (FDA).
- *Clinical Data Acquisition Standard Harmonization (CDASH)*: CDASH defines a standard way to collect data in a similar way across studies and sponsors so that data collection formats and structures provide clear traceability of submission data into the Study Data Tabulation Model (SDTM).
- *Analysis Data Model (ADaM)*: ADaM specifies the principles and standards to follow in the creation of analysis datasets and associated metadata.

The National Library of Medicine Value Set Authority Center (VSAC) is a repository and authoring tool for public value sets created by external programs. *Value sets* are lists of codes and corresponding terms from NLM-hosted standard clinical vocabularies (such as SNOMED CT, RxNorm, LOINC, and others) that define clinical concepts to support effective and interoperable sharing of data.

The Object Management Group has created a set of standards that would be of interest to this community as well. These standards are:

- Business Process Maturity Model (BPMM)
- Case Management and Notation (CMMN)
- Decision Model and Notation (DMN)

## MEANINGFUL USE OF ELECTRONIC HEALTH RECORDS

The HITECH and Recovery Acts authorized the Centers for Medicare and Medicaid Services (CMS) to develop and manage a certification procedure for electronic health records (EHRs) used by eligible health care professionals and hospitals and created lawful financial incentives to those who implemented certified EHRs for meaningful use (MU).[4] MU is using certified EHR technology to improve health care quality and cost through care coordination of an individual and for population and public health monitoring and surveillance. Here, *population health* refers to how an eligible professional or hospital performs for a clinical quality measure for the population of patients served. (For example, a population health MU for hypertension would be the ability of the EHR to track the proportion of patients in a practice with hypertension whose blood pressure is controlled.) By comparison, public health refers to the population of a jurisdiction and how data from a certified EHR contributes to surveillance activities conducted by government public health agencies. (For example, a public health MU is the ability of the EHR to transmit childhood vaccine administration data to a state immunization registry.) The use of certified EHR technology for electronic exchange of health information between health care and public health is the critical component of MU discussed here.

## ELECTRONIC CASE AND LABORATORY REPORTING

The two MU cases discussed here are electronic laboratory reporting (ELR) and electronic case reporting (ECR), chosen because they are excellent examples of using data standards for information exchange, interoperability, and automation. Both are based on states' legal requirements for laboratories, hospitals, and licensed providers to report to public health agencies certain conditions that pose a public health threat because of communicability or environmental exposure. Although the list of conditions is long (at least 74 using the Nationally Notifiable Condition List[5]), this regulatory feature of public health is central to the government's role in health security and is the foundational backbone of the authority of a public health agency. The disease-reporting mandate is an important incentive for the health care sector to implement ELR and ECR into their office workflow and EHR certification because it will lessen the burden of current telephonic or paper-based exchanges.

Automating a WNV case report utilizing ECR and ELR can be accomplished by originating an electronic initial case report using standardized names and codes that correspond to nationally accepted case definition narratives. Since WNV neuroinvasive disease is reportable, a provider might suspect the diagnosis in a patient presenting with fever, headache, encephalopathy, or neuropathy during the typical summer season when mosquito activity is high and WNV transmission peaks. The provider would enter the diagnosis in the EHR diagnosis field (International Classification of Diseases, 10th Revision, Clinical Modification [ICD-10-CM]), order laboratory tests by code (Logical Observation Identifiers Names and Codes [LOINC]), and receive results from laboratory testing (Standardized Nomenclature of Medicine Clinical Terms or [SNOMED CT]).

For ECR and ELR to work, an updated list of ICD-10-CM, LOINC, and SNOMED CT codes must reside within the EHR and laboratory information management system (LIMS); these codes can be compared using algorithms in real time to data elements entered in the EHR and LIMS. Hence, for WNV, codified entries such as "rule out WNV encephalitis" or "serologic blood test order for acute WNV infection" would trigger an initial case report to public health. The system must also be bidirectional and must report back to the EHR the fate of the initial case report, notifying the provider that the case did or did not meet criteria for reporting (Box 21.2). (Of note, ELR has been in place for many years, and ECR is under development, but an ELR report from a LIMS

## Box 21.2 | Data Transport and Exchange

A number of standards-developing organizations (SDO) have created data exchange standards. Health Level 7 International (HL7), created in 1987, is a leader in the field and has created a continuing progression of standards. The first standard for the exchange of data is known as v2.n; the current version is v2.8. More than 95% of hospitals and clinics use HL7 v2 today. The most commonly used version is v2.5.1. A second HL7 standard in wide use today is based on the v3 model-based standard and is known as the Clinical Data Architecture (CDA). An Implementation Guide based on this standard is in wide use to transfer Patient Summary data. This standard is known as the Continuity of Care Document (CCD). CDA is a popular, flexible markup standard developed by HL7 that defines the structure of certain medical records, such as discharge summaries and progress notes, as a way to better exchange this information between providers and patients. The Consolidated CDA is required by the Office of the National Coordinator for Health Information Technology (ONC) for Meaningful Use—Phase 2.

The most recent HL7 data transfer standard is called the Fast Healthcare Interoperability Resource (FHIR) standard. It is a web-based standard and uses the REpresentational State Transfer (REST). REST is an architectural style that defines a set of constraints and properties based on HTTP. Web services that conform to the REST architectural style, or RESTful web services, provide interoperability between computer systems on the Internet. Facebook, Google, and others use this standard. RESTful systems typically communicate over HTTP verbs (Create/Post, Read/Get, Update, and Delete). FHIR provides interoperability between computer systems over the Internet.

FHIR is built on logical, related compound structures called *resources*. Resources consist of small logically discrete units of exchange with defined behavior and meaning. Resources have a known identity and location identified by a Universal Resource Identifier (URI). All exchangeable content is defined as a resource. There are more than 150 different resources that are intended to cover 80% of health care. Examples include Patient, Practitioner, Family History, Care Plan, and Allergy Intolerance. Resources are defined using XML, JSON, or RDF. The core resources reside in a repository that is open and free for all to use.

Resources are combined into groups called *profiles* to identify packages of data to address clinical and administrative needs. Parties exchanging data define the specific way they want to use resources and their relations using profiles. FHIR is service-driven. Profiles define what a particular application needs to communicate based on resources and *extensions* (self-defined data elements that are not part of the core set). Only data that are required for specific purposes are sent. Profiles are used to constrain resources—that is, to define specifically what data is to be sent. Examples of profiles are those used for referral of a patient, for populating registries, for adverse event reporting, for ordering a medication, and for providing data to a clinical decision support algorithm, such as a risk assessment calculation.

to a public health agency contains very little information, often just the patient and provider identification and the lab order and/or the laboratory result, necessitating time-consuming follow-up by public health.)

## INNOVATION: THE DIGITAL BRIDGE APPROACH

Achieving automation of bidirectional information exchange between public health and health care for a WNV case requires more adjudication than is provided by the EHR-triggered initial case report. A single national solution required the vision and innovation of a public–private partnership of private funders and business consultants, government public health and related nonprofit organizations, health care, and the commercial EHR vendor communities. The Digital Bridge project emerged from these partners to establish a mechanism for a unique, single ECR solution using data standards and the innovative decision support intermediary (DSI) between public health and health care.[6]

The DSI is simply a software application running on a platform that can consume an initial case report from an EHR, determine if it matches reportability requirements for a jurisdiction, deliver a reportability response back to the EHR (and thus to the provider), and send the case to public health if criteria are met. The software, known as the *reportable condition knowledge management system* (RCKMS), developed by the Council of State Territorial Epidemiologists (CSTE) and the CDC, uses standardized codes and logic derived from narrative case definitions, and it has an interface that allows jurisdictions to author RCKMS to align with their unique reporting laws and rules.[7] The platform was developed by the Association of Public Health Laboratories (APHL), known as the APHL Informatics Messaging Services (AIMS). It is a secure, cloud-based environment that accelerates the implementation of public health messaging solutions by providing shared services to aid in the transport, validation, translation, and routing of electronic data.[8] The use of the DSI with existing local and regional health information exchanges is also being explored.

## CHALLENGES AND FUTURE DIRECTIONS

This chapter has sought to provide an overview of automated data exchange between public health and health care, highlighting ECR and ELR use cases and how health data are standardized and messaged. The WNV example demonstrates how health data can be used to lessen the burden of mandated disease reporting for health care and improve the timeliness, completeness, and accuracy of surveillance for public health. The Digital Bridge project was introduced as a national single and scalable solution emphasizing the importance of the public–private partnership.

Challenges facing the Digital Bridge approach include ensuring ongoing investments in all sectors for automation and data exchange, especially information technology infrastructure maintenance and a prepared workforce of engineers, epidemiologists, and data scientists (Figure 21.1). Significant investments have been made in the public health sector to improve surveillance

**Figure 21.1** ▼

The *Digital Bridge* approach to automated data exchange.

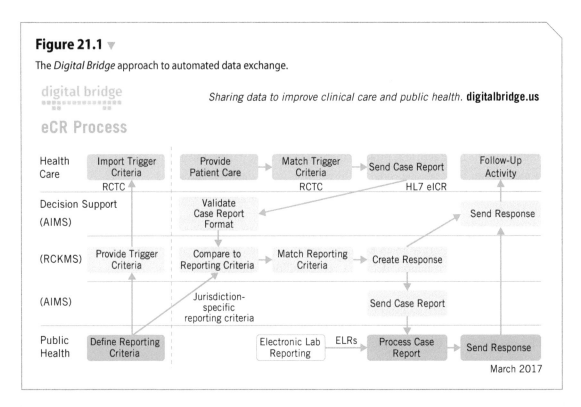

and health security from the lessons learned from bioterrorism and emerging infectious diseases (such as WNV). Health care continues to invest in more efficient and safer delivery of care addressing quality, safety, and cost. MU of the certified EHR is an incentive to providers and can be leveraged by government public health agencies.

Challenges will always exist around data security and the privacy of protected health information. The Digital Bridge and similar health exchanges build in compliance with the Health Insurance Portability and Accountability Act (HIPAA) using legal instruments such as business associate and data use agreements, as well as technical firewalls in the cloud environment. However, the Robert Wood Johnson Foundation, main funder of the Digital Bridge, has said it best in its "Better Data for Better Health" collection: "Data moves at the speed of trust."[9] Ultimately, exchange of health data will succeed when a community works together to improve health care and security in the Information Age. Key examples of this work include data exchange between healthcare and public health that work inside of HIPAA requirements. (Boxes 21.3 through 21.4). One source of data that public health has to offer is survey based data found in the Behavioral Risk Factor Surveillance System, which the 500 Cities Project is modeling to help government agencies, communities, and all partners to identify and work on emerging health issues (Box 21.5).

---

**Box 21.3 | Use Case 2: Where Are Housing Conditions Triggering Childhood Asthma?**

*Joshua Sharfstein*

*Purpose.* Research has shown that ambient conditions and hazards at home—including mold, cockroaches, mouse urine, and other allergens—can trigger asthma attacks.[1] Moreover, housing interventions can reduce the severity of asthma among children at risk.[2] The county health department is interested in identifying specific residential blocks in the county with high burdens of childhood asthma to assess environmental conditions and consider a range of potential interventions.

*Data request.* The health department requests a regular data file from each area hospital with information about county residents younger than 21 years diagnosed with asthma during an emergency department (ED) visit or hospital admission. For each ED visit and hospital admission for asthma, the data file should include the following fields: specific street address, date, age in years, gender, and race/ethnicity. The data file should not include name, social security number, or other demographic information. The health department asks that hospitals provide this data file at least weekly with a lag of 2 weeks or less.

*Plan for data use.* The health department will combine and analyze the data on a weekly basis to identify specific geographic areas of highest risk.

Once identified, the health department will assess the external air quality in the vicinity and offer the services of environmental inspectors to assess home hazards to all in the area. The services provided will not involve releasing specific health care data publicly.

As the need for services is identified, the health department will coordinate with the housing authority and other agencies to arrange for the remediation of hazards. This may include community-based rodent control programs, promotion of the tobacco quitline, small home repairs, and access to legal aid for renters to obtain corrective action by landlords. The health department will not disclose any personally identifying medical information to other public sector departments involved in remediation efforts.

The health department will also use geocoded data to construct a "heat map" of areas with high asthma burden in the city. This map will allow the health department to monitor whether and how areas of highest asthma burden change over time. The construction of a heat map will also be instrumental for the health department in determining where to deploy neighborhood-based services, such as environmental monitoring. The heat map will be maintained by the health department and will not be released in a way that permits identification of any geographic areas with fewer than 10 cases because the health department has concluded that this would preclude identification of any individual.

*Health Insurance Portability and Accountability Act (HIPAA) analysis.* As explained later, the health department's plan to combine and analyze patient data, including specific street addresses, on a weekly basis to identify specific geographic areas of highest risk is permissible under HIPAA. It would be legal for the hospitals to share the requested data for this purpose.

In this use case, the health department has clearly articulated a need for health information, including geographic data, related to a public health activity—assessment of home hazards related to asthma and the provision of remedial services to address health risks. This clear articulation gives the health department the legal authority to request and receive protected health information from local hospitals and health care providers under HIPAA.

The health department has carefully described the data elements that are necessary for fulfilling the public health activity. It also carefully limits the data elements to only those that are necessary to fulfill the public health activity. This careful inventory of data elements meets the HIPAA minimum necessary requirement and allows hospitals or health providers to voluntarily share the requested information with the health department.

The health department may maintain and use the identifiable health data collected from hospitals and health care providers for the internal home hazard program. The health department may also release necessary information to the housing authority and other agencies to arrange for the remediation of hazards in furtherance of the health department's public health activity. In this case, the health department is not disclosing information to other agencies about the health of an individual, and, therefore, these disclosures do not fall under HIPAA regulation.

*Additional applications.* Using electronic health data to find hot spots of illnesses can have positive benefits for health conditions beyond asthma.[3] For example, a health department can map concentrations of opioid overdoses to conduct outreach to specific parts of the city to provide naloxone and access to effective addiction treatment. In Baltimore, the health department is using electronic health data to develop maps of older adults suffering from serious falls; the goal of the city's B'FRIEND initiative.

**References**

1. Matsui EC. Environmental control for asthma: Recent evidence. *Curr Opin Allergy Clin Immunol.* 2013;13(4):417–25.
2. Krieger J, Jacobs DE, Ashley PJ, et al. Housing interventions and control of asthma-related indoor biologic agents: A review of the evidence. *J Public Health Manag Pract.* 2010;16(5 Suppl):S11–20.
3. Comer KF, Grannis S, Dixon BE, Bodenhamer DJ, Wiehe SE. Incorporating geospatial capacity within clinical data systems to address social determinants of health. *Public Health Rep.* 2011;126(Suppl 3):54–61.

**Box 21.4 | Use Case 3: Would You Like a Home Visit?**

*Joshua Sharfstein*

*Purpose.* Health departments often run programs to improve the health of individuals with chronic or recurring conditions. In the case of asthma, health departments can send nurses and other professionals to the home to support families in reducing allergens and in properly monitoring and managing a child's asthma.[1] The health department is interested in identifying children with severe asthma who could benefit from evidence-based services at home.

*Data request.* The health department requests a regular data file from each area hospital with identifying information for all individuals younger than 21 years admitted to the hospital with a discharge diagnosis of asthma. For each hospital admission for asthma, the data file should include the following fields: name, date, date of birth, address, phone number, gender, and race/ethnicity. The file should not include social security number or other demographic information. The health department asks that hospitals provide this data file at least weekly, with a lag of 2 weeks or less.

*Plan for data use.* The health department will combine these data to develop a registry of children admitted to the hospital for asthma. Those most frequently admitted will be contacted by the health department and offered home visits and care coordination. The health department will work with other city agencies to address housing conditions.

*Health Insurance Portability and Accountability Act (HIPAA) Analysis.* The health department's plan to combine and analyze patient data, including names and specific street addresses, on a weekly basis to identify specific children for the registry of those admitted for asthma is permissible under HIPAA. It would be legal for the hospitals to share the requested data for this purpose.

In this use case, the health department has clearly articulated a need for health information, including identifiable demographic data, related to a public health activity—reaching out to offer important health services to children and families. This clear articulation gives the health department the legal authority to request and receive protected health information from local hospitals and health care providers under HIPAA.

The health department has carefully described the data elements that are necessary for fulfilling the public health activity. It also carefully limits the data elements to only those that are necessary to fulfill the public health activity. This careful inventory of data elements meets the HIPAA minimum necessary requirement and allows hospitals or health providers to voluntarily share the requested information with the health department.

The health department may use the information collected to reach out and contact the families to offer them home-based services. Then, consistent with HIPAA, the health department may use this information to support the provision of home-based services with the consent of the families.

*Additional applications.* Health departments can offer different types of support to high-risk individuals with a range of medical conditions. For example, a health department can use electronic health data to identify individuals who suffer from nonfatal overdoses to offer peer support and referral to addiction treatment.[2] A health department can develop a program for high utilizers of emergency department care or individuals suffering from preventable complications of chronic illnesses. Finding candidates for these programs through electronic health data can help assure that limited resources are assisting those most in need.

### References

1. Le Cann P, Paulus H, Glorennec P, Le Bot B, Frain S, Gangneux JP. Home environmental interventions for the prevention or control of allergic and respiratory diseases: What really works. *J Allergy Clin Immunol Pract.* 2016;pii:S2213–2198(16)30313-0.
2. Pollini RA, McCall L, Mehta SH, Vlahov D, Strathdee SA. Non-fatal overdose and subsequent drug treatment among injection drug users. *Drug Alcohol Depend.* 2006;83(2):104–10.

## Box 21.5 | The 500 Cities Project: Model-Based Estimates of Health Measures for 500 Cities and Census Tracts

*Yan Wang, Jennifer LeClercq, Hua Lu, James B. Holt, Janet B. Croft, and Kurt Greenlun*

Effective planning for improving the health of residents within the nation's largest cities requires high-quality, small-area data for the current health status and behavioral risk factors that influence health. Until the release of the 500 Cities data, no data were available on a large scale for cities and for small areas within cities. In 2016, the Centers for Disease Control and Prevention (CDC), in collaboration with the Robert Wood Johnson Foundation and the CDC Foundation, first released model-based estimates for a select number of chronic disease measures for the 500 largest American cities and the approximately 28,000 census tracts within these cities. Measures include 5 unhealthy behaviors, 13 health outcomes, and 9 prevention services that have a substantial impact on public health. The method of generating small-area estimation is multilevel regression and post-stratification[1] using data from the CDC's Behavioral Risk Factor Surveillance System (BRFSS). The other data sources included the Census 2010 population and the American Community Survey data. These model-based estimates show strong or good consistency with direct survey estimates at state, county, and city levels from BRFSS and other external surveys.[2,3]

The data, map books, and iterative maps are available through a public "500 Cities" website (www.cdc.gov/500Cities) that allows users to view, explore, and download city- and tract-level data. High-quality small-area estimation data from the 500 Cities Project are being used to inform the development and implementation of effective and targeted public health prevention activities, the identification of emerging health problems, and the establishment and tracking of health objectives in many American cities. In addition, government, local health departments, nonprofit organizations, academic institutions, and others have been greatly aided by using the data to make decisions, allocate funding, develop proposals, and investigate research questions of interest.

### References

1. Zhang X, Holt JB, Lu H, Wheaton AG, Ford ES, Greenlund KJ, et al. Multilevel regression and poststratification for small-area estimation of population health outcomes: A case study of chronic obstructive pulmonary disease prevalence using the Behavioral Risk Factor Surveillance System. *Am J Epidemiol* 2014;179:1025–33.
2. Zhang X, Holt JB, Yun S, Lu H, Greenlund KJ, Croft JB. Validation of multilevel regression and poststratification methodology for small area estimation of health indicators from the behavioral risk factor surveillance system. *Am J Epidemiol* 2015;182:127–37.
3. Wang Y, Holt JB, Zhang X, et al. Comparison of multilevel regression and post-stratification estimation and local survey estimates for small area chronic diseases and health behaviors: Boston validation study, 2013. *Prev Chronic Dis* 2017;14:170–281.

## REFERENCES

1. The Bush Health Information Technology Plan was started in April 27, 2004 by Executive Order. https://georgewbush-whitehouse.archives.gov/news/releases/2004/04/20040427-4.html. Accessed on 1/16/2019.

2. The American Recovery and Reinvestment Act of 2009 Act. https://www.gpo.gov/fdsys/pkg/BILLS-111hr1enr/pdf/BILLS-111hr1enr.pdfHITECH and ARRA. Accessed on 1/16/2019.

3. The Public Health Security and Bioterrorism Preparedness and Response Act. https://www.gpo.gov/fdsys/pkg/PLAW-107publ188/pdf/PLAW-107publ188.pdf. Accessed on 1/16/2019.

4. CDC. Certified eHR and meaningful use incentives. https://www.cdc.gov/ehrmeaningfuluse/introduction.html. Accessed on 1/16/2019.

5. CDC. The national notifiable conditions. https://wwwn.cdc.gov/nndss/conditions/notifiable/2017/. Accessed on 1/16/2019.

6. The Digital Bridge Project. http://www.digitalbridge.us/. Accessed on 1/16/2019.

7. CSTE. The Reportable Condition Knowledge Management System program. http://www.cste.org/members/member_engagement/groups.aspx?id=154895. Accessed on 1/16/2019.

8. APHL. The APHL Informatics Messaging Services program. https://www.aphl.org/programs/informatics/pages/aims_platform.aspx. Accessed on 1/16/2019.

9. Ross D. https://www.rwjf.org/en/library/articles-and-news/2015/04/report-highlights-publics-hopes-fears-about-using-data-to-improve-health.html. The Better Data for Better Health Collection. https://www.rwjf.org/en/library/collections/better-data-for-better-health.html. Accessed on 1/16/2019.

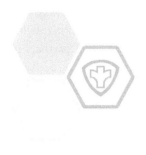

# Chapter 22

# How to Draft Successful Memorandums of Understanding and Data-Sharing Agreements

MATTHEW PENN AND RACHEL HULKOWER

With an increasing emphasis on cross-sector collaboration with Public Health 3.0,[1] working with government and community partners is becoming an integral part of public health practice at the state, tribal, local, and territorial levels. "Public health departments should engage with community stakeholders, from both the public and private sectors, to form vibrant, structured, cross-sector partnerships designed to develop and guide Public Health 3.0–style initiatives and to foster shared funding, services, governance, and collective action."[1] Cross-sector collaborations and community partners are also key elements of a Health in All Policies (HiAP) approach to public health improvements. "[T]he basic components [of HiAP] are community engagement, cross-sector collaboration, and government involvement."[2] The current attention on the role of cross-sector collaboration has encouraged new research, which has shown that communities with healthy cross-sector collaboration have better health outcomes among all of their population.[3]

Improving and increasing cross-sector collaboration in public health can be facilitated through the use of a *memorandum of understanding* (MOU). MOUs are written agreements that outline the relationship between two or more parties. MOUs describe the identity of the parties, the reasons why an agreement is necessary, a description of the parties' roles and responsibilities, and underlying assumptions about applicable laws. An MOU is a tool that can strengthen coordination between partners that have not traditionally been seen as public health collaborators, enabling stakeholders to combine resources and reduce redundant efforts to address the same public health problem.

Public Health 3.0 stresses that "public and private sectors should work together to enable more real-time and geographically granular data to be shared, linked, and synthesized to inform action while protecting data security and individual privacy."[1] But, under the limitations imposed by federal and state privacy law, such an exchange of data across sectors will often require a formalized agreement among collaborators. This tension highlights why MOUs are so important: using an MOU enables potential partners to identify similarities and differences in their priorities and goals, available resources (time, money, and expertise), project timelines, and expected outcomes prior to collaboration.

*Data use agreements* (DUAs) are a type of MOU, used when one party wants to receive and make use of data held by another party. MOUs and DUAs have many common aspects, and this chapter will use the terminology "MOU" when talking about these commonalities. The term "DUA" will be used when discussing things specific to agreements that involve data.

## BENEFITS

MOUs can play an important role in creating action-oriented and long-lasting collaborations. They are useful across all public health programs, including preparedness, injury control and prevention, immunization, and chronic diseases. They can define many activities, such as creating a stakeholder committee or workgroup, exchanging equipment and supplies, sharing data, sending personnel to work with a partner, and providing disease and injury prevention and control services. The primary benefit of an MOU is to bring clarity and specificity to the parties' roles and responsibilities. MOUs answer the question "Who is going to do what?" MOUs also offer an opportunity to create a common language among parties that will help avoid miscommunications and minimize the risk of missteps throughout the collaboration. This is especially true given the increasing complexity of community partnerships and work on the social determinants of health. MOUs can help partners clearly articulate their expectations for the division of shared work.

This leads to another benefit of MOUs: they are made with organizations, not individuals. As a result, these agreements can elevate individual ideas—something that may have started as an idea shared between colleagues at a conference—to the level of institutional policy. The named parties are the organizations; consequently, the agreements become an organizational responsibility that can last longer than the tenure of a particular staff person, even the person who initiated the agreement.

MOUs also provide a process through which community relationships can be built and maintained. The MOU is the documentation of what the parties have agreed to after the parties have each proposed, discussed, and negotiated the details of their ideas. This leads to increased communication through emails, calls, and meetings, and, in the process, the parties get to know each other and their values, missions, leadership, and capacities. Also, as will be discussed in more detail later, MOUs have a life span, so the parties must occasionally come back together and go through the process to renew agreements and work together with each other again.

## DRAWBACKS

One potential drawback of MOUs is that a good one takes time to create. Creating an MOU requires a time commitment internally and externally. One of the most important considerations when creating a good MOU or DUA is defining your organization's goals and capacity for participating in the partnership. You and your team must go through your own process of outlining what it is you need from the partnership, and this can take time. It's also a good idea to involve leadership and legal counsel early. Although beneficial, more people can increase the preparation time needed to get a draft MOU ready to share. Once you're ready to involve your prospective partner organization, the emails, calls, and meetings that allow partners to get to know each other also take time. The negotiations are time well spent, but it must be factored into project timelines so as not to impede overall progress.

MOUs can also expose weaknesses in a request or a partnership. You may have a programmatic idea that is unrealistic, exceeds the public entity's legal authority, or is too far ahead of the community. For example, your organization may want to organize a stakeholder workgroup and data-sharing arrangement around better utilizing the regional health information exchange while your partners, local health care providers, are just getting accustomed to their electronic health record (EHR) systems. In this circumstance, it is unlikely that the local health care providers have the capacity or the expertise necessary for collaboration at a regional level. Or, your organization may be asking something of a partner that they do not have the capacity or the authority to do. For example, your organization might believe that release of certain data fields are necessary for new behavioral health initiatives in the community, but then you may learn that federal, state, tribal, or local laws prevent the release of this type of data. Also, a public health department may be simply asking the wrong partner for the wrong thing. Finally, MOU negotiations may also expose other reasons that the two entities cannot enter into an agreement that are unrelated to the common purpose for engaging in the MOU process. For example, other jurisdictions and organizations may be prohibited by law from complying with indemnity or insurance requirements that you may have. Though these limitations may exist independent of the MOU, the negotiation process can bring them into the open.

## SUCCESSFUL MOUS

Before dissecting MOUs and exploring how they are put together, there are a couple of overall considerations to keep in mind. First, the process of drafting

MOUs does not start with the law. MOUs are grounded in contract law, and most will address some legal issues, but the core of these arrangements begins with what the parties want from each other. The process of developing a successful MOU is best when it begins at the planning level rather than an assessment of what law may or may not apply. If your organization goes to a lawyer at the beginning of the project, the lawyer is going to start by asking questions about what it is you are trying to achieve with this agreement.

The second consideration to remember is that the creation of MOUs is a largely collaborative process. The first drafts of MOUs are rarely the final versions, and partners should remain flexible to requested changes from the parties. In fact, even after an agreement is executed, many MOUs allow for future amendments to the agreement to best meet the goals of the engagement.

## PARTIES

An MOU includes a description of each partner agency or entity engaged in the agreement. A description of the parties may be as simple as listing the name of each organization agreeing to the terms of the MOU ("The New York City Department of Health and Mental Hygiene and [NAME] Health Care Facility"). As noted earlier, the parties to MOUs are organizations, not individuals.

One of the most important things to keep in mind is that finding the right party for your MOU is an integral part of the planning process. One of the best ways to identify the appropriate party is to start the MOU-building process by considering the intended purpose of the agreement, the scope of needed services, and the roles and responsibilities of each party. This is especially true with DUAs. Having a good sense of the data that you would like to obtain (or release) will help you to identify the parties to approach and begin negotiating with, and having a thorough data plan may be crucial to moving forward (Box 22.1).

Another interesting angle to parties of DUAs is that the agreement will probably have a section that lists individuals who may access, use, release, and receive data under the agreement. The listed individuals become subject to the rules and restrictions that surround the data described in the DUA. Creation of the list should contemplate all uses of the data, including the primary purpose for the DUA and any potential secondary purposes, such as research and publication.

## PURPOSE, BACKGROUND, AND DEFINITIONS

The introductory provisions of an MOU often include a statement of purpose and background information that provides context for the agreement. This introduces the relevant subject matter and describes the relationship between the parties. It can provide justifications for the agreement or a description of a larger context in which a particular agreement may fit. A statement of the

## Box 22.1 | Data Plans and Data Use Agreements

Data have a life cycle all their own. Data are created, collected, transmitted, stored, released, used, and sometimes destroyed. The laws governing data privacy, confidentiality, and security will change as data moves along these pathways and changes hands. Having a data plan that describes the pathways that your data will follow is critical to building a successful data use agreement (DUA) because rules at any point in the pathway may affect how you plan to release and use the data subject to your DUA.

There is no single format or template for a data use plan; it could be a lengthy and narrative memo or a brief and visual logic model. Whatever the format or style, a data plan can help map the out the life cycle of the data you would like to include in your DUA. The critical parts of a data plan are the data fields, the information points, and the information pathways. A subway train ride is a good analogy: the people are the data fields, the stations are the points, and the tracks between stations are the pathways. These three aspects of data largely determine what can and cannot be done with data at any particular information point.

Creating a data plan should begin with identifying the data. There are two aspects of the data to keep in mind: the overall topic and the specific fields to be released and used. The topic of the data must be part of the plan because it will directly impact the amount of data that can be used or released; the amount of that data that the entities that can use, release, or receive; and the circumstances under which the release can occur. Some topics, such as HIV, tuberculosis, and behavioral health, may have heightened data protections. The specific data fields to be used or released are also important to include in your DUA. Certain data fields, such as name and address, may be considered highly protected personal information and may also have special rules. Specifying the data fields that parties intend to use, release, or receive can help to identify sensitive information and the rules that apply to that information. It can also facilitate discussions about how to handle them in the DUA, which might include either eliminating them or providing them special protections.

The next aspect of a data plan to consider is the information pathway. When data are released, they travel from one custodian to another. The route that data takes between custodians is an *information pathway*.[1] These pathways are different for every data release and, at a minimum, will determine what data fields can make the trip. In some circumstances, federal, state, tribal, or local laws protecting data could block an intended pathway. Data released under the rules of the Health Insurance Portability and Accountability Act (HIPAA), for example, have a different pathway when released from a health care provider to an insurance company than from that same health care provider to a law enforcement agency. Thoroughly identifying the trips your data will take can also help clear up confusion or misunderstandings about the nature of different pathways. Health data shared along a pathway between units in a health department, for example, may be seen as a permissible public health use rather than a cumbersome or impermissible release.

Finally, a data plan must consider the information points through which the data will travel. An *information point*—or *entity*—is a spot along a pathway where data are collected, secured, used, or released.[1] The activities that take place at an information point can affect a previous release and can create new and multiple subsequent pathways. Two significant considerations related to information points are *purpose* and *security*. An information point's purpose for using or releasing information could facilitate or prohibit the intended release. For example, release of personally identifying information from a housing authority to a health department may be allowed for public health purposes, such as an asthma mitigation program, but may not be releasable for other purposes. IT security is another issue to consider for each information point along the life cycle of data. At a minimum, each information point is going to transmit data, and most will also store it. The systems that transmit and store data are subject to myriad laws, and a data plan can help determine what security may be required at each information point.

### Reference

1. Association of State and Territorial Health Officers. Privacy & pandemic flu guide. 2007. http://www.astho.org/pubs/Privacyandpanfluguide1.pdf. Last accessed on 1/16/2019.

purpose of the agreement and a description of intended outcomes may be helpful for interpreting other sections of the agreement. For example, if the larger context of an MOU involved tribal, state, or federal grants that required community partnerships for the dispersal of funds or to complete required activities, the purpose could include a description of the public health burden that the MOU is intended to address. Alternatively, the purpose section could describe the goals of the partnership: "The purpose of this Agreement is to facilitate sharing of public health related data, both individually identified and population-related, between Parties for the purpose, and no additional purpose, of preventing, detecting, or responding to a public health event, thus assuring prompt and effective identification of infectious disease and other agents that could affect public health, and to prevent further spread of disease."[4]

This background information section may also include a recitation of the relevant federal, state, tribal, local, and territorial laws. This background information section is often called the "whereas" section, because it contains language such as: "WHEREAS, the MDCH is a Public Health Authority, as defined by the HIPAA Privacy Rule, which is authorized by the Public Health Code to collect or receive protected health information for the purpose of preventing or controlling disease, injury, or disability, and to conduct public health surveillance, public health investigations, and public health interventions. MCL

333.2221, 45 CFR 164.512(b)(1)(i)." Reference to legal authorities that enable the parties to enter into an agreement can help with later interpretations. For example, citations to laws that authorize data sharing, as in the preceding quote, could help mitigate later allegations of an improper release, use, or breach under implementation of a DUA.

Definitions can also help set the context of an MOU, bring clarity to the language used, and facilitate later interpretations. Parties can define some of their own terms. The parties may use some terms in a unique way in an MOU, and this specificity should be captured in a definition: "Health data: Written, electronic, oral, telephone, or visual information, identifiable or population based, that relates to an individual's or population's past, present, or future physical or mental health status, condition, treatment, service or products purchased and includes, but is not limited to, laboratory test data or samples."[4] Federal, state, or tribal laws may define some terms used, and the parties could expressly repeat those definitions or incorporate the legal provision by reference: "'Protected health information' as used in this DUA shall have the same definition found in 45 C.F.R Part 164.501." Regardless of how definitions are incorporated, they can be a critical part of an MOU between governmental and other community partners because definitions serve as the foundation for what is expected of partners.

By describing the purpose and background, as well as definitions for the agreement, the parties can set parameters around the agreement that help all involved entities to understand the scope of activities that will take place. This can be especially important during negotiations as a draft agreement works its way through leadership approval. Many people within a partner organization may have to read, review, and approve an agreement, although they may not have been involved with the creation of the agreement. Careful work on these sections has the potential to lead to a better understanding of the agreement, which could set the stage for a seamless approval process.

## SCOPE OF SERVICES

The scope of services section is the heart of an MOU. This section provides the space to describe the roles and responsibilities of each party. The scope of services also represents the best starting point for the creation of the agreement. This section will answer many important questions for the agreement and the partnership, including what each party will do, how they will achieve those activities, and when they must be done. The scope of services section should be action-oriented, specific, clear, and concise.

Presumably, the purpose of the MOU partnership is for the parties to complete a series of action-oriented items aimed at achieving a larger goal. Within that context, the scope of services section lists the tasks the parties are responsible for completing. Often these tasks are reciprocal, exchanged promises that form the backbone of the agreement. These commitments make MOUs largely "self-executing," as opposed to contracts that a party would seek to enforce in a court. For example, a health department may enter into an MOU with a local baby supply store to provide messaging about the correct installation of child safety seats. As part of the MOU, the health department may have the task of supplying point-of-sale messaging to the store, and the store agrees to hand out the messaging to each buyer. Enforcing such an agreement in a court would be expensive and time-consuming. However, the tasks self-execute: If the health department does not provide the materials, the store does not have anything to hand out, and the commitment does not attach.

The scope of services section must also be as specific as foresight will allow. Primarily, the MOU is the reference that the parties will consult when discussing implementation of the agreement. These discussions could occur well after the creation of the partnership, when memories of those negotiations have faded. Using specificity in drafting the scope of services section helps preserve the original intent and define the tasks each partner needs to complete. For example, many MOUs ask each partner to designate a point of contact for their organization. A generally worded provision, for example, "The Health Department shall appoint a point of contact for purposes of executing the agreement," is far less useful than a provision that actually lists the point-of-contact's identity, position, and contact information. Specificity in the scope of services section allows the parties to pinpoint the expectations each has about the who, what, where, when, and how of the agreement.

DUAs have a special circumstance that requires specificity: the data to be released and used. Public health data are granular and complex, and unless a party is granting a partner ongoing and unfettered access to an entire database, the agreement must be specific about content, transfer and storage, permitted uses, and the life cycle of the data. First, the content of the data to be released must be defined. Data definitions should include details, such as type, source, file-naming conventions, fieldname, data type, format, maximum character lengths, and narrative descriptions of each data field. The agreement can lay these details out in a bulleted list or format them into a table. However they are organized, these details are important for several reasons. Specific details allow the party holding the data to determine if the data can be released. Health data are surrounded by privacy, confidentiality, and security requirements. But, as is often said, the devil is in the details. A law or agency policy that applies to one type of data field may not apply in the same way to another. The releasing party can make these decisions only if the agreement specifies what data the partner would like to obtain. Specificity helps the receiving party to determine whether the data to be released will enable it to fulfill the intended purpose of the partnership. The data set may fit the needs of the partnership, or it may be lacking some data fields that are necessary for the intended use. Specificity in describing the content of the data allows for negotiation about intent and expectations.

Data transfer and storage are other important issues to consider in DUAs. Public health data are sensitive and may be personally identifiable, and how data are transferred, stored, and secured are critical issues to address in the creation of a DUA. Transfer and storage are information technology (IT) security issues, and the details can make the difference between a DUA that works and one that does not. For example, a health department may want to release community-level data to a nonprofit partner for disease or injury control purposes. However, if the nonprofit cannot match the health department's encrypted security requirements to receive and store the data, the parties may not be able to exchange the data without violating privacy laws. Unless the technology details are specified in the DUA, the parties may not be able to discuss, negotiate, and mitigate that risk. Open discussion of the transfer and storage details could lead the nonprofit to request IT hardware and software support from the health department to increase its capacity to assist with the public health work. These dynamics can also play in the other direction. For example, the purpose of a DUA might be to facilitate the creation of a regional syndromic surveillance network. With the network, health care facilities would send real-time symptom data to the health department. Upon review of a first draft, some heath care facilities may discover that their EHR system does not support the data transfer functions needed for the program and might then express a need for IT hardware capacity that will allow them to collect and transfer the data to the health department. The specifics of the syndromic surveillance data transfer and storage could lead to an amended DUA, in which the health department agrees to provide hardware support or recruit an additional community partner to the surveillance initiative to provide the needed capacity.

The proposed uses of data after release can affect the ability of health departments and other community partners to release data. Data have primary uses where they are created, saved, and stored for particular activities. A health care provider, for example, may record a patient's clinical test results in an EHR system for the primary purpose of diagnosing and treating that patient's ailments. Data also have secondary and tertiary uses, where the original raw data are used a second or third time for new activities, possibly released to an outside entity or to a partner and put to still further uses. The information contained in the patient's EHR may be transmitted to the local health department so that the health department can monitor disease prevalence or antimicrobial resistance of an organism within the local population (Box 22.2). State and federal laws and internal agency policies can significantly affect the data that government agencies and health care facilities can release.[5] The uses of the data should be spelled out in the scope of services for a DUA. For example, "The Health Department shall make available to Community Partner data from the immunization information system in the form of a Limited Data Set, to be used by Community Partner solely for purposes of the Get the Shot vaccination

## Box 22.2 | Use Case 4: Don't Forget to Check the Asthma Care Plan

*Joshua Sharfstein*

*Purpose.* Many children with asthma return time and again to the emergency department (ED) because they lack a consistent source of primary care.[1] It is difficult for families to follow asthma care plans when each visit brings about a new set of instructions. To address this problem, a health department might be interested in developing a tool to flag patients at highest risk and alert clinicians at the moment of care about the existence of care plans and the need for greater coordination.

The health department is interested in alerting EDs when children with severe asthma are present so that clinicians can check the asthma care plan and understand specific patient needs.

*Data request.* The health department requests that the hospital permit the local health information exchange to match, in real time, the Admission, Discharge, and Transfer (ADT) message created at the start of every ED visit with a list of children with asthma care plans and then alert both the hospital and the health department when a child with a care plan is seen in the hospital. The ADT message includes patient name, date of birth, and address, as well as chief complaint and insurance information.

*Plan for data use.* The health department will maintain a registry of children with severe asthma (following Use Case 3), which will be linked to an application containing a care management plan for each child. The health information exchange (HIE) will cross-check the ADT against the registry through an automated electronic process to identify a positive match. When there is a match, the HIE will send the ED an alert that will make the child's asthma care plan accessible to the clinician, and it will send the health department an alert to update the care plan. The health department will only receive the alert from the HIE for children in the registry.

*Health Insurance Portability and Accountability Act (HIPAA) analysis.* As explained in the following text, the health department's request is permissible under HIPAA. It would be legal for the hospitals to share the requested data for this purpose.

In this use case, the health department has clearly articulated a need for hospitals to permit the HIE, which has access to ADT feeds for clinical care, to make a match. (This exchange would need to be covered by a data-sharing or other relevant agreement.) The match both provides clinicians with access to a patient's asthma care plan to ensure proper treatment and coordination of care and allows the health department to track the needs of high-risk children This clear articulation gives the health department the legal authority to request and receive protected health information from local hospitals and health care providers under HIPAA.

In this case, the health department does not obtain information for patients not matched by the HIE.

The health department has carefully described the data elements that are necessary for fulfilling the public health activity. This meets the HIPAA minimum necessary requirement and allows hospitals or health providers to voluntarily share the requested information with the health department.

In this case, the health department is only sharing information back to a hospital for treatment purposes, which is a permitted disclosure under HIPAA. The health department is making no further disclosures that might implicate restrictions under HIPAA.[2] (There are other mechanisms for this match to take place besides through an HIE. These include match by the hospital itself or match by the health department. If the latter, the health department could establish a business associate agreement with the hospital for this purpose.)

*Additional applications.* Health departments can use electronic health data to enhance coordinated care for patients with a variety of conditions. In Louisiana, clinicians receive alerts when patients with HIV infection in need of treatment seek episodic care. Other potential examples include efforts to assist high-risk patients with sickle cell disease, high-risk pregnancy, and risk of serious falls.[3]

### References

1. Behr JG, Diaz R, Akpinar-Elci M. Health service utilization and poor health reporting in asthma patients. *Int J Environ Res Public Health*. 2016;13(7):pii:E645.
2. Herwehe J, et al. Implementation of an innovative, integrated electronic medical record (EMR) and public health information exchange for HIV/AIDS. *J Am Med Inform Assoc*. 2012;19(3):448–52.
3. Ahmed L, Jensen D, Klotzbach L, et al. Technology-enabled transitions of care in a collaborative effort between clinical medicine and public health: A population health case report. March 31, 2016. National Academy of Medicine. https://nam.edu/wp-content/uploads/2016/03/Technology-Enabled-Transitions-of-Care-in-a-Collaborative-Effort-between-Clinical-Medicine-and-Public-Health.pdf. Accessed July 10, 2017.

awareness campaign." The party releasing the data may use the DUA to prohibit the recipient from using or further disclosing the information outside of the uses described in the agreement: "Any other uses of the Data are strictly prohibited." Because DUAs are generally self-executing agreements, an express prohibition of additional uses could trigger an "enforcement" provision that would terminate the agreement and require the partner that received the data to destroy or return all remaining data and stop all agreement-related activities.

As discussed earlier, health care and public health data have "life cycles" or time periods between their creation and when they are permitted or required to be destroyed. In fact, all states have laws that govern the retention and destruction of government and health care records and the data contained in those records. As an organization begins to create a DUA for the structured release of data it holds or wants to obtain, it may intend for the released data to end its life once the parties achieve the purposes of the DUA. This life cycle should be specifically defined with the scope of services. For example, a health department may use DUAs to release public health data for research purposes. The DUA would allow researchers to analyze the data and publish their results. At the same time, the DUA could require the researchers to destroy or return the data once the research project is completed.

## TERMS AND CONDITIONS

MOUs can contain an almost unlimited variety of terms and conditions. To a large extent, these terms and conditions have little to nothing to do with the subject of the agreement and are, instead, standard contract language. They will not vary as much as the topics of the agreements vary. As a result, organizations will often write the same terms and conditions provisions into all of their MOUs. This repetition of provisions across agreements is often called "boilerplate." Terms and conditions provisions tend to fall into two different categories: (1) provisions that govern the underlying mechanics of the agreement and (2) provisions required by federal, state, tribal, local, or territorial laws or policies.

Provisions that govern the underlying mechanics of an MOU first include the effective dates of the agreement that determine when and how parties may or must begin the agreed-upon activities and when the agreement ends. The "effective date" of many preparedness agreements is framed by an emergency or public health emergency declaration, and they are only exercised when a governor or other chief executive of a jurisdiction issues a declaration: "Upon the Proclamation by the Chief Executive of the Tribe that an emergency situation has descended upon the nation, this agreement shall become effective."

A second underlying mechanism of agreements is termination. A provision could contain a list of conditions under which a party may terminate or withdraw from the agreement. For example, preparedness agreements may terminate with the end of an emergency declaration.

Third, the parties may want to allow for future amendments to be made to the agreement once the collaboration begins and the reality of what can be accomplished under the terms of the agreement are realized. Thus MOUs often include a description of the methods for amending the agreement: "This MOU may be amended by agreement of all parties." Or, "Amendments to this agreement may be made by simple majority vote of the parties and will take effect immediately upon passage."[4]

One term that is unique to DUAs is "breach procedures." A breach occurs when unsecured data provided to a DUA party under certain conditions are released to an individual or entity not authorized under the DUA. Such a breach would violate the DUA and may violate applicable tribal, state, or federal laws. DUAs should be drafted to anticipate breaches, to describe the parties' expectations about how a breach will be handled, and to establish what the consequences of the breach will be. The core aspect of a breach provision should be what constitutes a breach and what process the breaching party should follow. A breach should be specifically defined. For example, "A data breach under the terms of this DUA occurs when an individual or an entity not listed under the Authorized Users section receives and is able to access data defined under the DUA." The process could cover issues such as mitigating the extent of the breach, if possible; notifying the other parties' to the DUA; notifying individuals whose data are released; specifying the content of any required notices; and termination of the DUA or other consequences.

Provisions required by federal, state, tribal, local, or territorial laws or policies include many of the terms and conditions provisions found in an MOU. It is imperative that the parties drafting an agreement include legal counsel who can represent each parties' best legal interest and ensure that the agreement covers the parties' intended outcomes. For example, collaboration under an MOU can and often does result in the creation and maintenance of records containing private information about people, such as patients or research participants. Jurisdictional laws may all impact whether and for how long parties must retain records, as well as how to dispose of records when the time comes. Therefore, drafting the roles and responsibilities provisions in an MOU, and particularly when considering a data use plan and accompanying DUA, should include consideration of the records to be created during implementation and whether and for how long those records should be retained.

Another important legal issue to address in the terms and conditions is the liability, or legal responsibility, of the parties. State, tribal, and federal constitutions and tort claims acts contain provisions that affect liability for governmental and sovereign actors. Additional state, tribal, and federal laws may affect how nongovernmental parties might be held liable for their actions under the terms of an MOU. Partners can identify how they would like to address their liability within the provisions of an MOU. For example, the MOU provisions can indemnify a party to exempt it from liability or provide compensation in the event that a party is sued: "Each Party . . . to this Agreement expressly agrees to hold harmless, indemnify and defend the Party rendering aid and its personnel from any and all claims, demands, liability, losses, suits in law or in equity which are made by a third party."[4] It is also important to note that laws will prohibit many jurisdictions from agreeing to an indemnification or hold harmless clause. A liability provision can also be used to ensure that each party retains liability for its actions under the agreement: "Each Party to this Agreement shall be responsible for its own acts and omissions and those of its officers, employees, and agents."[4]

## CONCLUSION

Cross-sector collaboration is an increasingly critical component of the public health system. Community partnerships can involve complex arrangements, with reciprocal promises to exchange goods and services, and MOUs can help organizations negotiate, organize, and maintain those relationships. For partnerships that need health care or public health data to function, DUAs can provide a mechanism to define the data needed and the parameters around the intended release and use of the data (see Box 22.2).

### ACKNOWLEDGMENTS

The authors would like to thank Will Britt, JD, and Dawn Pepin, JD, MPH, for their review, insights, and suggestions.

### REFERENCES

1. DeSalvo KB, WangYC, Harris A, Auerbach J, Koo D, O'Carroll P. Public Health 3.0: A call to action for public health to meet the challenges of the 21st century. *Prevent Chronic Dis.* 2017;14(E78). https://doi.org/10.5888/pcd14.170017.

2. Pepin D, Winig BD, Carr D, Jacobson P. Collaborating for health: Health in all policies and the law. *J Law Med Ethics.* 2017;45(S1):60–4. doi:10.1177/10731105177033273.

3. Mays G, Mamaril CB, Timsina L. Preventable death rates fell where communities expanded population health activities through multisector networks. *Health Aff.* 2016;35(11):2005–13. doi:10.1377/hlthaff.2016.0848.

4. Stier D, Thombley M. Public health mutual aid agreements—A menu of suggested provisions. Centers for Disease Control and Prevention. 2007. https://www.cdc.gov/phlp/docs/mutual_aid_provisions.pdf. Last accessed on 1/16/2019.

5. Begley EB, Ware JM, Hexem SA, Rapposelli K, Thompson K, Penn M, Aquino GA. (2017). Personally identifiable information in state laws: Use, release, and collaboration at health departments. *Am J Public Health.* 2017;107(8):1272–6. doi:10.2105/AJPH.2017.303862.

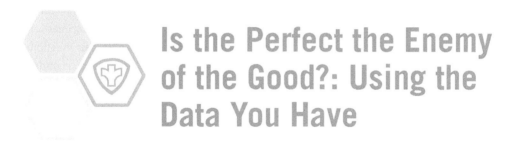

# Chapter 23

# Is the Perfect the Enemy of the Good?: Using the Data You Have

THERESA CHAPPLE-MCGRUDER, JAIME SLAUGHTER-ACEY, JENNIFER KMET, AND TONIA RUDDOCK

## DATA FOR DECISION-MAKING

To achieve its core functions—assessment, policy development, and assurance—public health relies on data. Public health professionals—practitioners, decision-makers, and researchers—utilize data to inform and drive decisions, actions, and policies. This occurs most often when undertaking public health program planning, management, and monitoring, and for creating local, statewide, or national policies that impact the population's health.[1] For example, data stemming from vital statistic records and child death review teams showed that motor vehicle accidents were the number one cause of childhood death in the United States. These data were then used to inform the public and to encourage individual behavior change around seat belt and car seat use. Additionally, data were used to advocate for state laws and federal regulations regarding child restraints. Currently, all 50 states plus Washington, DC, have some version of child restraint laws.[2–4]

Public health data are collected through two main efforts: primary and secondary data collection.[2] The distinction between primary and secondary data depends on the relationship of the person(s) analyzing or using the data to the person(s) who collected the data. If the individual(s) who collected the data are the same as those who are using them, the data are a result of primary data collection. If the data are collected by a person or group other than the person(s) who is analyzing them, the data are referred to as secondary data. Primary data collection is often seen as the gold standard, in part because the data were created to solely answer the question (e.g., research question, program evaluation question, policy question) that a person has in mind.[3,4] However, primary data collection requires time, monetary resources, and methodological and substantive expertise. In cases in which any one of the three stated requirements are not present, the use of secondary data sources should be considered. For example, public health practitioners and policymakers are often presented with public health problems or crises and have little time to make decisions that will impact the population's health. Therefore, collecting primary data is not an option in addressing questions with strict timelines or for driving decisions during public health crisis situations.

Secondary data, too, has its limitations; the main drawback to secondary data is that the data may not have been collected to specifically answer the question(s) at hand. Therefore, the data may lack specific details or particular information that would allow addressing question(s) in full. For example, with secondary data, it may only be possible to assess whether a relationship between two variables or concepts is present. However, the data may not contain enough detail to allow examination of the mechanisms linking the two variables or concepts, which would greatly assist in decision-making processes or program development. Additionally, the population surveyed may not exactly match the population currently in need, or certain variables may not have been collected in a way that matches the current project, leading to incomplete data. Another consideration when using secondary data is that available data may not always be the most current.[2–4] For example, most publicly available survey data are only collected every 3–5 years, vital records data take on average 2 years to become finalized, and administrative data sets are often updated with less frequency (e.g., the census, which is updated every 10 years). Despite these potential limitations, secondary data may still be advantageous to researchers, public health practitioners, and policymakers for public health decision-making.

## DATA SETS FOR COMMUNITY HEALTH DECISION-MAKING

*How do I decide on the secondary data source?* Deciding on the appropriate secondary data source depends on your question as much as it depends on your knowledge of what data sets exist. When choosing data sets for population health decision-making, some things to consider include the following:

1. Do you need community data or national data?
2. Does your question call for a data set that provides a specific level of detail in order to be applicable to your question? For instance, will race data alone be sufficient, or do you require race and ethnicity data?
3. Does your question require you to make comparisons, examine trends, or describe descriptive patterns within your community or population of focus?
4. Are the data needed at the individual level or community level?
5. Is the data set publicly accessible at no cost, or are data restricted and available to users at a cost?
6. Does the data set require necessary wait times or guidelines that dictate the use of the data sets (i.e., are the primary data owners allowed a certain amount of time to use the data before it becomes publicly accessible)?

7. Do any of the data sets identified have any limitations that could limit their usefulness in relation to your question and later public health decision-making?

In addition to these listed questions, it is also important to have an awareness of data sources that are frequently utilized for gathering evidence for public health decision-making.

This chapter provides an overview of data sets, categorized mainly by geography, and it details the frequency at which they are updated as well as the accessibility of state and national data sets. One thing to keep in mind is that most cities, counties, and small municipalities do not own their population health data outside of locale-specific programmatic data and notifiable disease surveillance. Population health data with relevancies at a substate level are often the result of abstracting relevant data from larger data sets, such as vital records data, hospital discharge data, surveys, and census data. For instance, cities often collect data that they do not have the authority to access, download, and analyze. Using vital records data as an example, the Philadelphia Department of Public Health does not issue or maintain birth or death certificate data; to obtain these data for the city of Philadelphia, it is necessary to request birth or death certificate data for Philadelphia from the state (the Pennsylvania Department of Health). This is not unique to Philadelphia; states own their vital records data as well as statewide public health programmatic data, even in the cases in which the cities are running the programs and/or entering the data into the data system.

State-level data sources come in the form of health outcome data and administrative data sets. Health outcome data collected at the state level include hospital discharge data and some state-specific household surveys. Administrative data collected at the state level include medical insurance claims data (some states that legislate all-payers claims data allow for private insurer claims data to be publicly accessible), hospital discharge (inpatient and ambulatory), vital events data (e.g., birth or death records), and state-run public health program data. Both claims and vital events data can take up to 1–2 years for a state to produce a final public file. The lag time for state-specific household surveys varies based on the complexities of the survey.

National-level data most relevant to decision-making include data that can produce state estimates. Nationals surveys such as the National Health and Nutrition Examination Survey (NHANES), National Health Interview Survey (NHIS), Pregnancy Risk Assessment and Management System (PRAMS), and Behavioral Risk Factors Surveillance System (BRFSS), are among the most frequently used, in part because they are routinely collected and they provide rich data into health behaviors and outcomes among the people surveyed. The advanced sampling methods used allow for these data to be extrapolated to those throughout the state, while also allowing for the combined data to provide a picture of health across the nation. Like state-level data, national-level data may also have a lag time from data collection to public use (i.e., 2–3 years).

## DECISION TO USE THE DATA YOU HAVE

The use of data to drive decisions, resources, and interventions is crucial to implementing effective public health strategies. There are vast amounts of rich data available for analysis, and the volume of available data continues to increase with the growth of information technology. Although population health data collected for purposes unrelated to your current question may have their drawbacks, a variety of methods can be employed to address these potential shortcomings in the analysis of the data and/or the interpretation of the findings. One of the previously mentioned problems with secondary data sets is that data available are frequently outdated. As technology has advanced, some improvement has occurred with preparing and making public health data available more rapidly[5,6]; however, untimely data are still problematic for most population health data sets. Depending on the data set, the most recent data available may be 6 months old, and more often is 12–24 months old. Despite this, these data can still provide insight for decision-makers, particularly in terms of examining trends in the data. Furthermore, projections based on these trends can be made to estimate the current and future burden of a public health problem assuming no intervention. When examined in the context of other information, it is possible to better interpret the noticeable trends and project future trends.

There are various statistical methods used to address missing data. There are no established cut-offs for what would be considered an acceptable percentage of missing data, although some have suggested less than 5–10%.[7] The reasons for data being missing should be assessed. If this is an issue, advanced statistical methods can be used to reduce bias and increase the likelihood of reaching valid conclusions.[8] When advanced statistical methods are required, appropriate consultation with an epidemiologist, statistician, or other individual with statistical expertise is advised.

## USING AVAILABLE DATA

The following sections describe several real-world examples from a local-level health department illustrating how some of these methods may be employed to make use of available data to drive decisions.

### Combining Administrative Data with Local Data to Identify Program Priorities

The City of Memphis in Shelby County, Tennessee, has consistently had infant mortality rates (IMR) that are among the highest in the nation. Although efforts to improve birth outcomes in Shelby County have been ongoing and some progress has been made, Shelby County IMRs remain substantially higher than the national average, and significant disparities exist. The Shelby County Infant Mortality Reduction Initiative (IMRI) was convened to develop a strategic plan to improve birth outcomes. During the most recent planning process, the primary data available included vital statistics data, Fetal and Infant Mortality Review (FIMR) recommendations, and child death review data. While much of these data, particularly vital statistics data, were not collected for the specific purposes of this initiative, and suffer from a lack of timeliness (e.g., the most recent strategic plan development was in 2013–2014, at which time the latest vital statistics data available were from 2012), the data were still useful to inform the plan and identify indicators for progress measurement. Trends were produced for factors and outcomes available from these data. Vital statistics data were also used for a perinatal periods of risk analysis (PPOR) (methods available from CityMatCH),[9] as well as mapping at the zip code level to help identify program targets. These data were used in combination with sleep-related infant death data from the child death review team and recommendations from the FIMR team. The IMRI core leadership team, which is a multisector collaboration, used all of these data (along with local community context, knowledge, and experience) to develop a plan that aligned with state priorities and identified performance measures as indicators of progress. Ten primary indicators were identified, and these measures are updated each year to identify progress and help inform efforts and priorities.

## Using Limited Data to Demonstrate Need, Target Efforts, and Justify Budget Requests for County-Level Response to Emerging Public Health Issues

In 2017, the US Department of Health and Human Services declared the opioid epidemic a public health emergency. The State of Tennessee has one of the highest opioid prescribing rates and one of the highest rates of prescription opioid overdose deaths (see https://www.cdc.gov/drugoverdose/data/index.html). While many counties in Tennessee have higher rates of opioid misuse than Shelby County, initial data analysis reveals an exponential increase in opioid-related events in Shelby County over the past several years. As a result of the epidemic, the Shelby County and City of Memphis mayors launched a joint plan and multisector task force to respond to the epidemic. The Shelby County Health Department Epidemiology Section is tasked with analyzing data to inform this plan, help justify a budget request, and demonstrate the need to establish additional data streams as well as data-sharing platforms.

At the time of this writing, limited data streams related to opioids were available to the health department. No data were currently being collected specifically for the purposes of this response and therefore desired details are lacking. Data currently available to the epidemiology section included death data (9- to 21-month data lag), hospital emergency room chief complaint/preliminary diagnosis data (current, but less precise), and hospital discharge data (more precise, but 18- to 30-month data lag). Some additional limitations of the available data were that these data represent only the most severe outcomes (death or hospital visits). Also, it is not possible to know to what extent opioids contributed to an event since, for most events, multiple drugs are indicated as contributing factors. The available data were analyzed using trends (examples are shown in Figures 23.1 and 23.2) as well as geographic choropleth mapping and hot spot analysis (examples are shown in Figures 23.3 and 23.4). Basic polynomial projections were used to illustrate the potential burden of this epidemic, assuming no change. The data have been used in presentations to the County Commission and the task force, as well as in discussions with other agencies regarding the need for additional data streams. The data have also been used to inform the development of public service announcements and other media,

## Figure 23.1 ▼

Drug overdose death trend data, Shelby County, Tennessee, 2007–2016.

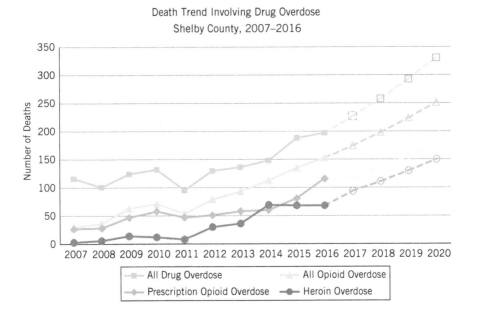

| Drug Overdose Death | 2007 | 2008 | 2009 | 2010 | 2011 | 2012 | 2013 | 2014 | 2015 | 2016 | 2017 (Projected) | 2018 (Projected) | 2019 (Projected) | 2020 (Projected) | Total (2007–2016) |
|---|---|---|---|---|---|---|---|---|---|---|---|---|---|---|---|
| All Drug Overdose | 116 | 101 | 124 | 132 | 95 | 130 | 136 | 148 | 188 | 197 | 227 | 258 | 292 | 331 | 1367 |
| All Opioid Overdose | 30 | 36 | 63 | 71 | 54 | 79 | 93 | 113 | 135 | 153 | 174 | 198 | 224 | 251 | 827 |
| Prescription Opioid Overdose | 27 | 28 | 47 | 58 | 47 | 51 | 58 | 60 | 81 | 116 | 118 | 136 | 155 | 177 | 573 |
| Heroin Overdose | 3 | 6 | 14 | 12 | 8 | 30 | 36 | 69 | 68 | 68 | 94 | 111 | 130 | 150 | 314 |

**Figure 23.2** ▼

Opioid-related emergency department visits, Shelby County, Tennessee, 2014–2017.

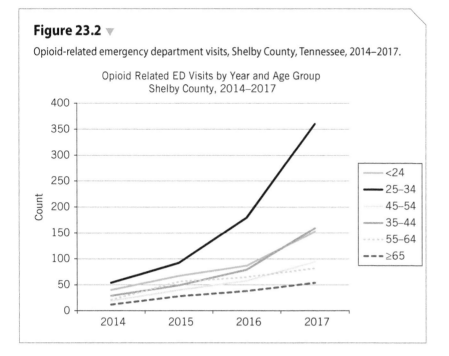

as well as for educational presentations to be used by the newly formed opioid education speaker's bureau.

At the national level, the lag in death data resulted in delayed awareness of the magnitude of the opioid misuse disorder epidemic. Shelby County is fortunate in that it is not among the counties with the highest rates of opioid misuse; however, given awareness of this public health issue, it was important to assess the extent of opioid misuse in Shelby County and provide information to guide effective prevention strategies. In order to address the lag in death data locally, basic projections were done to estimate the current and anticipated death burden. Additionally, counts of deaths suspected to be opioid-related were obtained from the medical examiner. Finally, the local syndromic surveillance system, which captures emergency room data with only a 24-hour time lag, was used to extract information about emergency visits possibly related to opioids. Data-sharing agreements are being developed with the medical examiner for direct access to more timely death data as well as with fire departments for emergency medical support (EMS) responses including administration of Narcan (naloxone, an opioid antidote medicine). Data from law enforcement agencies and other sources are also being investigated. This example illustrates multi-agency, multi-municipality collaboration, as well as expedient use of best available data—even if imperfect—to respond to an emerging health threat and inform a policy response while continuing to develop and refine more targeted data streams.

## Using Secondary Data for County and Subcounty Analysis

In 2016, chronic diseases accounted for 85% of deaths in the United States (https://www.cdc.gov/nchs/fastats/leading-causes-of-death.htm).

**Figure 23.3** ▼

Opioid-related emergency department visits by zip code, Shelby County, Tennessee, 2017.

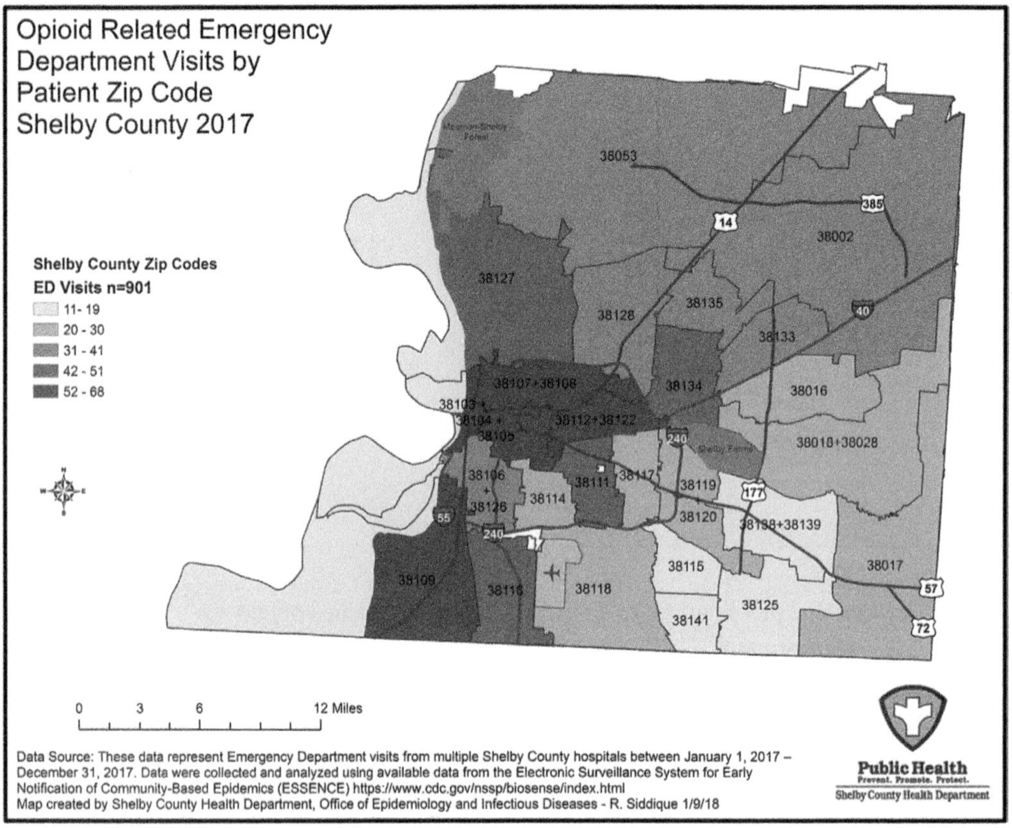

Opioid Related Emergency Department Visits by Patient Zip Code Shelby County 2017

Shelby County Zip Codes
ED Visits n=901
- 11- 19
- 20 - 30
- 31 - 41
- 42 - 51
- 52 - 68

0   3   6   12 Miles

Data Source: These data represent Emergency Department visits from multiple Shelby County hospitals between January 1, 2017 – December 31, 2017. Data were collected and analyzed using available data from the Electronic Surveillance System for Early Notification of Community-Based Epidemics (ESSENCE) https://www.cdc.gov/nssp/biosense/index.html
Map created by Shelby County Health Department, Office of Epidemiology and Infectious Diseases - R. Siddique 1/9/18

**Public Health**
Prevent. Promote. Protect.
Shelby County Health Department

Administrative data sets serve as the main data collection method, with the majority of our population-based knowledge about chronic diseases coming from death certificate data and/or hospital discharge data. These data represent the most severe outcomes of chronic disease, but the burden of chronic disease goes well beyond these extreme events. For a very limited number of diseases, registry data are available (i.e., cancer disease registry data are available). Surveys such as the BRFSS, NHANES, and NHIS are used to estimate prevalence and various risk factors; however data are self-reported, only reflect non-institutionalized populations, underestimate disease prevalence among the uninsured and those in health-professional shortage areas, and are often only representative at the national or state level and sometimes for large metropolitan areas.

In Shelby County, as in the nation, chronic diseases are recognized as a major population health problem. In order to inform community action, efforts have been made to use the data that are available at the county level, such as BRFSS, death certificates, and hospital discharge data. When trying to

**Figure 23.4** ▼

Opioid overdose death hot spot, Shelby County, Tennessee, 2013–2016.

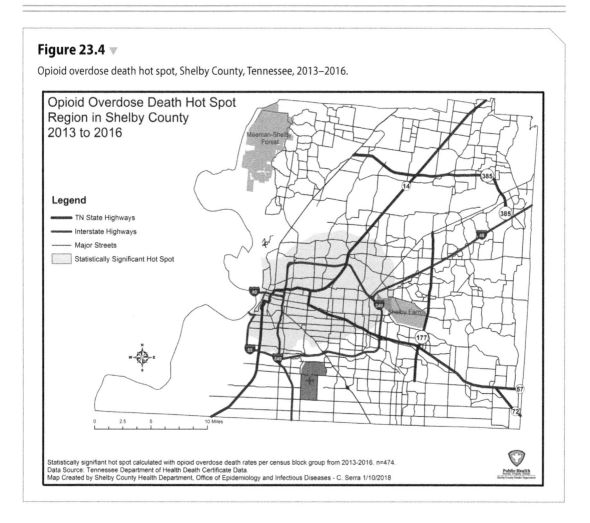

Opioid Overdose Death Hot Spot
Region in Shelby County
2013 to 2016

Legend

TN State Highways

Interstate Highways

Major Streets

Statistically Significant Hot Spot

0   2.5   5          10 Miles

Statistically signifiant hot spot calculated with opioid overdose death rates per census block group from 2013-2016. n=474.
Data Source: Tennessee Department of Health Death Certificate Data.
Map Created by Shelby County Health Department, Office of Epidemiology and Infectious Diseases - C. Serra 1/10/2018

design interventions in a county with a population of almost a million, analysis at a subcounty level is most useful for targeting resources. Thus, deaths and hospital encounters have been analyzed at zip code level for the leading chronic conditions, such as heart disease and cancer. Although these are not rare conditions, counts for extreme events such as deaths can still result in analytical problems resulting from a small number of events across zip codes or, especially, census tracts. For areas of the county that are less populated, denominators may also be too small. Numerator and denominator size are important for protecting privacy and producing stable rates. Simple tactics to overcome small numbers issues involve combining years of data and/or combining geographic areas. This zip code–level analysis has provided the county with useful information about chronic diseases; however, it is only the tip of the iceberg. For many of the leading issues affecting population health, such as asthma, diabetes, and hypertension, good prevalence data are not available since they are not reportable conditions. Refining methods and best practices for small-area analysis is work that is ongoing by academic and public health researchers across the nation (Box 23.1).

## Box 23.1 | Use Case 5: Are Children Filling Their Prescriptions for Needed Asthma Medications?

*Joshua Sharfstein*

*Purpose.* Children with moderate to severe asthma use "controller" medications, such as inhaled corticosteroids. However, studies have shown that doctors may underuse these medications, leaving children dependent on "rescue" medications.[1] A particular concern is that overuse of rescue medications by some children may increase the risk of death.[2] The health department is interested in helping promote medication adherence by working with physicians of patients with asthma.

*Data request.* The health department requests that hospitals add source of payment to the regular data file submitted by hospitals in Use Case 3 (see Chapter 21) (i.e., name, address, date of visit). For children with multiple emergency department (ED) visits and hospitalizations for asthma, the health department will request prescription fill data from a pharmacy data service (which is also covered by the Health Insurance Portability and Accountability Act [HIPAA]).

*Plan for data use.* For identified children who are not receiving a regular prescription for a controller medication, the health department will provide outreach to the families of patients and their primary care doctors to support improved access to therapy.

*HIPAA Analysis.* As explained in the following, the health department's data requests to hospitals for source-of-payment and prescription-fill data are permissible under HIPAA. It would be legal for the hospitals and pharmacy data services to share the requested data for this purpose.

In this use case, the health department has clearly articulated a need for health information related to a public health activity: promoting medication adherence by working with the physicians of patients with asthma to prescribe asthma "controller" medications. This clear articulation gives the Health Department the legal authority to request and receive protected health information from local hospitals, health care providers, and pharmacy data services under HIPAA.

The health department has carefully described the data elements that are necessary for fulfilling the public health activity. In this case, the data requested is limited to identifying information described in Use Case 3 (see Chapter 21) as well as source-of-payment data and prescription fill data for children with multiple ED visits. This meets HIPAA's minimum necessary requirement and allows hospitals, health providers, or pharmacy data services to voluntarily share the requested information with the health department.

In this case, the health department is only sharing information back to clinicians and/or patients for treatment purposes, which is a permitted disclosure under HIPAA. The health department is making no further disclosures that might implicate restrictions under HIPAA.

*Additional applications.* In addition to its use in asthma monitoring, use of electronic health data can facilitate public health oversight of other clinical conditions. In one study, researchers analyzed electronic health data from family medicine practices to identify and follow-up with patients with diabetes not receiving treatment according to guidelines.[3]

### References

1. Hasegawa K, Ahn J, Brown MA, et al. MARC-37 Investigators. Underuse of guideline-recommended long-term asthma management in children hospitalized to the intensive care unit: A multicenter observational study. *Ann Allergy Asthma Immunol.* 2015;115(1):10–6.e1.
2. Spitzer WO, Suissa S, Ernst P, et al. The use of beta-agonists and the risk of death and near death from asthma. *N Engl J Med.* 1992;326(8):501–6.
3. Crosson JC, Ohman-Strickland PA, Hahn KA, et al. Electronic medical records and diabetes quality of care: Results from a sample of family medicine practices. *Ann Fam Med.* 200;5(3):209–15.

## DATA USED ARE DATA IMPROVED

While scientific methods are constantly evolving to aid in addressing issues with data, data sets also have the opportunity to evolve. As previously discussed, most frequently used secondary data sets are routinely or continuously collected, which provides the opportunity for the data sets to be updated. Often, users of the data are provided with the opportunity to provide input to the primary data collectors about ways in which the data are used. For large national and statewide data sets, input is often systematic and comes in the form of data advisory groups consisting of data users and experts in the field. The process can be as simple as making decisions through consensus over a series of meetings, to processes codified in law, such as making changes to questions on vital record forms.

For an example, we can look to the 2003 revision of US vital records and improvements in the way that race and Hispanic ethnicity data were collected. The National Center for Health Statistics assembled a panel of state vital records registrars and organizations representing vital records data users and providers to evaluate the current variables and to propose changes. This process included surveys to the states evaluating the race and ethnicity variable for completeness and accuracy and searching for patterns within the missing data. Experts on the Panel to Evaluate the US Standard Certificates and Reports[5] noted inconsistencies in the way these variables were filled out and discussed potential explanations, such as the placement of the race variable before the Hispanic origin question. The final suggestions included a set number of races in a check box format, creation of categories for Hispanic origin (inclusive of a "not Hispanic or Latino" option), and asking both of these questions separately.

Another major change to come out of the Panel was that people were to be given the option to choose one or more races for the first time in US history. All changes proposed by the Panel were to be ratified by the US Secretary of Health and agreed upon by the states through the adaptation of the 2003 birth certificate.

## CONCLUSION

"Don't let the perfect be the enemy of the good." This well-known aphorism is as applicable to the analysis and use of data as it is to life in general. There is no such thing as perfect data, and tirelessly trying to achieve it can stymie progress. As this chapter has discussed, all data have limitations. Primary data, collected prospectively in a randomized controlled trial, are considered to be the gold standard, but even these data can be imperfect. The use of primary data in practice or policy decision-making is often constrained by resources and time because collecting robust data typically takes years. Although secondary data poses limits (e.g., data not being collected specifically for a particular health question, not being representative of the population of interest, or a lag in data availability), remember that data used are data improved.

The goal is to make evidence-informed or evidence-based decisions, actions, and policies with the best available data that provide information to prevent or reduce a health issue and to protect the population's health. Sometimes data are needed in real time or expeditiously; therefore, decisions must be made based on the highest quality data available. Analysts should always explore existing data in order to not "recreate the wheel." Existing data can be used to refine public health questions and incite a conceptual framework to understand the key determinants of health issues. With some data manipulation and statistical analysis experience, secondary data can be repurposed to answer your questions. Readers are encouraged to find the data that best suit their population and their questions. As a launching point, commonly used secondary data sets have been identified throughout this chapter, along with examples of real-world applications; a review of peer-reviewed articles can also be used to identify other existing data sources.

Become an engaged user of secondary data. Consider contacting the primary investigator to learn how the data were collected and share how you intend to use the data. Primary investigators can be a good resource and should be acknowledged for their consultation. Learning about the conditions under which the data were collected can explain the limitations of your findings. Critically assess and repurpose the data to answer your public health questions. Share the way in which you have used the data as well as your results. Express any further need for more robust or timely data streams. You can lead the change you need to see in order for secondary data to become your gold standard in practice or policy decision-making.

# REFERENCES

1. Boslaugh S. *Secondary Data Sources for Public Health: A Practical Guide.* New York: Cambridge University Press; 2007.

2. Safe Ride 4 Kids. Car Seat Laws by State—Find your state car seat laws. 2018. https://saferide4kids.com/car-seat-laws-by-state/. Accessed August 29, 2018.

3. Centers for Disease Control and Prevention. Child Passenger Safety. 2018. https://www.cdc.gov/features/passengersafety/index.html. Accessed August 28, 2018.

4. Bae JY, Anderson E, Silver D, Macinko J. Child passenger safety laws in the United States, 1978–2010: Policy diffusion in the absence of strong federal intervention. *Soc Sci Med (1982)*. 2014;100:30–7. http://doi.org/10.1016/j.socscimed.2013.10.035.

5. LaVenture M, Ross DA, Yasnoff WA. *Public Health Informatics: Biomedical Informatics.* Springer; 2014:503–16.

6. Dziura JD, Post LA, Zhao Q, Fu Z, Peduzzi P. Strategies for dealing with missing data in clinical trials: From design to analysis. *Yale J Biol Med.* 2013;86(3):343.

7. Howell DC. The treatment of missing data. In William Outhwaite and Stephen P Turner, eds., *The Sage Handbook of Social Science Methodology.* 2007:208–224. http://sk.sagepub.com/reference/the-sage-handbook-of-social-science-methodology/n11.xml

8. Yuan YC. *Multiple Imputation for Missing Data: Concepts and New Development (Version 9.0).* Rockville, MD: SAS Institute, Inc.; 2010:49, 1–11.

9. CityMatCH. Perinatal periods of risk approach. 2018. https://www.citymatch.org/perinatal-periods-of-risk-approach/. Accessed August 29, 2018.

# RESOURCES

National Center for Health Statistics. Report of the panel to evaluate the U.S. standard certificates. 2000. https://www.cdc.gov/nchs/data/dvs/panelreport_acc.pdf. Accessed August 29, 2018.

National Research Council (US) Committee on National Statistics. Vital Statistics: Summary of a Workshop. Washington (DC): National Academies Press (US); 2009. 4, Methodological Issues and the 2003 Revision of Standard Instruments. https://www.ncbi.nlm.nih.gov/books/NBK219875/.

Peck MG, Sappenfield WM, Skala J. Perinatal periods of risk: A community approach for using data to improve women and infants' health. *Maternal Child Health J.* 2010;14(6):864–74.

Sterne JA, White IR, Carlin JB, et al. Multiple imputation for missing data in epidemiological and clinical research: Potential and pitfalls. *BMJ.* 2009;338:b2393.

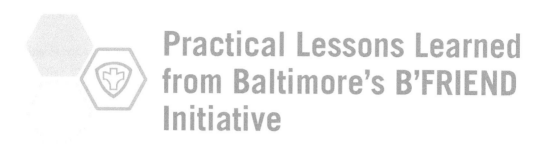

# Chapter 24

# Practical Lessons Learned from Baltimore's B'FRIEND Initiative

DARCY F. PHELAN-EMRICK, MICHAEL FRIED, HEANG TAN, MOLLY MARTIN, AND LEANA S. WEN

## BALTIMORE FALLS REDUCTION INITIATIVE ENGAGING NEIGHBORHOODS AND DATA

Falls among older adults (65+ years) are a growing public health problem, especially as baby boomers age and increase the proportion of older adults in the US population. Falls are the top cause of fatal and nonfatal injury among older adults.[1] Thirty-two percent of falls among older adults result in severe injury,[2] and such injury reduces a person's ability to live independently and get around as needed for daily activities. In 2015, 3 million older Americans visited an emergency department (ED) for a nonfatal fall.[3] That year, direct medical costs of nonfatal falls for the same group were estimated at $31.3 billion, and the costs for fatal falls were $637.5 million.[4] Despite their expensive public health burden, however, falls are preventable, and there are numerous effective evidence-based fall-prevention interventions. These include exercise (e.g., muscle and balance strengthening), home modification (e.g., reduction of physical fall risks), clinical programs (e.g., management of medication interactions and side effects, vision screening), and combinations of these approaches.[5]

Older adults in Baltimore City are at particularly high risk for falls. The rate of fall-related ED visits in Baltimore City is 22% greater than that of Maryland, and the rate of fall-related hospitalizations is 55% greater. In Baltimore City, 66% of injury-related hospitalizations among older adults are due to falls, and 52% of ED visits in the same group are due to falls.[6] Between 2009 and 2015, the fall-related mortality rate in Baltimore City increased by 13%.[7] The high risk of falls experienced in Baltimore City (vs. that in Maryland, for instance) may be driven by various factors, such as older housing stock (42.9% of the occupied housing units in Baltimore City were built before 1940 vs. 11.0% statewide[8]) and greater disability and poverty among older adults (84% of older adults in Baltimore City have a disability compared to 69% for Maryland older adults,[9] and 17% of Baltimore City older adults live below the federal poverty level vs. 8% for older adults statewide[10]).

To combat this rising public health threat, the Baltimore City Health Department (BCHD) created the Baltimore Falls Reduction Initiative Engaging Neighborhoods and Data (B'FRIEND). B'FRIEND builds on the long tradition at BCHD of convening and leading collective impact strategies to address critical public health challenges. B'FRIEND seeks to reduce fall-related ED visits and hospitalizations among older adults in Baltimore City by implementing a falls surveillance system with data from the state's health information exchange (HIE) and then using those data to target interventions.

B'FRIEND is a core group at BCHD of cross-departmental leadership, headed by the health commissioner. The group has expertise in IT, epidemiology, and older adult services. The core team convenes a community workgroup of representatives from more than a dozen local organizations involved in falls prevention, including representatives from the HIE and an advisory council of older adults from the community (details are discussed in the following section). By convening a spectrum of stakeholders, BCHD uses the analytical horsepower of a new falls surveillance system to activate community-level interventions with unprecedented speed and accuracy.

## PARTNERS AND INTERVENTIONS

Early commitment from leadership was critical to the project's success. The project team worked closely with leadership from BCHD, the HIE (Chesapeake Regional Information System for our Patients [CRISP]), and the primary data owner (the Maryland Health Services Cost Review Commission [HSCRC]). Demonstrating to this diverse group of stakeholders how the B'FRIEND model could be easily scaled across the state and then expanded to other public health topic areas was key to generating support from the start.

The B'FRIEND team prioritized community engagement early in the process, including soliciting input from various city agencies (e.g., housing), community-based nonprofit organizations, senior centers, academic institutions (e.g., schools of medicine, public health, and pharmacy), hospitals, and groups that specifically provide services to older adults (e.g., Meals on Wheels). The team formed a community workgroup to link stakeholders directly to the B'FRIEND core project team. This community workgroup provides valuable feedback, such as which types of information would be most useful to their organizations and which communities they feel are at greatest risk. This forum also provides the opportunity to survey which data sets are available from community providers that could be combined with core B'FRIEND data in future analysis.

The B'FRIEND team also receives input from an advisory council of older adults who have experienced falls themselves. These conversations are particularly useful for understanding how older adults would like B'FRIEND data to be used to prevent falls in Baltimore City. This group has helped to design the outreach strategy, particularly the use of existing trust centers for outreach to older adults (such as churches and senior centers).

Throughout the project, the B'FRIEND team keeps community input at the center of their work and looks to augment clinical data with practical information. For example, during a meeting with the community workgroup, B'FRIEND data indicated there was a falls "hot spot" in a certain neighborhood (Neighborhood A), and the ensuing discussion revealed that the closing of a nearby grocery store had likely led to an increase in falls. A community partner shared that "In that part of town, the grocery store located close by to four older adult housing complexes closed, and the housing residents can no longer easily buy groceries. Many are now walking to the next closest grocery store, which is located down a steep long hill. Older adults are falling and becoming injured while walking down and up the hill to get groceries." This type of practical, community-level awareness would be impossible to learn from health information exchange data alone (Figure 24.1).

B'FRIEND data are shared with stakeholders, and the focus is using the data to inform the implementation of falls prevention interventions. B'FRIEND team members present neighborhood-specific data findings at stakeholder meetings and discuss how the findings could be used. They also ask stakeholders what else they would like to know from the B'FRIEND data. Discussions among stakeholders at these meetings have quickly turned to addressing the falls hot spots identified in the data. In the example of Neighborhood A, stakeholders already working on older adult issues in that community decided to target collective falls prevention efforts to one of the older adult housing complexes for which the B'FRIEND data showed the greatest number of falls in the neighborhood. B'FRIEND data have also been used to guide investments by another city agency (details are discussed in the "Data" section, later in the chapter).

With respect to partnerships and interventions, there are two main obstacles faced by the B'FRIEND team. The first is lack (and timing) of funding for interventions. The lack of resources is a common problem in public health, but as real-time surveillance capabilities are established, new funding mechanisms that can rapidly redeploy resources are needed. The team is hopeful that using the near real-time B'FRIEND data for targeting resources and evaluation can provide new models for philanthropy. The B'FRIEND team has discussed with local funders and philanthropic organizations how they could use B'FRIEND data to inform their funding of falls prevention interventions in Baltimore City. BCHD is addressing funding challenges by convening groups of funders and community organizations to target investment and interventions in high-need

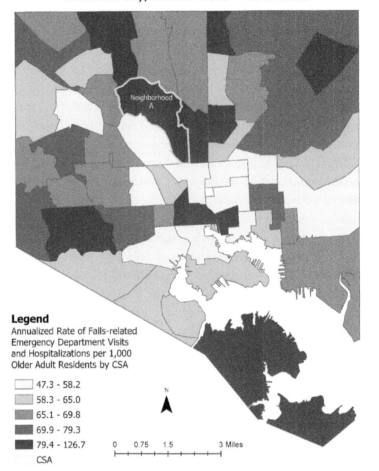

**Figure 24.1** ▼

Map of B'FRIEND data with "Neighborhood A" highlighted.

Annualized Rate of Falls-related Emergency Department Visits
and Hospitalizations per 1,000 Older Adult Residents (65+ years)
by Community Statistical Area (CSA),
Baltimore City, October 2015 - March 2018

Neighborhood
A

**Legend**
Annualized Rate of Falls-related
Emergency Department Visits
and Hospitalizations per 1,000
Older Adult Residents by CSA

☐ 47.3 - 58.2
▨ 58.3 - 65.0
▨ 65.1 - 69.8
▨ 69.9 - 79.3
■ 79.4 - 126.7
☐ CSA

N

0   0.75   1.5            3 Miles

Notes: A CSA is a grouping of census tracts. Rates were categorized by quintile. The
data source is the Maryland Health Services Cost Review Commission Inpatient and
Outpatient Case Mix Data with CRISP EID since October 2015 and the US 2010 Decennial
Census. Calculations and map were prepared by the Baltimore City Health Department.

areas. In addition, the mayor and health commissioner launched a citywide
strategy to reduce the rate of falls among older adults in Baltimore City.

The second partner obstacle was less anticipated: the degree of resistance
by other older adult stakeholders in the city to target falls prevention. These
stakeholders see other public health problems (e.g., behavioral health, nutrition) as more pressing than falls among older adults in Baltimore City, and
they are less interested in getting involved with B'FRIEND. This is an ongoing

challenge, and one that is addressed through the team's communications efforts. By focusing on the importance of falls with regard to an individual's independence, physical health, and social support, the team is able to work with stakeholders to understand the urgency of this critical issue.

## APPROVALS AND AGREEMENTS

B'FRIEND involves sharing of data across sectors, which has inherent challenges itself, and the data involved are covered by the Health Insurance Portability and Accountability Act (HIPAA) Privacy Rule, thus complicating matters further (Box 24.1). As such, the successful execution of approvals and agreements is key to B'FRIEND's success.

The B'FRIEND team worked with the Baltimore City Solicitor's Office to determine the most appropriate legal approach and justification for the disclosure of HIPAA-protected data with BCHD in the context of falls surveillance and prevention. The approach had to consider laws and regulations at the federal level (e.g., HIPAA), state level (e.g., Maryland Confidentiality of Medical Records Act, Code of Maryland Regulations [COMAR]), and local level (Baltimore City Charter). Because HIPAA includes "statutory carve-outs" where state law supersedes federal law, a thorough analysis of state and federal law was conducted to determine the most appropriate legal framework. This analysis then had to take into account local Baltimore City-specific laws and regulations. In the end, the Baltimore City Health Commissioner proposed a regulation through her authority as outlined in the Baltimore City Charter for the disclosure of the data. To be transparent, the B'FRIEND team posted the proposed regulation online and solicited public comment. The team incorporated feedback from the public and then filed the signed regulation with the city. The regulation is available on the Baltimore City Health Department's website (https://health.baltimorecity.gov/).

In terms of the key data partners (CRISP and the Maryland HSCRC), the B'FRIEND team reached out to their leadership to demonstrate how the B'FRIEND data-sharing approach would advance the goals of their organizations, could be scaled up to other jurisdictions in Maryland, and could be applied to other public health problems of interest. The CRISP Clinical Committee, which decides how the HIE's data may be used, approved data sharing for B'FRIEND, as did the Maryland HSCRC. The HSCRC and BCHD entered into a data use agreement wherein BCHD accesses aggregated HIE data via a secure online dashboard.

The B'FRIEND team faces three main legal challenges. First, the degree of legal expertise necessary for such data sharing is not common in local government. The team worked with the data partners to establish legal frameworks for data sharing, and a close partnership with the Baltimore City Solicitor's Office was critical to creating this new pathway. Second, there were changes in city leadership while this work was under way: a new mayor was elected and took

## Box 24.1 | Use Case 6: Is This Program Reducing Illness from Asthma?

*Joshua Sharfstein*

*Purpose.* The health department would like to initiate a quality-improvement project to assess the impact of specific interventions.

*Data request.* The health department requests from area hospitals a single data file that includes children in the county who have been seen in the emergency department (ED) or hospitalized for asthma in the previous 6 months. The data requested includes name, date of birth, street address, date of visit, gender, race/ethnicity, and ED visit or hospitalization.

*Plan for data use.* The health department will combine the data files from the hospitals to assess trends in hospital care for asthma for different groups of patients, including:

- Those who live in geographic areas that received specialized interventions compared to those who do not
- Those who were offered case management services compared to those who were not
- Those who have an updated asthma care plan compared to those who do not

The health department intends to employ these data to determine whether to continue or change specific intervention efforts.

*Health Insurance Portability and Accountability Act (HIPAA) analysis.* As explained in the following paragraphs, the health department's request to hospitals for data to use for program assessment is permissible under HIPAA. It would be legal for the hospitals to share the requested data for this purpose.

In this use case, the health department has clearly articulated a need for health information to assess a public health activity for the purpose of quality assurance and improvement. In this regard, hospital data enable the health department to determine whether to continue or change specific public health intervention efforts to improve the health of the community that it serves. This clear articulation gives the health department the legal authority to request and receive protected health information from local hospitals and health care providers under HIPAA.

The health department has carefully described the data elements that are necessary for fulfilling the public health activity. In this case, the data requested are limited only to the information necessary to complete the quality improvement project. This meets HIPAA's minimum necessary requirement and allows hospitals and health providers to voluntarily share the requested information with the health department.

In this case, the health department is only using the data for internal quality improvement activities and is not sharing this information outside the agency. In this case, it is clear that the health department is not conducting research, which might implicate other restrictions under HIPAA.

*Additional applications.* Many programs that seek to improve health outcomes are not regularly evaluated for effectiveness—but they should be. For example, a health department that refers to addiction treatment might be able to compare the rates of overdose by type of therapy or treatment provider. Similarly, community-based tobacco cessation programs, diabetes nutrition programs, and falls prevention efforts can be assessed using electronic health data.[1]

**Reference**

1. Wilson SR, Yamada EG, Sudhakar R, Roberto L, Mannino D, Mejia C, Huss N. A controlled trial of an environmental tobacco smoke reduction intervention in low-income children with asthma. *CHEST Journal.* 2001;120(5):1709–22.

office and the city solicitor departed, with an interim solicitor being appointed. Changes in staffing can lead to delays in making progress. Third, for groups interested in collaborating with B'FRIEND and sharing data, client consent forms lack sufficient information on how client information may be shared with third parties. Relationships and a collaborative approach are key to addressing each of these challenges. Having a strong core team augmented by community partners allows B'FRIEND to bring in outside expertise and translate that expertise locally. This thus enables the team to work with stakeholders and new staff to ensure that the project maintains momentum.

## DATA

The underpinning of the B'FRIEND approach is the use of HIE data for public health surveillance purposes. The CRISP Clinical Committee and Maryland HSCRC designated which variables would be available for these purposes. Using the HSCRC Inpatient and Outpatient Case Mix Data with CRISP unique patient identifiers (available for query through the CRISP dashboard), BCHD epidemiologists analyze aggregated data (i.e., fall-related ED visits and hospitalizations among older adults [65+ years], referred to as "falls" hereafter) by basic demographics such as age group, sex, race, insurance payer, residence zip code, and residence census tract. BCHD epidemiologists also calculate fall rates per population of older adults and "excess" falls (i.e., observed falls minus "expected falls": expected falls are calculated as the citywide falls rate multiplied by the number of older adults in the given geographic area—this is the number of falls expected to occur based on the number of older adults and the citywide falls rate). CRISP geocodes patient residence locations, and maps in the dashboard allow epidemiologists to identify falls "hot spots" in Baltimore City.

Public sharing of B'FRIEND data follows HSCRC cell suppression rules. The dashboard data are updated monthly.

B'FRIEND data have many uses, and stakeholders request data to inform their work. In one example, the Housing Authority of Baltimore City requested B'FRIEND data to guide its infrastructure investments in older adult housing complexes. The Housing Authority supplied BCHD with each complex location and number of units, and BCHD epidemiologists were able to calculate the rate of falls per unit for each of the complexes. The Housing Authority used this information to make decisions on how to spend its funds for improving older adult housing in the city.

The main data challenges are collaborating with the HIE to develop the dashboard and helping stakeholders to understand the limitations of B'FRIEND data. First, epidemiologists and technical HIE programmers generally operate in different settings and do not always understand the other's terminology. So, not unexpectedly, it takes continuous back-and-forth communication between BCHD and the HIE to make sure all are on the same page with the content of the dashboard and how each component should be calculated and visualized. Second, in sharing B'FRIEND data with stakeholders, the team encounters stakeholder frustrations that some data cannot be made public due to cell suppression rules of the Maryland HSCRC (i.e., the data "owner"). The team also works to help stakeholders understand other limitations of the data, such as that the data only contain falls that result in an ED visit or hospitalization (but not a regular visit to a primary care provider).

## LESSONS LEARNED

B'FRIEND seeks to reduce fall-related ED visits and hospitalizations among older adults in Baltimore City. The project pairs a cutting-edge surveillance system implemented in the statewide HIE with a set of on-the-ground interventions. This combination represents the future of public health. Prior to B'FRIEND, BCHD staff relied on data that were more than 1 year old to monitor fall-related ED visits and hospitalizations. Now BCHD is able to analyze in near real-time the same information, and the agency is able to advise community partners on where to locate interventions as well as to analyze whether the interventions are being effective.

### Public Health Innovation

B'FRIEND blazes a new path in public health: using HIE data for near real-time public health surveillance, establishing a legal framework for the use of this data within a local health department, and convening multisector stakeholders to address critical public health challenges. Public health is always difficult and underfunded, but innovation presents a unique set of challenges and opportunities for learning.

## Consistent Approach

One of the key lessons learned by the team is that a consistent approach to convening and communications can overcome leadership changes at specific agencies. Cross-sector projects that rely on partnerships will inevitably be challenged by the complexity of these relationships. The B'FRIEND approach to governance created a model that was more than the sum of its participants and allowed for confidence in the process.

## Complexity of Data Sharing

Another lesson learned is the complexity around sharing of protected health information and lack of formal guidance on how to handle these data-sharing partnerships. This is compounded by the data-sharing policies (of lack thereof) of each partner. The project has been successful by working to build a common understanding of data-sharing approaches and engaging support from experts to develop a shared comfort level among partners.

## Peer Learning

This type of cross-sector data collaboration can be accelerated by connecting with partners and peers doing similar work. The infrastructure of B'FRIEND was funded by the Robert Wood Johnson Foundation (RWJF) Data Across Sectors for Health (DASH), and DASH provided numerous ways for its funded projects to connect and learn from one another. In addition, it partnered with other funders to create the All In Network: Data for Community Health (http://www.allindata.org/). All In describes itself as "a nationwide learning collaborative that helps communities build capacity to address the social determinants of health through multi-sector data-sharing collaborations."[11]

## Hyperfocused Data and Interventions

Locally, B'FRIEND continues to bring a hyperfocus on falls hot spots in Baltimore City, with the first-of-its-kind citywide falls prevention strategy released by the health commissioner and mayor in April 2018. Paired with a set of interventions in the highest risk areas, the team will continue to use B'FRIEND data in collaboration with stakeholders to improve community health. Nationally, B'FRIEND is a model; other jurisdictions have reached out to the team about B'FRIEND's approach to legal frameworks, convening, and analysis.

B'FRIEND sets a new course for public health, one in which collective impact is fueled by real-time surveillance of cross-sector data, where partnerships prevail over bureaucracy, and where the local health authority becomes the catalytic point for data and action.

## REFERENCES

1. Bergen G, Stevens MR, Burns ER. Falls and fall injuries among adults aged ≥65 years—United States, 2014. *MMWR Morb Mortal Wkly Rep*. 2016;65:993–8. http://dx.doi.org/10.15585/mmwr.mm6537a2. Last accessed on 1/16/19.

2. Sterling DA, O'Connor JA, Bonadies J. Geriatric falls: Injury severity is high and disproportionate to mechanism. *J Trauma Injury Infect Crit Care*. 2001;50(1):116–9.

3. WISQARS. Leading causes of nonfatal injury reports, 2000–2015. Data query tool. https://webappa.cdc.gov/sasweb/ncipc/nfilead.html. Accessed March 3, 2018.

4. Burns ER, Stevens JA, Lee R. The direct costs of fatal and non-fatal falls among older adults—United States. *J Safety Res*. 2016;58:99–103. doi:10.1016/j.jsr.2016.05.001. Epub May 28, 2016: PMID:27620939.

5. CDC. *Compendium of Effective Fall Interventions: What Works for Community-Dwelling Older Adults* (3rd ed.). https://www.cdc.gov/homeandrecreationalsafety/falls/compendium.html. Accessed March 3, 2018.

6. PHPA. 2013 statistics on injury-related emergency department visits, hospitalizations and deaths. Maryland Department of Health. https://phpa.health.maryland.gov/ohpetup/Documents/Maryland%202013%20Injury%20Book_final.pdf. Accessed March 20, 2018.

7. SHIP. 2013–2015, Maryland state health improvement process, fall-related death rate, Baltimore City, Maryland overall. http://ship.md.networkofcare.org/ph/ship.aspx. Accessed March 20, 2018.

8. US Census Bureau. 2012–2016 American Community Survey 5-Year Estimates, Physical Housing Characteristics for Occupied Housing Units, Table S2504. https://factfinder.census.gov/faces/tableservices/jsf/pages/productview.xhtml?src=bkmk. Accessed 1/16/2019.

9. US Census Bureau. 2012–2016 American Community Survey 5-Year Estimates, Disability Characteristics, Table S1810. https://factfinder.census.gov/faces/tableservices/jsf/pages/productview.xhtml?src=bkmk. Accessed 1/16/2019.

10. US Census Bureau. 2012–2016 American Community Survey 5-Year Estimates, Selected Economic Characteristics, Table DP03. https://factfinder.census.gov/faces/tableservices/jsf/pages/productview.xhtml?src=bkmk. Accessed 1/16/2019.

11. All In Network. Data for community health website. About us. http://www.allindata.org/about-us/. Accessed March 3, 2018.

# Innovation: Enhancing Coordinated Impact Through New Roles and Tools

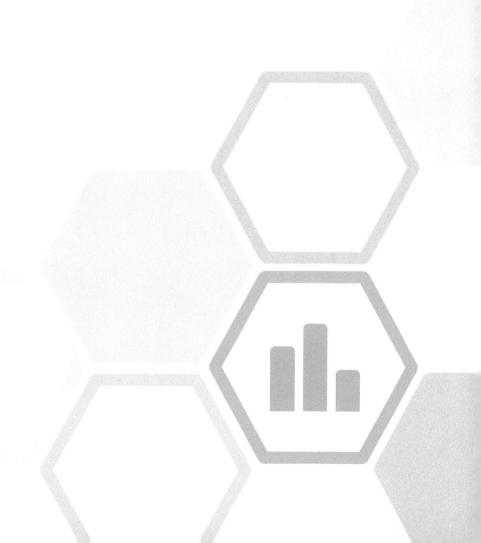

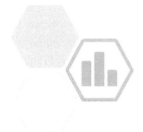

# Overview—Innovation: Enhancing Coordinated Impact Through New Roles and Tools

J. LLOYD MICHENER AND EDWARD L. HUNTER

D iscussions about innovation have become commonplace in the health fields as people and programs adapt to increasingly rapid shifts in funding, expectations, and relationships. But rarely do we have the opportunity to step back and consider innovation as a topic by itself, to see the changes we are facing as part of a larger picture. This section provides a concise overview of the types and forms of innovation, the factors driving it, guidance on some of the more successful innovations that are under way, and how to engage in those changes.

One of the first chapters in this section (Chapter 27 "The Role of Innovation in Improving Population Health") clarifies that innovation can be thought of as "The development of a new process, policy, product, or program that increase quality, impact, and efficiency."[1] Innovation can come in many forms: changes in current processes that make them more efficient or effective, shifts toward different processes to achieve the same goal, or larger changes that may include rethinking the task itself. While innovation can be part of the normal work flow, innovation is disruptive when it changes established roles and relationships.

Disruptive innovation is common outside of health care; for instance, film cameras have almost entirely given way to digital cameras, which in turn have been incorporated into smartphones. Health has begun a similar process of disruption as new forces engage in what is now the largest sector of our economy, and one for which the value is less than apparent. Public health approaches are disrupting the medical model as chronic disease becomes common, and health systems are disrupting governmental public health by taking on (and hiring people to take on) traditional public health roles of data gathering, analysis, and even planning and implementing community interventions to improve health.

Communities are disrupting both as they assert their fundamental ability to set priorities and processes for engagement, in many cases becoming the leaders of change.

Innovation need not be new: it can be an old idea rediscovered or repurposed. Although there is much discussion now about implementing community-wide prevention programs, in the 1970s, the residents of Franklin County, a rural community in Maine, decided to reduce their rates of chronic disease. Over the subsequent 40 years, they reduced mortality and hospitalization rates by implementing county-wide programs targeting hypertension, high cholesterol levels, and smoking, as well as diet and physical activity, work sponsored by multiple community organizations. Communities can form, find, and lead their own innovations and thus determine their own future.[2]

Innovation can come from any sector and may be most powerful when it arises from outside. We find innovation being led by communities (Chapter 28), fostered by foundations (Chapter 32), and focused on changes in partners and process (Chapters 29 and 32).

Innovation is facilitated by new tools. Data displays, such as maps of health outcomes across a region, can be powerful disruptors of current thinking as they display patterns for which the reasons are not clear and for which the intervention is likely not to be medical, but rather situated in the living conditions of the community. Increased attention to the social drivers of health is spurring development of new screening tools for health care providers that can help them become aware of the health-related needs of their patients and link them to local resources (Chapter 26).

Sometimes innovation comes from looking at current problems from a new perspective. Health equity is a powerful form of innovation because it is based on ethical principles of beneficence, fairness, and justice, which are fundamental to the health professions, and it helps us develop new tools for and ideas on how to improve outcomes with and for all, rather than for the average.

Multisector partnerships for health are growing rapidly and are tackling issues previously thought to lie within the domain of professional health care providers. The Maine example is an old illustration, whereas the partnership between hospitals and public health department in Chicago is a more recent example (Chapter 29). They may be so effective not because the interventions are new, but because they assemble the groups, data, and political will required to implement and sustain the needed changes. These partnerships can evolve to become systems for health (Chapter 29), and, in the process, roles are clarified and change, sometimes fundamentally (Chapter 32). In so doing they are innovating in one of the most powerful ways: by redefining the task and redefining the critical participants who are engaged in finding solutions.

But not all innovation is effective (Chapter 28). Innovation must be married to the need it addresses; it must be evaluated and results must be shared. Innovation that is not connected to the community will likely produce solutions that are disconnected from the problem. Innovations that are connected and successful need to be disseminated, adapted, and shared so they become the "new normal." The next stage for innovation in health will likely be learning and sharing what works in different settings, so that communites and their partners can draw from a mix of options, selecting those that best match their strengths and needs.

## REFERENCES

1. Public Health National Center for Innovations. *Innovation in Governmental Public Health: Building a Roadmap*. Alexandria, VA: Public Health National Center for Innovations; 2017. http://phnci.org/uploads/resource-files/Innovation-in-Governmental-Public- Health-Building-a-Roadmap-02-2017.pdf. Accessed April 10, 2018.

2. Record NB, Onion DK, Prior RE, Dixon DC, Record SS, Fowler FL, Cayer GR, Amos CI, Person TA. Community-wide cardiovascular disease prevention programs and health outcomes in a rural county, 1970–2010. *JAMA*. 2015;313(2):147–55. doi:10.1001/jama.2014.16969.

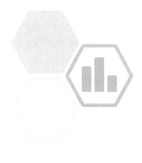

# Chapter 26

# Identifying and Addressing Patients' Social Needs in Health Care Delivery Settings

LAURA GOTTLIEB AND CAROLINE FICHTENBERG

In response to mounting evidence that patients' social and economic risk factors affect health and could be important targets for reducing health care costs, a wave of health care innovation has emerged around identifying and addressing patients' social needs as part of clinical care delivery.[1–8] This has been amplified by calls from health care professional organizations to include social needs assessments and interventions in primary care pediatrics, family medicine, obstetrics, emergency medicine, and other medical disciplines.[9–12] Simultaneously, interest from federal and state governments and other payers has led to the rapid proliferation of payment and policy experiments that incorporate social needs into health care delivery models.[13–18]

Innovation in this area has taken many forms, without clear consensus emerging on the best tools, workforce, population targets, partnerships, or payment strategies to facilitate identifying and/or addressing social needs in health care settings. There are almost as many approaches to incorporating social risk data into clinical care as there are clinical delivery settings. The field is ripe for more—and more rigorous—research and evaluation on effective and scalable strategies. In this chapter, we describe both patient- and community-level risk assessment tools and provide a framework for existing intervention models. We also highlight emerging payment models that may facilitate health care delivery–based social and economic needs screening and interventions, and we underscore outstanding knowledge gaps in this rapidly evolving field.

# SOCIAL RISK ASSESSMENT
## Multidomain Social and Economic Needs Screening Tools

Many health care professional organizations and individuals have developed tools for identifying patients' social determinants of health (SDH) needs using validated measures as available. These tools vary by SDH domains included, survey length, and target population (Table 26.1). Across tools, common social and economic needs topics include housing instability, food insecurity, transportation, and utility needs. Several tools also include topics related to intimate partner violence and social support. The Protocol for Responding to and Assessing Patient Assets, Risks, and Experiences (PRAPARE) has been adopted by almost 1,000 community health centers in the United States.[19] Developed and launched in 2016 for use in community health centers, it includes 21 questions covering a range of domains.[8] A second prominent screening tool is the Accountable Health Community (AHC) Health-Related Social Needs Screening Tool, which was developed by the Center for Medicare and Medicaid Innovation for the Accountable Health Communities Model demonstration.[20] The basic AHC tool includes 10 questions covering five domains (housing instability, food insecurity, transportation difficulties, utility assistance needs, and interpersonal safety). Optional questions cover eight supplemental domains (financial strain, employment, education, family and community support, physical activity, substance use, mental health, and disabilities). A third popular tool is the Health Leads Screening Toolkit, first published in 2016 and updated in 2018, which includes 10 questions on food insecurity, housing instability, child care, medical transportation, utilities, social isolation, and health literacy.

Other multidomain tools that have been published include social and economic needs screening measures such as WE CARE (pediatrics), WellRx, Health Begins Upstream Risk Screening Tool, The Online Advocate, Patient-Centered Assessment Method (PCAM), iHELP, HelpSteps, and Kaiser's Your Current Life Survey. Although these tools have been evaluated by national publications, many health care practices modify existing tools, choosing the questions that seem most relevant to their patient populations and the uses they foresee for collected data.

In addition to identifying needs, several screening tools (e.g., WE CARE, Health Leads, AAFP Toolkit) have added a question about patients' desire for help from clinic staff in addressing social or economic needs. This practice is driven by research studies that have found that not all those who screen positive for unmet needs will want help and, conversely, that some may want help who did not screen positive.[21]

**Table 26.1 ▼ Social and economic risk screening tools**

| | Recommended Social and Behavioral Domains and Measures for Electronic Health Records[49] | PRAPARE: Protocol for Responding to and Assessing Patient Assets, Risks, and Experiences[8] | Accountable Health Communities Screening Tool[50] | Health Leads Recommended Measures[51] | Kaiser Your Current Life Situation[52] |
|---|---|---|---|---|---|
| **Domain** | | | | | |
| Alcohol use | • | | | | •* |
| Child care needs | | • | | • | • |
| Clothing needs | | • | | | |
| Depression/mental health | • | | •* | | |
| Disabilities | | | •* | | |
| Education | • | • | •* | | •* |
| Employment | | | •* | | |
| Financial resource strain | • | | •* | | |
| Food insecurity | | • | • | • | • |
| Household income | | • | | | |
| Household size | | • | | | |
| Housing insecurity | | • | • | • | • |
| Incarceration history | | •* | | | |
| Insurance status | | • | | | |
| Interpersonal violence/safety | • | •* | • | • | • |
| Literacy/health literacy | | | | • | •* |
| Medicine/health care | | • | | | • |
| Migrant/seasonal farmworker | | • | | | |

(*continued*)

| | Recommended Social and Behavioral Domains and Measures for Electronic Health Records[49] | PRAPARE: Protocol for Responding to and Assessing Patient Assets, Risks, and Experiences[8] | Accountable Health Communities Screening Tool[50] | Health Leads Recommended Measures[51] | Kaiser Your Current Life Situation[52] |
|---|---|---|---|---|---|
| Neighborhood safety | | •* | | | |
| Neighborhood income | • | | | | |
| Physical activity | • | | •* | | |
| Primary language | | • | | | |
| Race/ethnicity | • | • | | | |
| Refugee status | | •* | | | |
| Residential address | • | • | | | |
| Social connections/ isolation | • | • | •* | • | • |
| Stress | • | • | | | • |
| Substance use | | | •* | | •* |
| Tobacco use and exposure | • | | | | |
| Transportation needs | | • | • | • | • |
| Utilities (phone, gas, electric) needs | | • | • | • | • |
| Veteran status | | • | | | |

**Table 26.1 ▼ Continued**

* Optional questions.

## IMPLEMENTING PATIENT-LEVEL SOCIAL SCREENING PROGRAMS

Practitioners implementing social screening programs need to identify the population targeted for screening, a screening (and intervention) workflow, and a strategy for tracking and using data. Although a growing number of health care delivery systems have developed social screening programs, little concrete evidence exists to guide implementation practices.

## Target Population

Early-adopting health systems have differed in choosing universal versus targeted patient screening. When screening is limited to a subset of the served population, patients are typically selected who are high-needs/high-cost in the health system. Although existing social screening programs are disproportionately described in primary care settings and emergency department settings, the actual prevalence of social screening practices across different medical settings/disciplines is currently unknown. Some social screening initiatives have been described in specialty clinics and inpatient settings.[22–26]

## Screening Workflow (Staff, Modality, and Timing)

Several technical assistance providers in this area have developed social screening workflow options.[8,27] These include having screening conducted pre-visit, by clinical staff and by nonclinical staff, each of which poses different advantages and challenges. Modes for screening administration vary considerably across settings (e.g., surveys can be paper or electronic, patient- or provider-administered). One randomized controlled trial among pediatric caregivers found that self-administered screening via self-administration (on electronic tablet) yielded higher reports of unmet social needs than questions administered by a research assistant.[28] Despite this finding, there are important barriers to implementing tablet-based, patient-facing screening in safety net settings, including concerns about literacy and the availability of technology to support information transfers. There is also little evidence available to provide information about the point at which an encounter should occur during screening, who should conduct the screening, or the ideal frequency at which screening should occur.

## Data Tracking

Once social needs data are collected, a major challenge facing clinical sites is how to capture and track social health data in electronic health records (EHRs). Documentation can help support patient and population health uses of the data, but it also is likely to be needed for payment and reimbursement requirements that are emerging in this area. Some screening tools have templates for EHR integration (e.g., PRAPARE), but this is not universal. Sites often need to develop their own processes for systematically recording SDH information in EHRs. An additional obstacle is the lack of standards for medical codes for SDH data. Codes exist in several of common medical terminologies (e.g., ICD, SNOMED, LOINC, CPT), but these codes are rarely used given the lack of incentives and guidelines for use.[29,30]

To address concern about the feasibility and actionability of patient-level social screening, some health care organizations have begun using neighborhood-level data to identify patients or populations with increased social risks.[31] The use of area-level data can inform patient- or community-level interventions, especially in cases in which universal patient-level screening is infeasible. Neighborhood-level data may facilitate risk stratification and targeting of screening resources toward populations most likely to benefit from interventions. Such data can also be used for risk adjustment to avoid penalizing providers who serve high-need populations.[32] They also can influence neighborhood-level intervention decisions. When being used to target patient-level interventions, individual risk assessments should be obtained to corroborate neighborhood-level data.[26]

## INTERVENING ON SOCIAL AND ECONOMIC HEALTH RISKS

Social risk assessments can be used to inform a wide range of interventions, including patient- and community-level interventions. Social risk assessments conducted in the context of clinical care delivery, however, typically lead to two types of interventions: (1) socially informed care, which focuses on how medical care access, diagnostics, and treatment can be altered to accommodate social and economic risk factors, and (2) socially targeted care, which includes interventions that more directly aim to change underlying social risk factors themselves. Both can be understood under the umbrella of "precision medicine," although this is using a definition of precision medicine that is expanded from tailoring medical decisions based on genetic or molecular profiles to one that also includes tailoring based on social, economic, and other contextual hardships. Social risk data can also inform community-level interventions that aim to change upstream social and structural determinants of health. All of these interventions take into account a broader array of risk factors and, in so doing, may provide new models for both improving health and decreasing US health inequities.

### Socially Informed Care

Across medical specialties, health care providers routinely make changes to care delivery that can improve access, diagnostics, and treatment for vulnerable populations. To improve access, an increasing number of clinics provide weekend and evening clinics and off-site services like mobile vans or school-based clinics; flu shots and HIV tests are now available in places as unconventional as the department of motor vehicles.[33] Information on social risks can also be used to inform medical diagnostics. For instance, the Mini-Mental Status Examination should be adjusted for literacy level,[34] and point-of-care diagnostics can be used to reduce phone or in-person follow-up visits. To improve treatment planning, social risk information should be used to improve access or adherence to clinically effective therapies. For instance, low income status qualifies patients for free drug programs, and patients who cannot easily take restroom breaks are not prescribed loop diuretics.

These types of socially informed care interventions have not traditionally been grouped together across disciplines or specialties, diseases, or populations

**Table 26.2 ▼ Examples of socially informed care at patient and system levels**

|  | Patient-level examples | System-level examples |
|---|---|---|
| Access | Interpreted visits for patients who do not speak English | Mobile vans provided to reach patients living in homeless encampments |
| Diagnostics | Scores for Mini-Mental Status Examination are adjusted for literacy | EHR alerts to ensure all homeless patients referred for TB testing |
| Treatment | Loop diuretics not prescribed for patients without convenient restroom access | Clinical decision supports recommend medication choices based on social risk factors |

(Table 26.2). This is critical to better understand the concrete strategies needed to maximize care effectiveness, including by improving access and adherence to recommended preventive care, diagnostics, and clinically effective treatment for vulnerable populations.

## Socially Targeted Care

A second bucket of social interventions involves more directly targeting patients' social and economic needs as a part of clinical care delivery (socially targeted care), rather than just using that information to change the delivery of care (socially informed care). This crop of interventions typically involves referrals to either internal programs or external agencies (Table 26.3) that can help reduce social risks and thereby improve health care access or medical treatment. To facilitate external referrals, some health care systems have developed relationships with intermediaries that provide community and social service resource directories and can enable electronic referrals, consultations, and both patient and provider follow-up. Each platform offers some unique features. These technology-based resource platforms include 2-1-1, but also many newer technology companies, such as NowPow, Healthify, REACH, Unite Us, and TAVHealth.

The expansion of medical care delivery to include social targets has been controversial. In some respects, social needs targets may be considered outside the purview of conventional care delivery, especially in times of limited resources and in the context of the many other demands of busy clinical workplaces.[35] Proponents argue that poor health status and large health inequities in the United States are in large part dependent on these social risk

**Table 26.3 ▼ Examples of socially targeted care**

|  | Internal programs | External referrals |
|---|---|---|
| Food | Onsite food pantry/pharmacy | Government food benefits program |
| Housing | Tenant eviction protection letter | Housing support agency |
| Transportation/utilities | Transportation vouchers | Low-income heat and energy assistance program (LIHEAP) |

factors and that traditional medical care models must change to achieve the Triple Aim of improved experience of care, improved population health, and decreased costs.[36,37]

## Payment Reform

The advent of value-based payment models has accelerated opportunities at federal and state levels to pay for both more systematic social screening and integrated care delivery interventions. At the federal level, examples of payment demonstration models that can be used to support integrated care have included the Comprehensive Primary Care Plus program,[16] Accountable Health Communities,[38] and health homes.[39] Other programs have been adopted under state Medicaid §1115 waivers, including California's Whole Person Care demonstration[40] and Oregon's alternative payment models for community health centers.[41] In Massachusetts, the state Medicaid agency is now incorporating social risk factors such as homelessness and neighborhood deprivation into per-member per-month capitation rates.[42] Similarly, in Hawaii, some Medicaid providers provide higher per-member per-month rates to providers who regularly document enabling services. In Oregon, the Oregon Health Authority is considering the use of food security screening and intervention as an optional quality improvement metric for regional coordinating care organizations to use in incentive payments.[43]

Because many of the socially targeted interventions rely on strong community partner agencies, increasing attention is being paid to strategies that could shift some financial resources to these non-health care partners. More research is needed to understand how to design these partnerships to maximize returns for all partners.[44] This will demand improving alignment more generally between the medical and social service sectors. To that end, the Center for Medicaid and Medicare Innovation (CMMI) has included a dedicated track of the Accountable Health Communities demonstration that requires resource pooling.

## Community-Level Interventions

In addition to patient-level actions to address social determinants, many health systems are increasingly engaging in activities to address social determinants at the community level. This work has been spurred by an increased focus on community benefits as part of nonprofit hospitals' tax exempt status, led by new requirements for community health needs assessments and implementation strategies that were part of the 2010 Patient Protection and Affordable Care Act.[45] These activities are also being driven by the country's new focus on value-based care and a critical emphasis on reducing costs for high-needs/high-cost patients, many of whom face social needs challenges. As a result, health systems and health centers are increasingly supporting community-based efforts to address SDH, for example by financing development of affordable housing, improving access to healthy foods, engaging in multisector collaborations to reduce violence or improve early childhood outcomes, or providing workforce training programs.[46] One model for health system engagement in community health is the "anchor institution model," which leverages health systems' economic power to improve the health of the communities in which they are located.[47] In this model, health systems can use inclusive hiring strategies, local sourcing, and place-based investing to improve local employment and economic opportunities. As part of place-based investing, health systems are progressively collaborating with community development organizations to help revitalize communities.[48] Although patient- and community-level interventions are usually carried out by different parts of a health system, they can often complement each other and, ideally, should be coordinated.

## THE FUTURE

There is mounting interest and innovation focused on social screening and interventions into health care delivery settings (Box 26.1). Opportunities to advance the field depend on better understanding of the impacts of these programs, but also on how to implement them in busy clinical settings. From a health

---

**Box 26.1 | System of Prevention: Checklist for Taking Action**

*Prevention Institute*

This checklist was developed to reveal the diverse range of valuable actions health care practitioners and organizations can take to advance prevention and community health and well-being as part of a system of prevention.

**Support Prevention in Clinical Practice**

- Implement preventive medicine protocols
- Provide health behavior education and coaching
- Establish systems to screen and refer patients to social and economic support services
- Foster connections between physical and behavioral health

**Share Insight on How Community Determinants Influence Health**

- Include assessment of community determinants in community health needs assessments/community health assessments
- Provide opportunities for patients and staff to share reflections on how community conditions are impacting community health
- Analyze patient data to identify patterns of illness and injury

**Collaborate to Improve Community Environments**

- Assess the community landscape to learn about community efforts under way
- Establish formal or informal partnerships with other organizations/coalitions

- Establish community engagement principles to guide activities in communities
- Partner with other health centers, hospitals, and health systems to complement integrated services with community-level prevention efforts

**Model Organizational Best Practices**

- Adopt and implement policies and practices in the health care site(s) to ensure safety, promote environmental sustainability, and encourage healthy behaviors
- Implement healthy, equitable, and sustainable contracting /procurement and disposal programs
- Offer high-quality employment opportunities and advancement, and support programs that expand access to health care careers in underserved communities
- Invest in surrounding communities via community benefits, core capital, and human capital

**Engage Patients and Local Residents**

- Activate patients through information-sharing practices and broader community planning and engagement activities
- Convene patient advisory boards regularly

**Speak Up for Improving Community Determinants and Decisions**

- Advocate for community improvements and policies with elected officials and decision-makers
- Generate data and stories, and communicate with the media to make the case for community-level changes
- Influence peers in the health care sector to be advocates of community-based prevention

services perspective, future work will need to explore the workforce needed to support social health screening and intervention programs, technology's role in facilitating these programs, and policy and payment reforms that can maximize intervention uptake. Both interventions and research in this field would be strengthened by more active engagement of patient and community stakeholders.[49–52]

## REFERENCES

1. Institute for Alternative Futures. Community health centers: leveraging the social determinants of health. 2012. http://www.altfutures.org/pubs/leveragingSDH/IAF-CHCsLeveragingSDH.pdf. Accessed May 1, 2018.
2. Bachrach D, Pfister H, Wallis K, Lipson M, Manatt Health Solutions. *Addressing Patients' Social Needs: An Emerging Business Case for Provider Investment.* New York: The Commonwealth Fund; 2014: http://www.commonwealthfund.org/

publications/fund-reports/2014/may/addressing-patients-social-needs. Accessed May 1, 2018.

3. The Menges Group. *Positively Impacting Social Determinants of Health: How Safety Net Health Plans Lead the Way*. Washington, DC: Association for Community Affiliated Plans; 2014: http://www.communityplans.net/Portals/0/Fact%20Sheets/ACAP_Plans_and_Social_Determinants_of_Health.pdf. Accessed May 1, 2018.

4. Alderwick HAJ, Gottlieb LM, Fichtenberg CM, Adler NE. Social prescribing in the US and England: Emerging interventions to address patients' social needs. *Am J Prev Med*. 2018. Epub ahead of print.

5. Ashbrook A, Hartline-Grafton H, Dolins J, Davis J, Watson C. *Addressing Food Insecurity: A Toolkit for Pediatricians*. Washington, DC: Food Research & Action Center and American Academy of Pediatrics; 2017. http://www.frac.org/wp-content/uploads/frac-aap-toolkit.pdf. Accessed April 30, 2018.

6. Pooler J, Levin M, Hoffman V, Karva F, Lewin-Zwerdling A. *Implementing Food Security Screening and Referral for Older Patients in Primary Care: A Resource Guide and Toolkit*. Columbia, MD: AARP Foundation and IMPAQ International; 2016. https://www.aarp.org/content/dam/aarp/aarp_foundation/2016-pdfs/FoodSecurityScreening.pdf. Accessed April 30, 2018.

7. Health Research & Educational Trust. *Social Determinants of Health Series: Food Insecurity and the Role of Hospitals*. Chicago, IL: Health Research & Educational Trust; 2017. http://www.hpoe.org/Reports-HPOE/2017/determinants-health-food-insecurity-role-of-hospitals.pdf. Accessed April 30, 2018.

8. National Association of Community Health Centers Inc., Association of Asian Pacific Community Health Organizations, Oregon Primary Care Association. *PRAPARE: Protocol for Responding to and Assessing Patient Assets, Risks, and Experiences*. Paper Version of PRAPARE for Implementation as of September 2, 2016. Bethesda, MD: National Association of Community Health Centers; 2016. http://www.nachc.org/wp-content/uploads/2016/09/PRAPARE_One_Pager_Sept_2016.pdf. Accessed April 30, 2018.

9. Daniel H, Bornstein SS, Kane GC. Addressing social determinants to improve patient care and promote health equity: An American College of Physicians Position Paper. *Ann Intern Med*. 2018;168(8):577–8.

10. American Academy of Family Physicians. Social determinants of health policy. 2013. http://www.aafp.org/about/policies/all/social-determinants.html. Accessed May 1, 2018.

11. Daniel H, Bornstein SS, Kane GC. Health and Public Policy Committee of the American College of Physicians. Addressing social determinants to improve patient care and promote health equity: An American College of Physicians Position Paper. *Ann Intern Med*. 2018;168(8):577–8.

12. Committee on Health Care for Underserved Women. ACOG Committee Opinion No. 729: Importance of social determinants of health and cultural awareness in the delivery of reproductive health care. *Obstet Gynecol*. 2018;131(1):e43–e48.

13. Alley DE, Asomugha CN, Conway PH, Sanghavi DM. Accountable Health Communities—addressing social needs through Medicare and Medicaid. *N Engl J Med*. 2016;374(1):8–11.

14. Fraze T, Lewis VA, Rodriguez HP, Fisher ES. Housing, transportation, and food: How ACOs seek to improve population health by addressing nonmedical needs of patients. *Health Aff (Millwood)*. 2016;35(11):2109–15.

15. National Academies of Sciences, Engineering, and Medicine. *Accounting for Social Risk Factors in Medicare Payment*. Washington, DC: The National Academies Press; 2017.

16. Centers for Medicare & Medicaid Services. *Comprehensive Primary Care Plus*. Baltimore, MD: Centers for Medicare & Medicaid Services; 2018. https://innovation. cms.gov/initiatives/comprehensive-primary-care-plus. Accessed April 30, 2018.

17. DHCS. *Whole Person Care Pilots*. Sacramento, CA: California Department of Health Care Services; 2017. http://www.dhcs.ca.gov/services/Pages/ WholePersonCarePilots.aspx. Accessed April 30, 2018.

18. Committee on Accounting Socioeconomic Status in Medicare Payment Programs. Accounting for Social Risk Factors in Medicare Payment. In: Kwan LY, Stratton K, Steinwachs DM, eds. Accounting for Social Risk Factors in Medicar Payment. Washington, DC: The National Academies Press; 2017. https://www.nap.edu/read/ 23635/chapter/1. Accessed April 30, 2018.

19. Jester M. *Strategizing Workflow Models to Implement PRAPARE to Collect Standardized Data on the Social Determinants of Health*. Bethesda, MD: National Association of Community Health Centers, Inc.; 2018. http://www.nachc. org/wp-content/uploads/2018/03/Strategizing_Workflows_for_PRAPARE_ Implementation_3.27.18.pdf. Accessed May 1, 2018.

20. Centers for Medicare and Medicaid Services. Accountable Health Communities Model. *CMS.gov*. Baltimore, MD: Centers for Medicare & Medicaid Services. https://innovation.cms.gov/initiatives/ahcm/.

21. Wylie SA, Hassan A, Krull EG, et al. Assessing and referring adolescents' health-related social problems: Qualitative evaluation of a novel web-based approach. *J Telemed Telecare*. 2012;18(7):392–8.

22. Kangovi S, Mitra N, Grande D, et al. Patient-centered community health worker intervention to improve posthospital outcomes: A randomized clinical trial. *JAMA Intern Med*. 2014;174(4):535–43.

23. Pettignano R, Caley SB, Bliss LR. Medical-legal partnership: Impact on patients with sickle cell disease. *Pediatrics*. 2011;128(6):e1482–8.

24. Rodabaugh KJ, Hammond M, Myszka D, Sandel M. A medical-legal partnership as a component of a palliative care model. *J Palliat Med*. 2010;13(1):15–18.

25. Fleishman SB, Retkin R, Brandfield J, Braun V. The attorney as the newest member of the cancer treatment team. *J Clin Oncol*. 2006;24(13) 2123–6.

26. Auger KA, Kahn RS, Simmons JM, et al. Using address information to identify hardships reported by families of children hospitalized with asthma. *Acad Pediatr*. 2017;17(1):79–87.

27. Center for Care Innovations. *Optimizing the Flow of Information and Work for Social Needs*. Oakland, CA: Center for Care Innovations; 2017. https://www. careinnovations.org/resources/optimizing-flow-information-work-social-needs/. Accessed May 1, 2018.

28. Gottlieb L, Hessler D, Long D, Amaya A, Adler N. A randomized trial on screening for social determinants of health: The iScreen study. *Pediatrics*. 2014;134(6):e1611–18.

29. Torres JM, Lawlor J, Colvin JD, et al. ICD social codes: An underutilized resource for tracking social needs. *Med Care*. 2017;55(9):810–16.

30. DeSilvey S, Ashbrook A, Sheward R, Hartline-Grafton H, Ettinger de Cuba S, Gottlieb L. *An Overview of Food Insecurity Coding in Health Care Settings: Existing and Emerging Opportunities*. Boston, MA: Hunger Vital Sign National Community of Practice; 2018. http://childrenshealthwatch.org/wp-content/uploads/An-Overview-of-Coding_2.15.18_final.pdf. Accessed April 30, 2018.

31. Bazemore AW, Cottrell EK, Gold R, et al. "Community vital signs": Incorporating geocoded social determinants into electronic records to promote patient and population health. *J Am Med Inform Assoc*. 2016;23(2):407–12.

32. Lines LM, Rosen AB, Ash AS. Enhancing administrative data to predict emergency department utilization: The role of neighborhood sociodemographics. *J Health Care Poor Underserved*. 2017;28(4):1487–508.

33. Steward N. D.C. brings HIV testing to the crowd at the DMV. *Washington Post*. September 30, 2010: District Politics.

34. Crum RM, Anthony JC, Bassett SS, Folstein MF. Population-based norms for the Mini-Mental State Examination by age and educational level. *JAMA*. 1993;269(18):2386–91.

35. Solberg LI. Theory vs practice: Should primary care practice take on social determinants of health now? No. *Ann Fam Med*. 2016;14(2):102–3.

36. Berwick DM, Nolan TW, Whittington J. The triple aim: Care, health, and cost. *Health Aff (Millwood)*. 2008;27(3):759–69.

37. Kaufman A. Theory vs practice: Should primary care practice take on social determinants of health now? Yes. *Ann Fam Med*. 2016;14(2):100–1.

38. Centers for Medicare and Medicaid Services. Affordable Care Act (ACA) funding opportunity: Accountable Health Communities (AHC). 2016. Funding Opportunity Number: CMS-1P1-17-001. https://www.grantsolutions.gov/gs/preaward/previewPublicAnnouncement.do?id=55237. Accessed May 1, 2018.

39. Health Home Information Resource Center. Baltimore, MD: Centers for Medicare & Medicaid Services. https://www.medicaid.gov/state-resource-center/medicaid-state-technical-assistance/health-home-information-resource-center/index.html. Accessed April 30, 2018.

40. California Department of Health Care Services. *Whole Person Care Program: Medi-Cal 2020 Waiver Initiative*. Sacramento, CA: California Department of Health Care Services; 2016. http://www.dhcs.ca.gov/provgovpart/Documents/WPCProgramOverview.pdf. Accessed April 30, 2018.

41. Cottrell E, Arkind J, Likumahuwa S. The alternative payment methodology in Oregon Community Health Centers: Empowering new ways of providing care. Bethesda, MD: Health Affairs Blog; 2014. https://www.healthaffairs.org/do/10.1377/hblog20140721.040242/full/. Accessed April 30, 2018.

42. Breslin E, Lambertino A, Heaphy D, Dreyfus T. *Medicaid and Social Determinants of Health: Adjusting Payment and Measuring Health Outcomes*. Princeton, NJ: Woodrow Wilson School of Public & International Affairs; 2017. https://www.healthmanagement.com/wp-content/uploads/SHVS_SocialDeterminants_HMA_July2017.pdf. Accessed April 30, 2018.

43. Oregon Health Authority. *Food Insecurity Screening Measure Specification Sheet*. Salem, OR: Oregon Health Authority; 2016.

44. Gottlieb LM, Tabbush V. Strategies for using healthcare dollars to support social services. *Generations*. 2018;42(1):36–40.

45. Rosenbaum S, Byrnes M, Rothenberg S, Gunsalus R. *Improving Community Health through Hospital Community Benefit Spending: Charting a Path to Reform*. Washington, DC: Milken Institute School of Public Health at George Washington University; 2016. https://hsrc.himmelfarb.gwu.edu/cgi/viewcontent.cgi?article=1825&context=sphhs_policy_facpubs. Accessed April 30, 2018.

46. Chen MA, Unruh MA, Pesko MF, et al. *The Role of Hospitals in Improving Non-Medical Determinants of Community Population Health*. New York: NYS Health Foundation; 2016. https://nyshealthfoundation.org/wp-content/uploads/2017/12/community-population-health-report-april-2016-1.pdf. Accessed April 30, 2018.

47. Democracy Collaborative. Hospitals aligned for healthy communities. http://hospitaltoolkits.org/. Accessed April 30, 2018.

48. Build Healthy Places Network. By joining forces, community developers and health professionals can have a more powerful impact. https://www.buildhealthyplaces.org/. Accessed April 30, 2018.

49. Institute of Medicine of the National Academies Committee on the Recommended Social and Behavioral Domains and Measures for Electronic Health Records. *Capturing Social and Behavioral Domains in Electronic Health Records: Phase 2.* Washington, DC: The National Academies Press; 2014.

50. Centers for Medicare & Medicaid Services. The Accountable Health Communities Health-Related Social Needs Screening Tool. Baltimore, MD: Centers for Medicare & Medicaid Services. https://innovation.cms.gov/Files/worksheets/ahcm-screeningtool.pdf. Accessed April 30, 2018.

51. HealthLeads. Social needs screening toolkit. Boston, MA: HealthLeads; 2018. https://healthleadsusa.org/tools-item/health-leads-screening-toolkit/. Accessed April 20, 2018.

52. Kaiser Permanente. Your Current Life Situation (Shorter Form) v.2.0. Oakland, CA: Kaiser Permanente; 2016. http://sirenetwork.ucsf.edu/sites/sirenetwork.ucsf.edu/files/Your%20Current%20Life%20Situation%20Questionnaire%20v2-0%20%28Core%20and%20supplemental%29%20no%20highlights.pdf. Accessed May 1, 2018.

Chapter 27

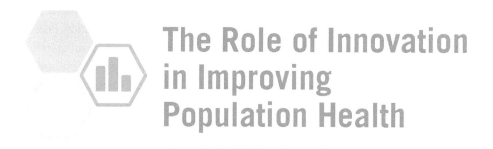

# The Role of Innovation in Improving Population Health

JESSICA SOLOMON FISHER AND KELLIE L. TETER

It can be disheartening to acknowledge that health care, including the provision of medical care, accounts for very little of what drives population health. Increasingly, health care providers want to contribute by "doing" population health work. At the same time, public health is increasingly moving to address upstream causes of inequities to get to the root causes of the so-called *social determinants of health* (SDHs). Across the public health and health care landscapes, common drivers are pushing for change, among them cost pressures, anxiety about the sustainability of traditional approaches, and the need to stay true to our mission while keeping the lights on. In our quest for population health, these and other drivers are pushing public health and health care toward a single tool: innovation. The process of innovating asks the question "How might we . . .?" For example, "How might we approach interrupting the major drivers of health?" The complex problems for which we are seeking solutions today could be characterized as "How might we use innovation to improve population health?" But first, what is innovation?

## INNOVATION

The term is used in many contexts today and implies different things to different people. If a product is new on the market (e.g., has just been invented), is it necessarily an innovation? If a technology exists elsewhere, but is newly applied in your sector, is that an innovation? If a process has been used by some businesses or agencies for years but is not yet pervasive, is its further dissemination an innovation? The answer to these and other questions depends on where you look. Myriad definitions and schools of thought relate to the term "innovation" as it applies to business, technology, solving social problems, and, of course, health. Add to that the need for a clear distinction between innovation and disruption, innovation and quality improvement, innovation and just plain change: the list goes on.

One perspective comes from the Public Health National Center for Innovations (PHNCI), a division of the Public Health Accreditation Board, which sought to bring clarity to these questions. To bring real meaning to the term innovation, for the field and its partners in the work of population health, PHNCI defines innovation in public health as "The development of a new process, policy, product, or program that increases quality, impact, and efficiency." The definition holds that the *power* of any innovation depends on the prevalence of certain characteristics, listed here, that, when present, support the definition:

- Is novel, new, or creative
- Reflects the dynamic state of change inherent in public health transformation
- Occurs by internal or cross-sector collaboration
- Involves co-production of the process, policy, product, or program with partners, stakeholders, and/or customers
- Has the potential to generate a new or improved means to create value
- Lends itself to adaptation and adoption/replication and diffusion
- Generates real-time information for evaluation and course correction
- Is open-source in some way (meaning that the process or the product, in its development and/or utilization, is publicly available for input, adaptation, adoption, or other use).[1]

## Co-production and Collaboration

Those who engage in co-production experience it as a dynamic, experimental, and reflective process sustained by different forms of engagement, including social interactions and relations that generate new forms of care that are outside of and beyond health care (e.g., inclusive relationships and authentic partnerships to achieve equity). This engagement revolves around values beyond economic value (e.g., equity, justice) and spawns new insights and research practices that are relevant to different disciplines and practices (e.g., community participation, patient advocacy, and collaborative research) (Box 27.1).[2]

## Design Thinking

In fact, both collaboration and co-production are key characteristics of *design thinking*, a common process used to support innovation. In design thinking, the situation is entirely viewed from the customer's perspective. We must be prepared to see things anew, including a change in what is, and is not, defined as problematic. For example, perhaps the customer sees the root cause of poor child health as the bias against men and fathers in nearly all health and human service settings. Looking at it from that point of view would take the design of problem-solving regarding child health in a whole new direction. Just imagine

> **Box 27.1 | Collaboration and Co-production in Innovation**
>
> Many aspects of innovation lead to success. Very often, collaboration, either internal to an industry or field or across sectors, can drive innovation.
>
> Co-production is another common characteristic that takes collaboration to the next level. Co-production is shared power and decision-making in the process of development. When we truly work alongside the community, not simply "on their behalf," we are engaging in co-production because power and decision-making are shared. Authentic co-production consistently produces solutions that look very different from typical population health approaches.
>
> An example of co-production is when staff from the health department, clinic, and schools come together with youth to form a Youth Sexual Health Collaborative to look at barriers and opportunities for young people (9–25 years) who need sexual health care. Such a group might, for example, apply a reproductive justice lens to traditional teen pregnancy prevention messages. They might determine that these messages are fundamentally shaming and do not honor the reproductive authority of young adults in their own lives.

what might be included in such a design. Innovation wells up from such new thinking—the type of thinking you can generate by applying certain tools and techniques. According to Tim Brown, CEO of the global design firm IDEO, "[d]esign thinking is a human-centered approach to innovation that draws from the designer's toolkit to integrate the needs of people, the possibilities of technology, and the requirements for business success."

Phases of design thinking are depicted in Figure 27.1 and Box 27.2. Although the figure illustrates a linear process, design thinking is iterative and flexible, with steps often occurring simultaneously or being repeated.

## Transformation via Innovation

Innovation is a process: a means to an end but not an end in itself. Ultimately, innovation can be transformational, such as public health and health care coming together to improve population health. Never has the need for this kind of transformation been more critical. According to a 2017 evaluation by the Commonwealth Fund, the US health care system is the worst among the 11 developed nations it analyzed as part of an evaluation conducted every 3 years.[3] Only through innovation, and ultimately system transformation, can individual and population health be assured as we, ideally, co-create the future.

## Emerging, Leading, and Prevailing

The journey to a transformed public health and health care system can be conceptualized as approaches, or practices, moving along three points on a spectrum: (1) emerging, (2) leading, and, ultimately, (3) prevailing.

# Figure 27.1 ▶

Phases of design thinking. Although the figure illustrates a linear process, actual design thinking is iterative and flexible, with steps often occurring simultaneously or being repeated.

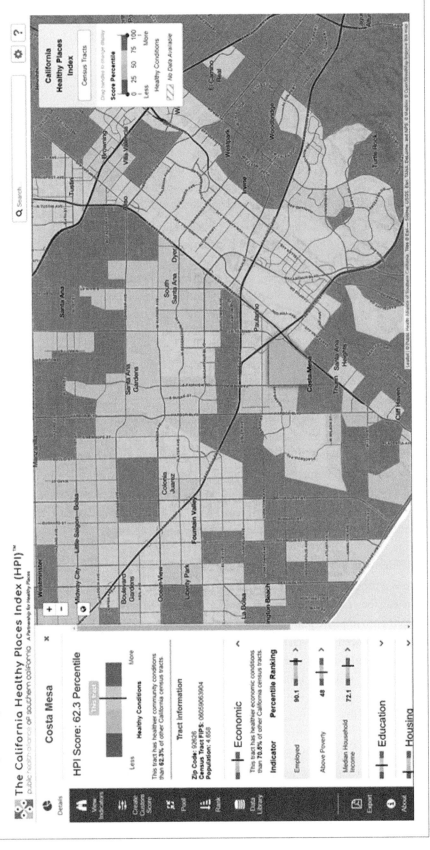

**Box 27.2 | California Healthy Places Index: Improving Population Health with Data in Action**

*Neil Maizlish, Helen Dowling, Tracy Delaney, Bill Sadler, Stephanie Caldwell, Derek Chapman, and Steve Woolf*

The California Healthy Places Index (HPI), developed by the Public Health Alliance of Southern California and Virginia Commonwealth University's Center on Society and Health, is a new tool that health care professionals can use to explore and address local conditions that influence life expectancy. The HPI provides overall scores for California communities and offers detailed data on specific policy actions that can improve population health, such as better housing, education, and health insurance. Because the index was derived from the statistical association between place-based factors and life expectancy, it quantifies the independent contribution of each policy action area across California. Put simply, it helps users identify policy areas with the greatest potential to impact population health.

The HPI is available online (http://healthyplacesindex.org) with user-friendly and actionable resources for health professionals and others working to improve health. The site includes the interactive HPI map and a thorough policy guide with practical solutions for improving local community conditions. The map includes robust features that allow users to view HPI scores, examine more than 40 health-related indicators for every census tract in California, create custom geographies, consider individual policy action areas, upload additional data, and prepare detailed reports.

Health care professionals, from frontline clinicians to CEOs, can use HPI information alongside input from community residents to prioritize investments to promote healthier community conditions. For instance, St. John's Health Center used HPI data for its 2016 Community Health Needs Assessment. The California Department of Public Health, and Los Angeles hospitals have used HPI to study community conditions that may explain high rates of pre-term births among African American women when developing their Community Birth Plan.

Marking the beginning of transformation, "emerging" practices are innovations. They come from one or a small group of practitioners and are brand new to the field. "Leading" practices are innovations that have been adapted and adopted or, perhaps, replicated by others. Although no longer considered innovative, they are not recognized as the usual way of doing business. Leading practices are widely viewed as best practices, and an increasing number of practitioners are likely to emulate them. Finally, "prevailing" practices are those that are accepted and are in play throughout the practice community. They are no longer considered leading practices because they have been diffused throughout the health care or public health community (Box 27.3). As an innovation first

**Box 27.3 | Examples of Emerging, Leading, and Prevailing**

Using electronic health records (EHR) to drive improved outcomes in primary care practice is an *emerging practice* in population health. Few are doing it, it is being used mostly as a pilot, and the technology and practice components are being innovated in real time. Today, across the patient care and public health landscapes and in medical research, we recognize patient voice/community input as a *leading practice*. It's still not the usual way of doing business, but we want it to be, and history upholds the promise. For example, when the HIV and AIDS epidemic came to the forefront 30 years ago, a strong tide pushed this change forward and patients began demanding a voice in everything from drug development to funding decisions. *Prevailing practices* are hard to see because they are prevailing. For example, patient consent for treatment or masking low-frequency events in a data set (to protect privacy) are prevailing practices that were once innovative, then emerging, later leading, and finally prevailing.

emerges, it may be transformative for the entity that develops the practice. "As evidence of the effectiveness of an innovation grows and it becomes a leading practice, and ultimately is recognized as a prevailing practice, it can transform the field."[1] This spectrum also exemplifies how an innovation can be diffused.[4] In regard to public health and health care coming together as a field to address population health, we are currently situated squarely in the emerging category, with agencies on both sides coming together to test new ways of doing business. Innovations themselves can be incremental or disruptive, and both can lead to transformation within an agency or field. To move along the spectrum toward leading and, ultimately, prevailing, we need to consider whether an innovation can be successfully diffused. Diffusion depends on variables related to the innovation itself, the characteristics of the adopters, and the social and political contexts, needs, and motivations of the potential adopter. Furthermore, opinion leaders' adoption of an innovation, often after careful study, leads to other organizations' adoption of an innovation without the same level of scrutiny.[5]

What then cultivates or suppresses innovation? Consider innovators located in governmental public health departments or in health care environments such as hospitals or clinics. Whether they are a small agency (61% of the nation's local health departments are considered small, serving populations smaller than 50,000[6]), a very large suburban or urban health department, an independent community clinic or private practice, or a gigantic health system or hospital, there are common traits.[6] For example, start-up businesses and businesses in general are less risk-averse than their public sector counterparts working in public health and health care. For the public sector, risk-taking seems riskier when lives are in the balance, and changes come at the notoriously slow speed of the scientific evidence base. And yet innovation clearly happens, often out of a kind of desperate necessity to solve stubborn problems. And as these fields increasingly intersect, there is a growing need to think creatively about how to innovate as a means to solve complex problems. Tom Kelley of the global design firm IDEO says "Fail often so you can succeed sooner." We would do well to take these words to heart. Innovation needs a protected space in any organization, as well as dedicated staff time, reporting at a high level, and no pressure to generate revenue. And these innovators need not only permission, but the very expectation that they will take risks and be rigorous in their scrutiny of every success and failure. They also need some kind of time pressure so that they will prototype, revise, and try again. Absent a deadline, they will work or plan forever on the perfect solution. If we know nothing else about innovation, we know this: If you put the same people in the same room for long enough, they will come up with the same solution (essentially) over and over again, absent some kind of disturbance in their routine. Changing the people, although straightforward, is not easy. Inviting new voices, assuring the power dynamics are such that all can speak and be heard, and taking the risk to act differently based on those ideas—including sometimes silencing old notions and ideas—is tricky work. Changing the room can be literal: get off your campus, out of your office, go over to the other side of town. Or it can be figurative: declaring (and then modeling) different methods of convening, decision-making, communicating, and evaluating and thus providing a new "space" to interact. Innovation processes also put an emphasis on moving more quickly than do traditional public health or health care approaches. Use of the evidence base and careful planning are important and valuable, but taking wild ideas and testing them on a small scale—not as a means to prove a hypothesis but as a means to learn from them—will result in a faster moving process and one that builds supporting evidence through prototyping along the way.

Public health and health care are dynamic fields, constantly adapting to the context of the community and issues that surround them. For public health, it might be changes in community health status or in the understanding of what impacts health outcomes (e.g., SDHs) that change practice. For health care, it might be a discovery about how disease works or a shift in how payments are reimbursed. With innovation as a tool in our toolkit, we have uncommon potential for success, especially with public health and health care overlapping in how we think about both the "problems" and the "solutions."

Innovations in public health practice are happening at agencies small and large. In public health, from promising work in the rural Garrett County Health Department in Maryland, where an open-source, online community engagement tool is being used to increase participation in community health improvement planning, to DuPage County, Illinois, where a sheriff's office and local health department are working together to reduce recidivism among those with mental illness in the criminal justice system, the time is ripe to improve population health. On the health care side, we have the concept of hospitals as anchor institutions leveraging assets as a means of improving community health, including hiring, purchasing, and investment for equitable, local economic impact.[7] To the extent that we appreciate the social SDHs as fundamental drivers of health, we must address the determinants in a fundamental way. Efforts by large institutions to go beyond living wages, for example, and begin to support wealth-building in the community through mechanisms such as capital investment in employee-owned businesses, are essential. (An example of this is the Cleveland Clinic, where they transformed from a contract with a national laundry service to an investment in an employee-owned laundry, providing wealth-building, jobs, and improved service for their hospital.[8]) This is a luminous example of population health efforts by health care to coalesce with public health strategies at the highest level. Through the coming together of public health and health care to advance innovations, those innovations can be amplified to address SDHs and further improve population health.

## INNOVATION AND IMPROVEMENT

What drives (or stifles) innovation in public health? What drives (or stifles) innovation in health care? And what challenges are inherent in being innovative in addressing population health?

Health care at the systems level is filled with uncertainty, especially at this moment. It might seem unfair to characterize the industry as risk averse, but neither is it a hotbed of innovation. Public health, often located in local and state government, is also a containing environment for innovators. Why is this?

When we think about performance or quality improvement in health care and in public health, we subscribe to improvement processes such as the plan-do-check-act cycle. Regardless of the model, the process will include collecting data and information, demonstrating a willingness to change, experimenting, and general use of a deliberate approach. From that perspective, innovation sounds familiar. "Quality improvement (QI) is used to improve existing processes, products, programs, or policies through technical solutions, whereas design thinking is used to solve complex problems for which there is not an existing process, product, program, or policy and, while taking the emotional state of the end user into account." [9] Innovation is distinct from QI in another important way: its starting assumption. QI starts with an assumption of the current state as imperfect and aims to improve it (i.e., create an ideal or more ideal state). Innovation (sustaining and, especially, disruptive innovation) seeks an entirely new approach, finding what is entirely inadequate for whatever reason. It is the difference between adjusting the recipe and reconsidering what items should constitute the food or the ingredients. For example, to address pregnancy-related depression, we can improve screening, assessment, referral, and treatment in dozens of ways, making it faster, easier, more universal, and less biased. Adding integrated behavioral health in primary care settings begins to look like innovation. Using design thinking to bring a community of women in recovery together to create what would have worked best for them as new moms might yield an innovation, such as training moms to be mentors.

To support cultures of quality that also foster innovation, leadership must continue to strongly support quality while at the same time actively protecting a space for innovation. The ability to take risks and to fail is inherent in innovation. Without leadership support, innovation can take place, but it may require being carried out "under the radar" or on a smaller scale.

## DISRUPTIVE INNOVATION

Considering the definition and characteristics already listed, we would argue that change is not necessarily innovation. Similarly, not all innovation is disruptive. Sustaining or incremental innovation—that which is novel or new, flowing in and improving, and becoming integrated into practice—is essential to transformation. Sustaining innovation is the most frequent condition for innovation. Disruptive innovation is less common and plays its own role. First identified as a phenomenon of markets and widely described (and debated) in business literature, disruptive innovation is evidenced by certain hallmarks. Among them is a threatened "incumbent"—those associated with the existing policy, process, or product—fighting to keep the status quo. In this condition, claims that change is too big a risk and that subpar quality will prevail under the (disruptive) innovation are a response to innovation that will disrupt the position of the incumbent. In business, this means losing business or, in the extreme, being pushed out of the market altogether.[10] In the business of population health, where we presumably want to "work ourselves out of a job," what is the role of disruption and our response to it?

Looking through a wide lens, we view the very existence of governmental health departments as a disruptive innovation—entering the market of health care when traditional methods of medicine and disease control were ineffective and at least partially inattentive to the well-being of specific segments of the population.[9]

Equally, health care, by moving into the population health space, is disrupting what for years has been traditional public health practice. If at first this perspective does not ring true, consider how you and your colleagues, as the incumbents positioned in public health, primary care, community health, or elsewhere, respond to the entrance of others into your area of mission and performance.

However, another way to look at the disruption would be to capitalize on the new entrant and champion a new provider to an overlooked segment of the market. If we can elegantly and with careful design promote disruption and protect and support innovation with regard to population health, then the result would be a new process, policy, product, or service that addresses a stubborn population health concern and unaddressed segment of the market.

*Disruption describes a process whereby a smaller company with fewer resources is able to successfully challenge established incumbent businesses. Specifically, as incumbents focus on improving their products and services for their most demanding (and usually most profitable) customers, they exceed the needs of some segments and ignore the needs of others. Entrants that prove disruptive begin by successfully targeting those overlooked segments, and gaining a foothold by delivering more suitable functionality—frequently at a lower price. Incumbents, chasing higher profitability in more demanding segments, tend not to respond vigorously. Entrants then move upmarket, delivering the performance that incumbents' mainstream customers require, while preserving the advantages that drove their early success. When mainstream customers start adopting the entrants' offerings in volume, disruption has occurred.[10(p. x)]*

How then does each of us promote and protect such (disruptive) innovation? What can public health and health care do together that is unprecedented? How do we create something new that sneaks into the cracks of what has been unaddressed by the existing approach? We believe we must use our most refined tools in a new way, including meaningful cross-sector partnerships, data sharing, and combined community health improvement planning processes. Innovate in the way you interface with the people and the community, insert design thinking into the dynamic, and put the "user" at the center of the process. Disrupt the power dynamic and co-create with shared decision-making. Consider that the same people, in the same room, for long enough, will produce essentially the same answer over and over again. Insist that something be different, whether it is the space (literally or figuratively), the people, or the time allotment. Commit to taking much more risk, failing much more often, and understanding your work in a way that is truly responsive to those you serve, even when it threatens your incumbency.

## TRANSFORMATION DEPENDS ON INNOVATION

The value that an innovation lens, and process, can add to population health practice is the point at which true transformation can take place. Embracing the characteristics of innovation, in particular collaboration, co-production, and the notion of "failing often to succeed sooner," can be incorporated into existing public health or health care practice. Innovation is occurring in population health practice. We are moving in the same direction and need to continue to come together to advance population health practice. The very idea of such a collaboration is driving transformation through building trust, balancing the tension between losing incumbency versus the mission of community health improvement, and addressing upstream causes to health inequities. The chapters that follow provide examples of innovation in practice.

### REFERENCES

1. Public Health National Center for Innovations. *Innovation in Governmental Public Health: Building a Roadmap*. Alexandria, VA: Public Health National Center for Innovations; 2017. http://phnci.org/uploads/resource-files/Innovation-in-Governmental-Public-Health-Building-a-Roadmap-02-2017.pdf. Accessed April 10, 2018.

2. Filipe A, Renedo A, Marston C. The co-production of what? Knowledge, values, and social relations in health care. *PLoS Biol*. 2017;15(5):e2001403. http://journals.plos.org/plosbiology/article?id=10.1371/journal.pbio.2001403. Accessed April 10, 2018.

3. Schneider EC, Sarnak DO, Squires D, Sha A, Doty MM. Mirror, mirror 2017: International comparison reflects flaws and opportunities for better U.S. health care. The Commonwealth Fund website. July 2017. http://www.commonwealthfund.org/interactives/2017/july/mirror-mirror/. Accessed April 12, 2018.

4. Rogers EM. *Diffusion of Innovation*. 5th ed. New York: Simon & Schuster; 2003.

5. Dearing JW, Cox JG. Diffusion of innovations theory, principles, and practice. *Health Aff*. 2018;37(2):183–90.

6. National Association of County & City Health Officials. 2016 National Profile of Local Health Departments. Published 2017. http://nacchoprofilestudy.org/wp-content/uploads/2017/10/ProfileReport_Aug2017_final.pdf. Accessed April 12, 2018.

7. Healthcare Anchor Network. About the Healthcare Anchor Network. Healthcare Anchor Network website. http://www.healthcareanchor.network/about.html. Accessed April 12, 2018.

8. Trent S. Turning health care into community wealth in Cleveland. *Next City*. May 10, 2018. https://nextcity.org/daily/entry/turning-healthcare-into-community-wealth-in-cleveland. Accessed May 16, 2018.

9. Fisher JS. Public Health Accreditation Board's innovation center continues the mission to advance the quality and performance of health departments. Supplement, impact of public health accreditation. *J Public Health Manag and Pract*. 2018;24(suppl 3):S117–9.

10. Christensen CM, Raynor ME, McDonald R. What is disruptive innovation? *Harv Business Rev*. December 2015. https://hbr.org/2015/12/what-is-disruptive-innovation. Accessed September 14, 2017.

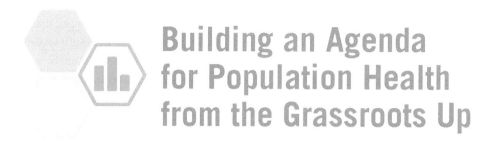

# Chapter 28

# Building an Agenda for Population Health from the Grassroots Up

TYLER NORRIS AND ASHLEY HILL

It may seem like a misplacement for a chapter on building an agenda for population health to be in the *Practical Playbook* section on "innovation." Building an agenda that creates "health for all" from the grassroots up hardly seems to fit the common mental model of "innovation" as something new, technology-based, or disruptive. Much of this work is nothing new: the Healthy Communities movement has been advancing for some 30 years, initially catalyzed by Healthy Boston, California Healthy Cities, and a collaboration between the US Department of Health and Human Services and the National Civic League.[1] It's not especially technology-based, although mapping and story tools such as Community Commons (https://www.communitycommons.org/) have made it easier to advance place-based health improvement work by giving users the ability to collect, see, and share publicly available data while shaping solutions-based narratives of communities' health.

Turning to communities to build an agenda for population health that goes beyond "doing good things" and instead is "accountable for outcomes," though, holds massive potential to be disruptive. Frankly, the current approaches in many places, including those that feature "collective impact" framing, must be disrupted. Despite promising work, a measurable and sustained improvement in population health outcomes has not occurred over the past few decades. Findings on diseases and deaths of despair, such as those reported in Pain in the Nation (www.paininthenation.org) initiative, demonstrate trends moving in the wrong direction and remind us that, as a nation, we have a long way to go.

A disruptive, community-created agenda must address chronic fragmentation and move toward comprehensiveness. This means operationalizing a "health in all practices, all policies, and all investments" approach, addressing all community systems concurrently and taking actions with sufficient "dose" (reach, intensity, and duration)[2] to assure the conditions for intergenerational well-being.

## WHERE ARE WE NOW? MAJOR OBSTACLES TO POPULATION HEALTH IMPROVEMENT

The path to population health improvement faces a litany of challenges, many of which are detailed throughout this book. Most notably, the US health system exists as a marketplace for care (not health, per se) where resources are by and large dedicated to the provision of medical care services, mostly treating people after they become sick. Only at the margin does the sector address the factors that keep people from becoming sick in the first place. With persistent—and often profitable—market incentives that favor volume over value, less than 4% of the US health care dollar goes toward creating the environments, incentives, and behavior change that underlie improvement in population health outcomes.

Furthermore, the health- and medical care-centric system we do have is severely fragmented. We have disassociated physical from mental health, despite both being vital elements of overall well-being. Even the federal agencies that research and resource health treat the two separately: mental health is segmented within the National Institutes of Health (NIH), distinct from other institutes that address physical health. The Substance Abuse and Mental Health Services Administration (SAMHSA) provides funding distinct from the Centers for Medicare and Medicaid Services (CMS) and Centers for Disease Control and Prevention (CDC) funding, with money going to separate agencies at the state level for largely disassociated interventions. Attempts to integrate physical and behavioral health in multidisciplinary health settings have been underfunded and generally ignored.[1] Generations of general practitioners, frontline clinicians, and public health practitioners have not been taught to value the mind–body connection or given practical training on how to treat behavioral health as attentively as they would treat their patients' physical health.

The greater societal context in which our health system is situated is also deeply troubled. The scars of genocide and displacement of native peoples, slavery, internment, sexism, racism, nativism, classism, and systematic disenfranchisement all cast long shadows. These issues have left terrible legacies of inequitable opportunities and disparate health outcomes between different groups of people, legacies that are not easily erased.

## OVERCOMING THE OBSTACLES

The United States spends much and gets little in terms of population health from the care system we have. To complicate matters even further for health care providers, there remains much uncertainty around reimbursement models as providers enter into more arrangements putting them "at risk" for the outcomes of their patients and covered lives.

In the face of this misaligned and scarred system, the innovation challenge is this: How do we transition from the "dose-insufficient," shorter term, single-issue programs, projects, and initiatives that are too often typical of philanthropic and governmental approaches to collaboratively addressing community health via a comprehensive, longer term approach that is a well-being investment and policy *strategy* for the community? In other words: *How do we amplify comprehensiveness?*

Across the nation, pockets of promise and solutions are rising like an immune response to meet this innovation challenge. Since the late 1980s, thousands of independent, multisector, collaborative partnerships have gradually but steadfastly arisen in communities across the country. These partnerships—between hospitals and health systems, local and national businesses, neighborhood and faith-based groups, social service organizations, philanthropic partners, community members, and others (many of which are referenced throughout this book, and two of which are detailed in the following text of this chapter) are the antibodies to the current system. By coming together to address the complex network of factors that lead to population health and health equity, our communities are beginning to do what it takes to move from a system of *health care* to a system of *health* (and associated well-being). They are attending to the minds and spirits as well as the bodies of their communities and focusing on whole-person health. And they are addressing the deep scars left on their populations by adverse community experiences.

## EXAMPLES: PARTNERSHIPS IN OAKLAND AND OKLAHOMA CITY

### Oakland

In 2016, the city of Oakland, California, launched Oakland Promise, using a "cradle-to-career" approach to significantly increase college graduation levels. The initiative includes the Brilliant Baby program, where $500 is set aside in a college savings account for every baby born into poverty in the city. Parents of these babies who enroll in financial coaching programs receive an additional $500. Kindergartners and first-graders in poverty are also eligible for college scholarships and parent engagement activities, and "Future Centers" at local high schools help high schoolers apply for financial aid and connect them with mentors. The program is unique in its multisector approach; spearheaded by the city of Oakland government, it is largely funded by private philanthropy. Services are provided through the local public school district, and families can sign up for the Brilliant Baby program at clinics and newborn support programs throughout the city. Other community partners provide wraparound services, such as legal rights education. Over its first 2 years, the Oakland Promise program has resulted in $5.5 million in scholarships and 670 students enrolled in college with scholarships and mentors. The initiative serves African American, Asian, and Latino children at equal or higher rates than those of the overall local public school population.[3] To those who claim that college graduation is not a health issue, consider that people who have not attended college are living shorter, less healthy lives and reporting higher levels of stress compared with college graduates.[4]

### Oklahoma City

In 2009, then-mayor of Oklahoma City, Mick Cornett, created an agenda for a healthier city through a series of comprehensive improvement projects. The city initiated a 1% sales tax to fund improvements in public transit, sidewalks along major city streets, and the completion of a citywide system of biking and walking trails. The city created an Olympic-class rowing complex and added lighting along the Oklahoma River to light up after-dark rowing races.[5,6] They created new senior wellness centers.[7] Partners in the effort included local foundations, local businesses, and local tribal groups. The positive business effects of a healthy community were a major highlight of the overall effort. Mayor Cornett emphasized the importance of employee livability for potential employers, as well as the potential health care costs and absenteeism costs of an unhealthy population.[8] The effort resulted in 1 million pounds of weight lost community-wide and the lowest unemployment levels in the United States.[9]

Part of what makes these examples so compelling is that these communities faced the same challenges that all communities face, a system focused on health care instead of health, fragmentation, and rooted health inequities, as well as additional localized challenges, and yet they still were able to act and improve health for their community members. But why? Why were these changes able to come from community-led collaboratives and not mandates or policy changes?

One reason may be the beautifully simple fact that community members aren't siloed by sector. An individual "community member" is a family member, a friend, an employee, a boss, a shopper at the local grocery store, a voter, a Frisbee player in the local park, a pet owner, a neighbor, and a concerned citizen rolled into one. Community emphasizes the connections between people and between all the different forces that affect people's daily lives. Similarly, addressing population health also requires an emphasis on the connections between all the different factors that affect people's daily lives: housing, transportation, education, public safety, relationships, social connections, and behavioral as well as physical health.

## THE PATH FORWARD: BUILDING A POPULATION HEALTH AGENDA

The true innovation here—the disruptive idea—is not that communities are addressing health in a way that the federal and many state governments seem unable to do, it is in how we might build on the foundations that communities are laying. If we do nothing but step back and applaud these efforts, we will ultimately fail in achieving population-level health impacts.

All partners need to commit to more than short-term, small-scale grants and pilot initiatives. We need to start by applying sufficient "dose"—reach, intensity, and duration of the interventions—to achieve population-level impacts.[10] As long as sectors "stay in their own lanes" and organizational practices, public policies, and investment priorities stay disconnected from one another, our efforts will continue to be insufficient.

One place to start is with collaboration between sectors. Arthur Himmelman describes inter-organization or inter-sector work as being on a spectrum: coordination, cooperation, collaboration. Collaboration "is a relationship in which each organization wants to help its partners become the best that they can be at what they do . . . when organizations collaborate they share risks, responsibilities, and rewards, each of which contributes to enhancing each other's capacity to achieve a common purpose."[11] In other words, working in collaboration helps each organization to use resources differently and achieve more together than they could alone. Community partnerships across the nation are all over the board on degree of collaboration; there is a wide degree of variation in what they do, how they work, and their efficacy. Moving toward more collaboration will require overcoming the barriers of time, trust, and turf.[12]

We also need to view healthy communities from the lens and the lived experience of the most vulnerable. Vulnerable populations need to be involved at every stage of a healthy community design process because they understand the nature of what their needs are. As communities move toward collaboration and build a comprehensive system of practices, policies, and investments, they also need to build in comprehensiveness of experience for those in the system. Programs and policies need to be knitted together not just to provide adequate dose, but also to create a seamless experience for those who need it most. Services for newborns should be connected to services for mothers. School services should be connected to job training for youth and then job placement for those youth as they age. Clinical services in a doctor's office should be connected to social services and programs in the community. Think from the view of a community member, from the view of vulnerable populations, across life stages—*are we regularly assessing the social, economic, and environmental needs of individuals? Are we making warm referrals from one program to another? Are we leveraging anchor institution strategies?*[12] *Are we leading for comprehensiveness?*

Just as it took generations to build our way to the dysfunctional health system that we have, it will likely take time to rebuild the system that we want from the grassroots up. There is reason for optimism, though. In a recent poll, both Republicans and Democrats named the same priorities when it comes to community health: affordable housing, access to healthy food, and affordable childcare.[13] If we can create a common agenda for population health, we have an unusual, unifying opportunity to hold elected officials across political persuasions to that shared agenda.

Moving from individual projects to whole-person, whole-community, dose-sufficient strategies will require an "all-in" approach, in which multisector collaboration is not optional but required. Hospitals, insurance companies, and health services providers can contribute leadership and direction and fund incentives in alignment with whole-person health. Policymakers can break down legal and bureaucratic barriers to collaboration and incentivize, enact, and fund what works. Some of the other unique and shared roles that various stakeholders should prepare to take on are detailed in the following sections.

## SUGGESTED ACTIONS FOR EACH SECTOR
### Health Care Providers

- Make social needs assessments a standard of care; systematically assess the social needs of patients and build such assessments into care tools, such as electronic medical records.
- Make referrals to community-based organizations a standard of care, and build these organizations' capacities.
- Encourage multidisciplinary health approaches wherever possible. Educate clinicians on mind–body linkages and incentivize appropriate integrated prevention and treatment for both behavioral and physical health.
- Examine inequities in the populations that you serve, and change any practices, policies, or investments that may be perpetuating those inequities, intentionally or unintentionally.
- Lead by taking on data- and risk-sharing where appropriate.
- Adopt anchor institution strategies to address the economic, social, and environmental conditions that impact health.[14]

### Health Care Payers

- Pay for multidisciplinary approaches to health, not just medical approaches, wherever possible. Provide incentives for providers and individuals to focus on health rather than health care.
- Support providers who educate clinicians on mind–body linkages, and incentivize appropriate treatment for integrating behavioral and physical health.
- Where possible, quantify the benefits and costs of upstream and community-based interventions and share these with other potential funders to incentivize co-investment.
- Examine inequities in the populations that you serve and change any practices, policies, or investments that may be perpetuating those inequities, intentionally or unintentionally.

### Health Policymakers (Federal, State, and Local)

- For federal payers (i.e., Centers for Medicare and Medicaid Services [CMS]), continue efforts that allow state Medicaid programs flexibility in addressing social needs of covered patients.
- Enhance connectivity across health, other social programs, and other government services by supporting comprehensive approaches, such as "Health in All Policies" resolutions.[15]

### Health Care Investors

- Seek out investment opportunities that promote health, not just health care.
- Examine inequities in investments you make and the stakeholders they work with (e.g., consumers, workforce, suppliers, leadership) and encourage changes in any practices, policies, or investments that may be perpetuating those inequities, intentionally or unintentionally.

### Academic Institutions

- Engage in community-based participatory research (CBPR) (for more on CBPR training, check out the CBPR Partnership Academy, led by the Detroit Community-Academic Urban Research Center, a 20-year-old CBPR partnership[16]).
- Adopt anchor institution strategies to address the economic, social, and environmental conditions that impact health.

### Community Organizations

- Resist the mindset of "stick to what you know" or "stay in your own lane." Continuously improve your programs, but also seek to make connections between your sector and others. Look for shared interests and seek out opportunities for collaboration.
- Examine inequities in the populations that you serve and change any practices, policies, or investments that may be perpetuating those inequities, intentionally or unintentionally.

### Business Community

- Encourage whole-health community approaches rather than narrow, traditional workplace wellness programs.
- Examine inequities in your external and internal stakeholder populations (e.g., consumers, workforce, suppliers, leadership) and change any practices, policies, or investments that may be perpetuating those inequities, intentionally or unintentionally.
- Adopt anchor institution strategies to address the economic, social, and environmental conditions that impact health.

**All**

- Understand the difference between "health care" and "health." Reiterate this difference—and the importance of focusing on health and well-being—to others.
- Educate yourself on existent inequities in your communities: Which groups of people are disproportionately unhealthier than others? Which groups of people have inequitable access to opportunities to become healthy or stay healthy? Which groups of people have inequitable access to the factors that determine health, such as safe neighborhoods, good education, and strong relationships?
- In times of potential disagreement, emphasize the shared values underlying a focus on health. Remember, most people already agree that these are priorities!
- Be persistent. Come at this work with the energy of a sprinter, but understand that it's going to take the endurance of a marathoner to accomplish lasting population health improvement.
- Remember that you yourself cross sectors and roles. Walk the walk. If you have a choice, seek care from clinicians who participate in community health efforts. Vote for politicians who put community health at the top of their agenda. Purchase from businesses that commit to community health and equitable wealth-building in local communities. Help break down stigma between mental and physical health with your language and presence with others. Educate and encourage your loved ones, neighbors, coworkers, and friends to do the same.

No matter who you are or what role you play within the health system, you can take a leadership role in crafting and spreading this agenda. The role of the leader is to ask yourself the following questions: Is there an understanding of the outcomes from current efforts? Is there clarity about what you're getting from your current efforts? And if your current efforts aren't generating the outcomes, then what is it going to take to do so, and how are you going to do that?

The fundamental disruption needed to advance population health in a way that results in significantly improved health and well-being for all is one of up-leveling civic leadership. This asks more of each of us, wherever we serve. Nothing less than the well-being of our nation is on the line.

### REFERENCES

1. Norris T. Healthy Communities at Twenty-Five: Participatory democracy and the prospect for American renewal. 2014. *National Civic Rev.* Winter 2013. doi:10.1002/ncr.21142.

2. Schwartz P, Rauzon S, Cheadle A. Dose matters: an approach to strengthening community health strategies to achieve greater impact. Discussion paper, National Academy of Medicine. Washington, DC. Published August 26, 2015. https://nam.edu/wp-content/uploads/2015/08/Perspective_DoseMatters.pdf. Accessed March 20, 2018.

3. Kaiser Permanente Center for Community Health and Evaluation. Population dose: understanding, measuring, and boosting the impact of community health interventions. Published July 2015. https://share.kaiserpermanente.org/wp-content/uploads/2015/08/DoseOverview.pdf. Accessed March 20, 2018.

4. Case A, Deaton A. Mortality and morbidity in the 21st century. Brookings Papers on Economic Activity. Spring 2017. https://www.brookings.edu/wp-content/uploads/2017/08/casetextsp17bpea.pdf. Accessed April 20, 2018.

5. Nellenbach M. Economic growth and better health in Oklahoma City. Bipartisan Policy Center. October 2, 2013. https://bipartisanpolicy.org/blog/economic-growth-and-better-health-oklahoma-city/. Accessed April 29, 2018.

6. Godfrey E. Eight OKC-area schools compete in rowing, kayaking championships. NewsOK. November 16, 2011. http://newsok.com/article/3623885. Accessed April 29, 2018.

7. Snyder T. Oklahoma City mayor Mick Cornett: We have to build this city for people. Streetsblog USA. January 24, 2013. https://usa.streetsblog.org/2013/01/24/oklahoma-city-mayor-mick-cornett-we-have-built-this-city-for-cars/. Accessed April 29, 2018.

8. Gardner A. Oklahoma City attracts businesses, gets healthy with smart growth principles. Smart Growth America. March 23, 2011. https://smartgrowthamerica.org/oklahoma-city-attracts-businesses-gets-healthy-with-smart-growth-principles/. Accessed April 29, 2018.

9. Cornett M. Interview transcript. Smart Growth Stories: common sense smart growth investments in Oklahoma City. April 4, 2012. Smart Growth America. https://smartgrowthamerica.org/app/legacy/documents/smart-growth-stories_cornett-transcript.pdf. Accessed April 29, 2018.

10. Schwartz P, Rauzon S, Cheadle A. Dose matters: an approach to strengthening community health strategies to achieve greater impact. Discussion paper, National Academy of Medicine. Washington, DC. Published August 26, 2015. https://nam.edu/wp-content/uploads/2015/08/Perspective_DoseMatters.pdf. Accessed March 20, 2018

11. Himmelman AT. Collaboration for change. 2002. https://depts.washington.edu/ccph/pdf_files/4achange.pdf. Accessed April 28, 2018.

12. Norris T, Howard T. Can hospitals heal America's communities? 2016. The Democracy Collaborative. https://democracycollaborative.org/sites/clone.community-wealth.org/files/downloads/CanHospitalsHeal AmericasCommunities.pdf. Accessed April 28, 2018.

13. Onie R. Why don't we deliver the health we should? Oral presentation at: NEJM Catalyst event Expanding the Bounds of Care Delivery: Integrating Mental, Social, and Physical Health; January 25, 2018; Nashville, TN. Accessed April 2, 2018.

14. Norris T, Howard T. Can hospitals heal America's communities? 2016. The Democracy Collaborative. https://democracycollaborative.org/sites/clone.community-wealth.org/files/downloads/CanHospitalsHeal AmericasCommunities.pdf. Accessed March 25, 2018.

15. Rudolph L, Caplan J, Ben-Moshe K, Dillon L. *Health in All Policies: A Guide for State and Local Governments*. Washington, DC and Oakland, CA: American Public Health Association and Public Health Institute; 2013. Accessed April 29, 2018.

16. Coombe CM, Israel BA, Reyes AG, et al. Community-Based Participatory Research (CBPR) Partnership Academy: A national initiative to promote health equity by enhancing CBPR capacity. Oral presentation at: American Public Health Association Annual Meeting; November, 2015; Chicago, IL. https://apha.confex.com/apha/143am/webprogram/Paper327332.html. Accessed March 27, 2018.

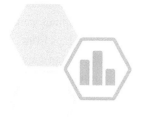

# Case Study—The Alliance for Health Equity: Hospitals, Health Departments, and Community Partners Working Together for Health Equity in Chicago and Suburban Cook County

JESS LYNCH, MEGAN CUNNINGHAM, AND JULIE MORITA

Chicago and suburban Cook County epitomize a complex health care and public health landscape, consisting of more than 40 hospitals, dozens of Federally Qualified Health Centers (FQHCs), six certified local health departments, and hundreds of community-based organizations, all serving 5.2 million residents living in more than 130 municipalities and 77 Chicago community areas. There is no doubt that the landscape can seem daunting, especially with the layering on of political jurisdictions; however, there is also extraordinary potential to align and coordinate resources to positively impact community health.

In 2015, several factors converged, resulting in opportunities to tap into that collective community health potential:

- *Community health needs assessment (CHNA) and common priorities.* Hospitals were gearing up to start CHNAs and also recognizing that there was substantial overlap in community health priorities.
- *Health department leadership on health equity.* The Chicago Department of Public Health (CDPH) started off 2015 under new leadership, and Commissioner Julie Morita was steadfast in centering health equity as the core principle for Healthy Chicago 2.0. The Cook County Department of Public Health (CCDPH), serving nearly all of suburban Cook County,

was simultaneously building its community health WePLAN 2020 on a core principle of health equity.

- *Leaders within hospitals and health systems.* Key leaders from community hospital systems, academic medical centers, and safety net hospitals were willing to get involved in the messy work of building partnerships from the ground up, with a commitment to taking a community-engaged approach to their work and to finding ways to harness the potential impact of collaborative work.
- *Community organizations seeking a more unified approach to working on health equity.* Key community-based organizations helped to lead the way in pushing for a more unified approach to addressing social and structural determinants of health (SDHs).
- *A public health institute with a mission to align public health systems for greater health improvement.* The Illinois Public Health Institute (IPHI), with expertise in community health improvement, sought to promote efficiency and impact through collaborative approaches. IPHI worked closely with several hospital partners, CDPH, and CCDPH to shepherd the idea of a collaborative from concept to initiation.
- *A common recognition that the major issues driving health inequities cannot be solved by any one institution on its own and a willingness to put aside competition to work on them.*

This alchemy of factors in 2015 resulted in the launch of two hospital collaboratives with similar goals and even several hospital members in common. In 2017, the two collaboratives merged to form the Alliance for Health Equity. The success of this merger is a testament to the commitment of the hospital and public health leaders to a common vision of health equity and their opposition to letting competition or individual interests undermine the collective potential.

As of March 2018, the Alliance for Health Equity partnership includes 35 hospitals, 6 certified local health departments, and nearly 100 regional and community partners, with the IPHI as the backbone organization. All of those stakeholders collaboratively developed the Alliance for Health Equity's collective purpose, vision, and values, which have been particularly instrumental in holding us accountable to our health equity purpose and in prioritizing the work of the Alliance for Health Equity (Figures 29.1 and 29.2).

The most significant financial support comes from the hospitals, whose membership contributions support the core infrastructure and staffing for the Alliance for Health Equity, ongoing implementation design, and CHNA. Several foundations helped to launch the work and support implementation initiatives. The Otho S. A. Sprague Memorial Institute was instrumental in launching one of the collaboratives and continues to provide support to ensure that the merger is effective and also to underwrite participation by safety net hospitals. The Robert Wood Johnson Foundation funded an early developmental evaluation

## Figure 29.1 ▼

Collective purpose, vision, and values of the Alliance for Health Equity.

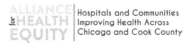 Hospitals and Communities
Improving Health Across
Chicago and Cook County

**Collective Purpose:**
Improve population and community health by:

- Promoting **health equity**
- **Capacity building**, shared learning, and connecting local initiatives
- Addressing **social and structural determinants of health**
- Developing broad city/county wide initiatives and **creating systems**
- Engaging community partners and **working collaboratively** with community leaders
- **Developing data systems** for population health to support shared impact measurement and community assessment
- Collaborating on **population health policy and advocacy**

**Vision:** Improved health equity, wellness, and quality of life across Cook County

**Values:**

1. We believe the highest level of health for all people can only be achieved through the pursuit of social justice and elimination of health disparities and inequities.
2. We value having a shared vision and goals with alignment of strategies to achieve greater collective impact while addressing the unique needs of our individual communities.
3. Honoring the diversity of our communities, we value and will strive to include all voices through meaningful community engagement and participatory action.
4. We are committed to emphasizing assets and strengths and ensuring a process that identifies and builds on existing community capacity and resources.
5. We are committed to data-driven decision making through implementation of evidence-based practices, measurement and evaluation, and using findings to inform resource allocation and quality improvement.
6. We are committed to building trust and transparency through fostering an atmosphere of open dialogue, compromise, and decision making.
7. We are committed to high quality work to achieve the greatest impact possible

that was based on a collective impact framework and helped the Alliance for Health Equity understand successes and identify areas for improvement. Other funding partners for initiatives described in this chapter include the Chicago Community Trust, Chicagoland Workforce Funders Alliance, Michael Reese Health Trust, Polk Brothers Foundation, and the J. B. and M. K. Pritzker Family Foundation.

The Alliance for Health Equity is intentionally working both to (1) form direct partnerships for large-scale systems change and collective impact and (2) align and connect across local collaborative efforts for health equity. As a result, the Alliance for Health Equity partners with collaboratives such as West Side United, South Side Health Collaborative, and Proviso Partners for Health to share and scale efforts.

SDHs and substance use are the two primary implementation priorities for the Alliance for Health Equity. The following sections highlight three key areas of implementation: (1) housing, (2) mental health and substance use, and (3) community safety through community development.

**Figure 29.2** ▽

Structure of the Alliance for Health Equity.

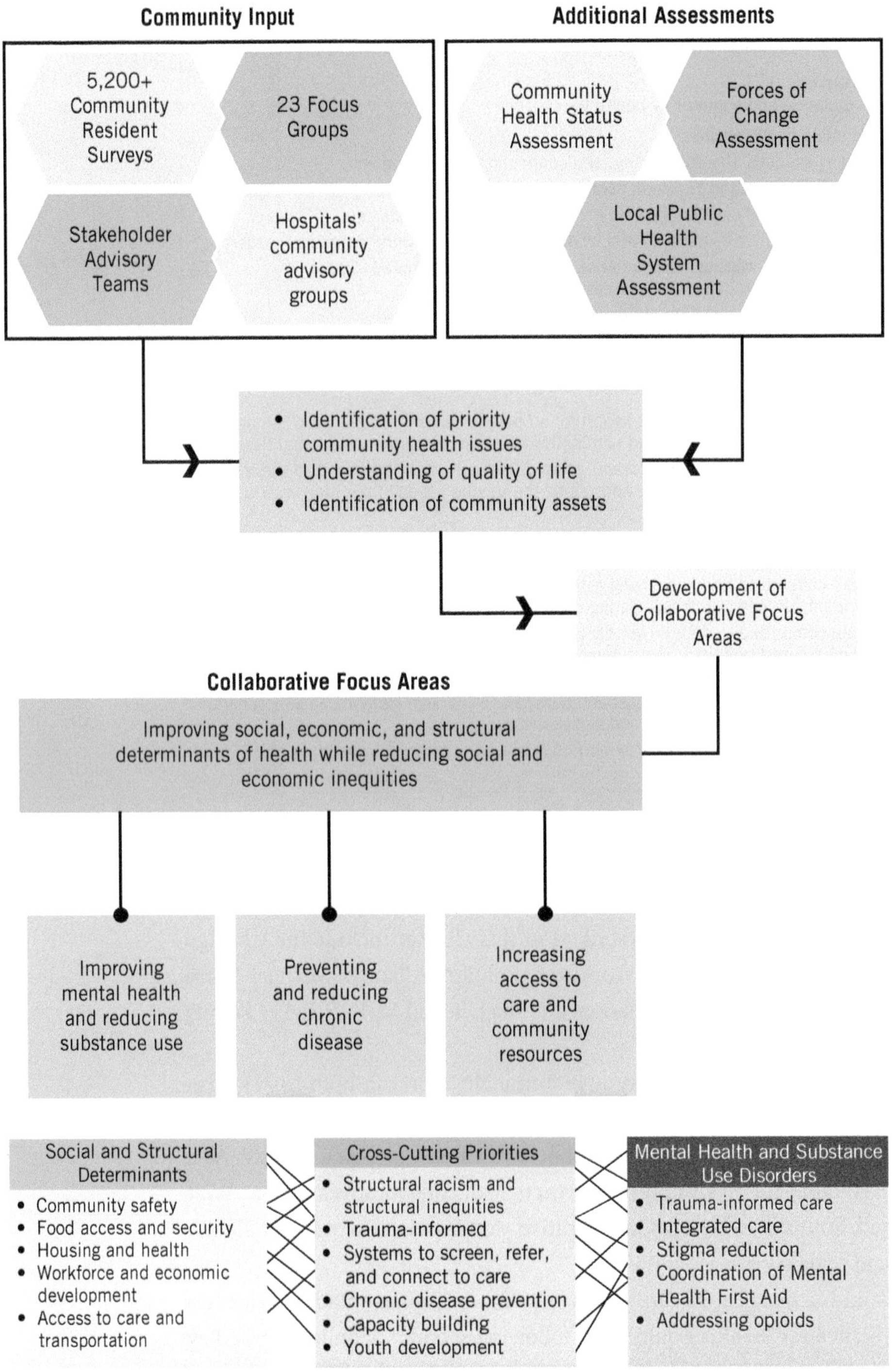

**Community Input**

5,200+ Community Resident Surveys

23 Focus Groups

Stakeholder Advisory Teams

Hospitals' community advisory groups

**Additional Assessments**

Community Health Status Assessment

Forces of Change Assessment

Local Public Health System Assessment

- Identification of priority community health issues
- Understanding of quality of life
- Identification of community assets

Development of Collaborative Focus Areas

**Collaborative Focus Areas**

Improving social, economic, and structural determinants of health while reducing social and economic inequities

Improving mental health and reducing substance use

Preventing and reducing chronic disease

Increasing access to care and community resources

**Social and Structural Determinants**

- Community safety
- Food access and security
- Housing and health
- Workforce and economic development
- Access to care and transportation

**Cross-Cutting Priorities**

- Structural racism and structural inequities
- Trauma-informed
- Systems to screen, refer, and connect to care
- Chronic disease prevention
- Capacity building
- Youth development

**Mental Health and Substance Use Disorders**

- Trauma-informed care
- Integrated care
- Stigma reduction
- Coordination of Mental Health First Aid
- Addressing opioids

## HOUSING

Healthy Chicago 2.0, Suburban Cook County WePLAN 2020, Alliance for Health Equity, and the CHNA, all identify housing as an area with substantial partnership opportunities in Chicago and Cook County. As a result, the Alliance for Health Equity started a Housing and Health Workgroup in partnership with CDPH. Fifteen hospitals, several FQHCs and health care associations, and numerous housing stakeholders participate in the workgroup.

- The University of Illinois (UI) Hospital and Health Sciences System piloted a "Better Health Through Housing" initiative to pay for supportive housing for homeless individuals using emergency department (ED) services, in partnership with the Center for Housing and Health. For the 18 people who were housed through the pilot, UI Health saw a 62% decrease in ED visits, 60% decrease in inpatient days, and 21% decrease in the participants' cost to the health system. As a result of the collaboration in the Alliance for Health Equity Housing Workgroup, three additional health systems are now funding Better Health Through Housing programs for homeless people frequenting their EDs.
- As a next stage in this work, the Corporation for Supportive Housing (CSH) is working with health and housing partners to establish a "flexible housing pool" (FHP) as a sustainable collective solution to the shortage of permanent supportive housing in Chicago and Cook County. Design of the FHP began in 2017, and the first individuals will be housed in 2018. The FHP will allow for funders across sectors—government, philanthropy, health care, and business—to invest in permanent supportive housing units for people with comorbidities and high use of multiple systems (e.g., hospital EDs, jail, emergency medical services [EMS]). The FHP aims to raise $12 million during the first two phases of implementation to establish 750 new units of permanent supportive housing.
- In addition to these initiatives, hospitals and health systems in Chicago and suburban Cook County are involved in a number of healthy homes initiatives, including a pay-for-performance pilot focused on environmental triggers for asthma, medical respite programs, and efforts to build data-sharing systems between health and housing. The Housing and Health Workgroup provides a forum to share the progress of these initiatives and identify new partnerships and ways to scale success.

## MENTAL HEALTH AND SUBSTANCE USE

Mental health and substance use are also top priorities for CCDPH and CDPH. Throughout 2016–2018, CDPH, the Cook County Health and Hospitals System and CCDPH, and the Cook County Medical Examiner's Office have demonstrated unprecedented levels of collaboration across jurisdictions to establish more complete data related to opioids in Cook County through yearly joint data briefs.

The Alliance for Health Equity has established six areas of impact for mental health and substance use that align with Healthy Chicago 2.0 and WePLAN 2020: reduced stigma, increased access, increased coordination, increased integration and quality of care for both mental health and opioids, increased trauma-informed institutions and communities, and increased peer employment roles.

Through the Alliance for Health Equity, hospitals and other health care partners are working with public health, community mental health providers, policy leaders, and individuals with lived experience to implement strategies to make positive change in these areas of impact.

As shown in Figure 29.3, several of the Alliance for Health Equity's committees and workgroups are working on these strategy areas, including the Mental Health and Substance Use Committee and the Trauma-Informed Hospitals Collaborative Committee, Policy Committee, and Housing Workgroup. The Alliance for Health Equity and partners are currently at the stage of developing metrics to assess the impact of these strategies.

The Trauma-Informed Hospitals Collaborative Workgroup includes 16 hospitals and health systems in the Chicago area that have been actively working for the past year to become trauma-informed organizations. This collaboration is convened by the Illinois ACE Response Collaborative and Health & Medicine Policy Research Group in partnership with CDPH and leaders from participating hospitals, including physicians, behavioral health directors, hospital managers, administrators, and hospital leadership, to join CDPH in achieving its goal of making Chicago a trauma-informed city. Building on foundational ACE/Trauma 101 training, workgroup participants have inventoried existing trauma-informed efforts at their institutions, begun to explore existing institutional priorities through a framework of understanding trauma as a root cause and trauma-informed care as a solution, and identified project teams and project management resources. They have also begun to adapt a CDPH tool for organization-wide surveying in preparation for training and staff development, and they are preparing to focus on supporting staff wellness and resilience.

## COMMUNITY SAFETY AND COMMUNITY DEVELOPMENT

Community safety is a top priority for many of the hospitals participating in the Alliance for Health Equity. Many of them have long-standing violence prevention partnerships, implementing programs such as the Cure Violence/CeaseFire model, and are interested in building out partnerships to have more impact on reducing violence and increasing community safety. Many organizations across the city have been working to develop a holistic, multifaceted

## Figure 29.3 ▼

Alliance for Health Equity strategy and impact areas.

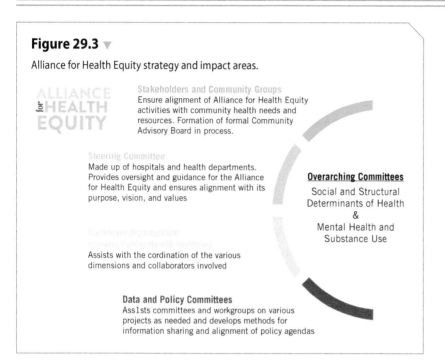

**ALLIANCE for HEALTH EQUITY**

**Stakeholders and Community Groups**
Ensure alignment of Alliance for Health Equity activities with community health needs and resources. Formation of formal Community Advisory Board in process.

**Steering Committee**
Made up of hospitals and health departments. Provides oversight and guidance for the Alliance for Health Equity and ensures alignment with its purpose, vision, and values

**Backbone Organization Illinois Public Health Institute)**
Assists with the cordination of the various dimensions and collaborators involved

**Data and Policy Committees**
Ass1sts committees and workgroups on various projects as needed and develops methods for information sharing and alignment of policy agendas

**Overarching Committees**
Social and Structural Determinants of Health
&
Mental Health and Substance Use

approach for health care to engage in violence prevention and community safety (Figure 29.4).

The Alliance for Health Equity is participating in collaborative initiatives on health care–focused workforce and economic development initiatives led by the Chicagoland Healthcare Workforce Collaborative, West Side Anchors/West

## Figure 29.4 ▼

Multifaceted framework for health care engagement in violence prevention.

| Strategy Areas | Impact Areas | | | | | |
|---|---|---|---|---|---|---|
| ALLIANCE for HEALTH EQUITY — Hospitals and Communities Improving Health Across Chicago and Cook County | ↓ Stigma | ↑ Access | ↑ Integration & Quality Care for Both MH + Opioids | ↑ Coordination of Systems | ↑ Trauma-Informed Communities | ↑ Peer Employment Roles |
| Anti-Stigma Initiatives with Providers and Faith Communities | ✓ | ✓ | ✓ | | ✓ | ✓ |
| Partnerships for Peer Support Services and "contact strategies" to engage individuals with lived experience | ✓ | ✓ | ✓ | ✓ | ✓ | ✓ |
| Mental Health First Aid (MHFA) Coordination | ✓ | ✓ | | ✓ | | |
| Housing Workgroup - Flexible Housing Pool | ✓ | ✓ | ✓ | ✓ | | |
| Trauma-Informed Hospitals Committee | ✓ | ✓ | | | ✓ | |
| Explore Policy Opportunities | | | | | | |
| Identify Partnership Strategies to Address Opioids | | ✓ | ✓ | ✓ | | ✓ |

Side United, and the Safer Foundation. In addition, the Alliance for Health Equity has identified an opportunity to develop better data to understand and address prevention opportunities through data sharing between health care and law enforcement. To that end, the Alliance for Health Equity Data Committee and Community Safety Workgroup are planning a pilot implementation of the Cardiff Model for Violence Prevention.

## DATA COMMITTEE

Because data are a critical component to all of the partnership initiatives, the Alliance for Health Equity has established a Data Committee to work in conjunction with many of the other workgroups. The Data Committee, as co-chaired by CDPH and Ann and Robert H. Lurie Children's Hospital, has four goals:

1. Pilot initiatives for connected data systems and/or data sharing
2. Develop shared metrics for tracking community health initiatives
3. Promote access to public health data
4. Facilitate collaboration on community health needs assessment and implementation strategies

## POLICY COMMITTEE

It's become clear that policy change is one of the key action levers for the Alliance for Health Equity. Leaders in government relations at 15 health systems and policy staff from three health departments participate in the Policy Committee. This committee focuses on population and community health policy issues aligned with the Alliance for Health Equity priorities. The Policy Committee undertakes advocacy and engagement, policy development, policy implementation, monitoring and tracking, and sharing best practices and information. The committee is working on local policy (aligned with health departments' Health in All Policies efforts), state policy in the Illinois General Assembly, federal policy, and institutional policy.

Currently, the policy committee has endorsed two legislative priorities: Tobacco 21 (raising the age for buying tobacco to 21 years) at the state level and Trauma-Informed Communities (supporting teachers, health care providers, and community-based service providers in addressing trauma and resilience in communities) at the federal level. In addition, the committee is tracking and sharing action opportunities on 26 state-level community health–focused bills.

In 2018, the policy committee is investigating three areas for future policy development and advocacy: (1) Supplemental Nutrition Assistance Program (SNAP) and food security policy, (2) institutional and legislative policy to protect immigrants, and (3) policy to address opioids. The policy committee also responds to policy issues that bubble up from the Alliance for Health Equity committees and workgroups, such as working with the Steering Committee to submit a letter to support the Flexible Housing Pool in the Chicago City Council.

## LESSONS LEARNED

- Working in a large geography with vast inequities is complex in terms of understanding the landscape in different parts of the city and county, navigating institutional dynamics, and supporting community-led initiatives. Nesting partnerships and finding ways to operationalize alignment and connection between local and regional efforts is key for collaborative success. Two specific lessons learned in this regard are (1) it requires substantial time and effort to build needed trust and to facilitate communication and coordination between local and regional efforts, and (2) the partners must be open to iterative development of initiatives and continuous improvement to build a collaborative structure that has meaningful impact to advance health equity.
- Leveraging existing organizational and individual relationships is a key to success, and trust-building at all levels in the collaborative allows for relationships to grow.
- Hospital and health system participation on multiple levels facilitates buy-in from other partners. Most importantly, most hospitals involved in the collaborative did not have a "check-the-box" mentality, but were interested in investing resources to do this work in a meaningful way. Particularly in working on SDHs, finding ways to link broader initiatives to the clinical work and to other strategic imperatives of health systems is key to success.
- Health department leadership is instrumental in forging public health and health care partnerships for SDHs. Health department leaders and staff have been ready and willing to step up and be co-creators of the collaborative, particularly by providing data collection capacity, sharing data, and showing the commitment to work on developing shared data systems. Their commitment to a health equity focus really helped to solidify the health equity focus of the hospital collaborative as well.
- Community stakeholder representatives are consistently engaged and committed to the effort. They have invested real leadership and have engaged in a process that included "building the plane while flying it," even though they have no requirements to do so. We acknowledge that there are structural barriers and power imbalances that must be addressed if we want to truly work for health equity, and there is no easy or quick fix. As

part of our health equity purpose, the Alliance for Health Equity strives to go further to create clear avenues for communities to participate in decision-making, address power imbalances, and be partners in assuring a more sustainable environment for community-based organizations and service providers. This is still very much a work in progress.

- As we work toward more equitable solutions, the Alliance for Health Equity staff and Steering Committee have identified cross-cutting issues (Figure 29.5)—structural racism and other structural inequities, trauma-informed care, systems to screen/refer/connect, chronic disease prevention, capacity building, and youth development—that we infuse into the development of projects and initiatives across topic areas.
- The backbone organization (IPHI) balances multiple roles as neutral convener and relationship manager; it holds the group accountable to the vision, establishes ways to measure value and impact, is responsive to individual partners' needs and strategic priorities, and keeps the work moving so everyone can feel that collaboration is resulting in action and progress.
- Communications to and among such a broad network is a challenge. The Alliance for Health Equity is working to develop and implement a communications strategy to make sure partners know and understand what the Alliance for Health Equity is working on.
- Different partners within the Alliance for Health Equity will lead different efforts, and the backbone organization (IPHI) does not need to lead or convene all of those efforts. For example, food insecurity is recognized as a region-wide challenge, and, because a countywide infrastructure is in place, it makes sense to work through that infrastructure. Different levels

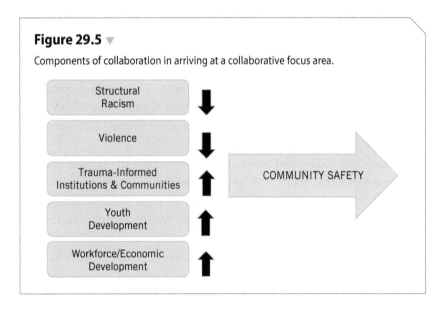

**Figure 29.5** ▼

Components of collaboration in arriving at a collaborative focus area.

of infrastructure exist for different issue areas, so the Alliance for Health Equity has to be open to playing different roles on different issues.

- Champions with expertise, trusted relationships across professions and sectors, and access to data and resources that are willing to leverage those assets for the collective good are essential for successfully implementing pilots and scaling those initiatives.

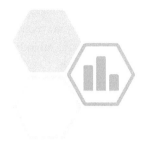

# Chapter 30

# The Health System's Role in Community Health Improvement: The Work of Three Insurance Providers

BRIAN C. CASTRUCCI, ELIZABETH CORCORAN, LOEL S. SOLOMON, CARALINE COATS, ALYSE B. SABINA, LAMOND DANIELS, AND AMY A. CLARK

W e are fortunate to live in a nation where our health care system is filled with dedicated providers offering cutting-edge, innovative clinical practice, but clinical efforts alone are no longer enough. Our communities experience complicated health challenges that are the result complex, interdependent economic, social, educational, and environmental factors.

When treatment was episodic and quick, the system worked. A patient could show up at the doctor's office with an infection, receive treatment, and likely be cured. Increasing costs were somewhat contained. Today, with chronic diseases like asthma, heart disease, and diabetes much more prevalent and 40% of our adult population obese,[1,2] care is continuous, and the bills start adding up. After correcting for inflation, total US health care expenditures rose 65% between 1990 and 2000, then another 83% between 2000 and 2016.[3]

America is dealing with diseases that have more to do with our zip codes than our genetic codes.[4] Concentrated poverty, struggling schools, and unsafe neighborhoods create very different opportunities—and health—than those available to people with stable incomes living in thriving communities. Yet, we still pressure clinicians to achieve outcomes for problems that originate far beyond their reach. Medicine can help manage the symptoms of these diseases, but it will never address the root problems. The bottom line is: If we want to live healthier lives, we are going to have to build healthier communities.

To improve the health of populations and reduce health care costs, American health care needs to transform beyond a focus on the individual patient and recognize that the health of the patient and the health of the community are indelibly linked. This change will not come easily. It will take leadership like that demonstrated by the three insurers highlighted in this chapter. Each is engaging in thoughtful upstream interventions targeted in communities they serve, beyond their specific members. This is the difference between addressing an individual patient's need and addressing the social determinants of health.

These health care leaders are moving beyond the clinic to tap into a wide range of skills, relationships, resources, and even policy, which results in more robust and effective community health improvement. They are all working toward systems-level partnerships and community-based solutions to our health care problems. As these efforts take root, we will have the opportunity to develop a body of evidence to propel us from great ideas and programs to a sustainable movement to improve health. Public and private insurance industry reforms, like pay for performance and value-based payments, are eliminating financial incentives for unnecessary tests and procedures and instead rewarding hospital systems and practice groups that reduce the total cost of care for a group of patients. However, until the promise of these reforms can be realized, these vignettes demonstrate that there are steps that everyone interested in promoting health can take today to reorient their own work, the work of their institutions, and the communities in which they live toward achieving health for everyone.

## KAISER PERMANENTE: POLICY PIONEERS

*Loel S. Solomon*

Public policy can be a powerful and highly effective primary prevention strategy, as evidenced by some of the most successful public health efforts of the 21st century. As part of multicomponent public health strategies, policy has played a prominent role in declining rates of motor vehicle deaths, vaccine-preventable diseases, lead poisoning, tobacco addiction, and other significant causes of morbidity and mortality.

Accordingly, public policy is a long-standing and foundational element of Kaiser Permanente's community health strategy. Kaiser Permanente was founded as a prepaid, integrated delivery system for shipyard and construction workers 75 years ago. Today, the system covers 12.3 million members across eight states and the District of Columbia. Kaiser Permanente's focus on policy as a primary prevention strategy is driven by an organizational structure that integrates care, coverage, and community health; a payment model that creates financial incentives for investments in prevention; an imperative to achieve scale and impact across its service areas; and a mission to improve the health of its members and the communities it serves.

In 2003, Kaiser Permanents embraced an explicit focus on policy change in the design and execution of its comprehensive, place-based approach to obesity prevention. Over the following decade, the organization funded and participated in more than 60 multisectoral Healthy Eating/Active Living (HEAL) collaboratives. Collectively, these sites implemented more than 730 separate community change interventions. Fifty-one percent of those strategies were policy or environmental change interventions; 31% were programmatic interventions, and 18% focused on capacity building. A cross-site evaluation of the initiative published in 2018 concluded that 69% of these strategies had evidence of a positive impact on population-level behavior change.[5]

Complementary efforts focus on advancing HEAL-related policies in schools and supporting state and federal policy efforts. These efforts include the HEAL Cities Campaign, an initiative that supports the adoption and implementation of municipal policies across Kaiser Permanente's footprint through partnerships among state municipal leagues and state-wide public health advocacy groups. Since its inception in 2009, more than 350 cities have joined the HEAL Cities Campaign, passing more than 1,000 local policies that reach more than 20 million people, including Kaiser Permanente members and nonmembers alike.

Encouraged by the success of the HEAL Cities Campaign, and seeking to broaden its local policy change efforts to address other social determinants of health, Kaiser Permanent joined the de Beaumont Foundation as a co-sponsor of CityHealth. CityHealth assesses the 40 largest US cities' progress across nine specific policy areas including high-quality universal pre-K, food safety in restaurants, healthy food procurement, "complete street" policies that promote more biking and walking, establishing 21 as the minimum age for purchase of tobacco products, clean indoor air laws, limiting the density of outlets selling alcohol, and earned sick leave. Policy has also been a focus of Kaiser Permanente initiatives to address other public health issues including support for the health care safety net providers, environmental sustainability, mental health and wellness, and, most recently, advocacy for increased investments to address the shortage of affordable housing.

Like other health care organizations, Kaiser Permanent has found that it can have a substantial impact on public policy due to its sizable social, economic, and political influence. While most policymakers and the public at large expect health care organizations to advocate for policies related to health care quality and access, Kaiser Permanente has effectively leveraged the "the power of the white coat" to advance the social determinants of health by framing those issues as health issues and by drawing the line to their impact on population health, health care affordability, and overall well-being.

Across its policy change efforts, Kaiser Permanent has deployed a number of influence strategies. Formal endorsement of legislation and associated advocacy efforts can be a powerful lever, but it is not always the most effective or the most viable lever to pull given the complex set of stakeholders that any health plan or health care delivery systems must manage. The broader array of policy influence tools, and examples of how those strategies have been deployed, is depicted in Table 30.1.

| Strategy category | Examples |
|---|---|
| **Table 30.1** ▼ Policy influence tools and strategies | |
| Endorsement of legislation | Endorsement of school nutrition standards; regional bond measures for parks, trails, and open spaces |
| Public testimony | Testimony by physicians and other health care providers on the health impacts of physical education programs and school nutrition standards on student health and academic performance |
| Participation in coalitions and collaboratives | Sponsorship of 60 place-based HEAL collaboratives advancing policy and environmental approaches to obesity prevention and related issues |
| Framing and communications | Partnership with NIH, CDC, and other funders in *Weight of the Nation*, an HBO series that helped frame obesity as a problem requiring policy and environmental changes |
| Convening | Creation of the Everybody Walk Campaign, a collaborative of more than 100 organizations that came together to advance policy and programmatic approaches to creating safe, walkable communities; an annual Walking Summit has played a major role in building momentum for the movement |
| Strategic grant-making | Funding of the Safe Routes to School National Partnership policy coordinators to advance safe routes and complete street policies with a focus on state transportation agencies and regional planning organizations |
| Organizational practice change | Adoption of nutrition standards for inpatient food service, vending machines, and cafeterias on hospital campuses |

## HUMANA'S BOLD GOAL AND POPULATION HEALTH STRATEGY

*Caraline Coats, Vice President, Population Health, Office of the Chief Medical Officer*

Humana Inc., headquartered in Louisville, Kentucky, is committed to helping our millions of medical and specialty members achieve their best health, and the best health of the communities they live in. Our successful history in care delivery and health plan administration is helping us create a new kind of integrated care ecosystem with the power to improve health and well-being and reduce costs. Our efforts are leading to a better quality of life for older adults, families, individuals, military service personnel, and communities at large.

Four years ago, we announced our Bold Goal, Population Health Strategy—which is to improve the health of the communities we serve by 20% by 2020 because we help make it easier for people to achieve their best health. We are tracking our progress using the US Centers for Disease Control and Prevention (CDC) population health tool, Healthy Days, which takes into account the whole person by measuring both mentally and physically Unhealthy Days over a 30-day period. This allows us to show a direct link between improved health, positive business results, and social impact.

To accomplish this, we support physicians and other health care professionals both inside and outside of the clinical setting. Inside the doctor's office, we are elevating the provider experience with a wide-range of clinical capabilities, resources, and tools such as in-home care, behavioral health and pharmacy services, data analytics, and wellness solutions.

Outside the doctor's office, we are working with nonprofit organizations, government, and business leaders to address barrier to health and to co-create solutions to better health at a local level. Together, we are creating evidence-based, scalable, and financially sustainable solutions. By targeting priority conditions and social determinants of health, we are finding ways to make it easier for people to achieve their best health.

Our goal is to increase freedom and relevancy for our members, their families, and communities. We may not be able to reverse a clinical diagnosis, but, through our diverse set of health plans and Bold Goal, we can focus on making sure a patient maintains a healthy lifestyle and has access to care and community resources so that he or she can live their best life.

Part of our commitment also involves supporting policies that will lead to healthier places and people. For instance:

- We are working to build a compelling body of evidence showing that addressing social determinants of health—like food insecurity and social isolation—positively impact the Healthy Days of our members, as well as clinical outcomes and utilization. Our aim is to leverage these data to advocate for policy and benefit change.
- We are filing innovative new benefits—leveraging the Center for Medicare and Medicaid Services' (CMS) expanded definition of "health related supplemental benefits"—to improve or stabilize health conditions of members while addressing their health-related social needs.

Cross-sector partnerships are important to Humana, as is evident through our Bold Goal population health strategy. Together, we are helping to drive better health outcomes and quality and benefit improvements, as well as create better relationships between our industry and the communities we serve. We believe in doing well by doing good, which means that good health is good for everyone. For more information or to partner with Humana, visit www.humana.com/BoldGoal.

## HEALTHIEST CITIES & COUNTIES CHALLENGE: AN AETNA FOUNDATION INITIATIVE TO BUILD HEALTHY COMMUNITIES

*Alyse B. Sabina, Lamond Daniels, and Amy A. Clark*

The Aetna Foundation, the American Public Health Association (APHA), and the National Association of Counties (NACo) launched the Healthiest Cities & Counties Challenge (the Challenge) in 2016. The purpose of the Challenge is to support small to mid-sized US cities and counties in their efforts to build multisectoral collaborations and develop evidence-based strategies promoting health, equity, and social interaction.

The Aetna Foundation is investing in this Challenge as part of its broader efforts to build healthier communities. The Challenge recognizes that health is much more than just health care and that, when it comes to health, place matters. Therefore, to participate in the Challenge, communities must build strong cross-sector teams focused on public health issues of critical importance to their communities.

The vision for the Challenge is to:

- Support communities in their collaborative efforts to become healthier places to live, work, learn, play, and pray
- Recognize excellence in achieving a measurable impact as a result of these efforts
- Identify models of effective collaboration that can be sustained and replicated throughout the United States

Underlying this vision is a belief that to improve economic vitality by moving the needle on health and wellness, cities and counties also must address issues of health equity and what happens outside the doctor's office.

In 2016, the Challenge named 50 cities and counties from across the country (the HealthyCommunity50) as Finalists to compete for a grand prize recognizing achievements in improving community health. Along with APHA and NACo, the Aetna Foundation selected these 50 programs because of their ability to tackle social and environmental conditions that frequently lead to chronic health issues. Finalists are positively impacting their communities throughout the Challenge, as these early accomplishments demonstrate:

- In Chatham County, North Carolina, the Chatham Health Alliance has succeeded in embedding a Health in All Policies approach into the Chatham County Comprehensive Plan which sets the vision for the county over the next 25 years. Through the inclusion of a Health Element in the Comprehensive Plan, recommendations, policies, strategies, examples of implementation, and action items around health and equity are explicitly stated in the 25-year vision for Chatham's growth. Select strategies include addressing infrastructure gaps to promote healthier living and promoting cross-sector partnerships for safe routes to school and tobacco-free grounds and policies.
- Danville, Virginia, and Caswell County, North Carolina, have created a Health Collaborative that focuses on policies, systems, and environmental changes. This work has resulted in the City of Danville passing an internal complete streets policy, and Caswell County passing a Health for All Resolution in June 2017. County Administration and Commissioners see it playing a role in several decisions that are upcoming in 2018.

- In Waco-McLennan County, Texas, a community survey identified three zip codes within the county that suffer from increased rates of obesity. To help improve nutrition in the community, the Waco-McLennan Public Health District partnered with local organizations to create awareness and access to fresh local produce through healthy cooking demonstrations, a mobile farmers' market, and a new nonprofit grocery store in an identified food desert.

Through the Challenge, $1.5 million in prizes will be awarded to cities and counties that are able to show measurable improvements in health outcomes over 2 years through cross-sector partnerships. As part of its commitment to share successful health improvement strategies, the Challenge will publicize the prize winners' stories and facilitate adoption of their effective practices in other communities.

For more information on the Challenge, visit www.healthiestcities.org and join the conversation at #HealthiestCitiesChallenge.

## REFERENCES

1. Hales CM, Carroll MD, Fryar CD, Ogden CL, et al. *Prevalence of Obesity Among Adults and Youth: United States, 2015–2016. NCHS Data Brief.* Hyattsville, MD: National Center for Health Statistics; 2017.

2. Frieden TR. Asleep at the switch: Local public health and chronic disease. *Am J Public Health.* 2004;94(12):2059–61.

3. Kamal R, Cox C. How has US spending on health care changed over time? December 20, 2017. https://www.healthsystemtracker.org/chart-collection/u-s-spending-health care-changed-time/#item-state. Accessed August 31, 2018.

4. Graham GN. Why your zip code matters more than your genetic code: Promoting healthy outcomes from mother to child. (1556-8342 (Electronic)). https://www.ncbi.nlm.nih.gov/pubmed/27513279. Accessed 1/16/2019.

5. Schwartz PM, Kelly C, Cheadle A, Pulver A, Solomon L. The Kaiser Permanente Community Health Initiative: A decade of implementing and evaluating community change. *Am J Prevent Med.* 2018;54(5s2):S105–S9. doi:10.1016/j.amepre.2018.02.004.

# Chapter 31

# Community-Centered Health Homes: Bridging Health Care Services and Community Prevention

LESLIE MIKKELSEN, REA PAÑARES, AND LARRY COHEN

P reventing illness and injury in the first place has the potential to be a powerful component of the nation's strategy to improve population health while strengthening access to quality health care and reducing costs. In 2010, the Community Clinics Initiative (now the Center for Care Innovations, or CCI) commissioned Prevention Institute to analyze how safety net providers might maximize patient and community health by incorporating a community prevention approach into the development of medical homes. (The CCI began as a unique collaboration between Tides and The California Endowment in 1999 to provide grants, evidence-based programming, and training for community health centers. Since then, it has served as a place for the health care safety net to connect and collaborate, learn from one another, and explore creative solutions).

The resultant publication, *Community-Centered Health Homes: Bridging the Gap Between HealthServices and Community Prevention,* introduced the term *community-centered health home* (CCHH) to describe health care organizations that took an active role, in partnership, to improve community conditions that impact patients' health (e.g., supporting rental housing code enforcement, building septic systems, and improving community access to healthy food and places for physical activity).[1] The CCHH model was developed by synthesizing promising practices from these different health care organizations into a systematic approach. The model rests on the evidence and practice base of the social determinants of health (SDHs) and community-level prevention that elevates the fundamental power of community conditions in shaping population health status and fostering health equity[2-5]

The CCHH model is aligned with the evolution toward a value-based system that emphasizes quality health care and improvement in population health outcomes.[2] There is increasing awareness among health care professionals of the influence of SDHs on health outcomes.[3-4] To improve patient outcomes, health care quality improvement efforts have promoted stronger care coordination and consideration of the whole person, including nonmedical needs, as well as consideration of the social and community context of their patients.[5,6] Health care providers feel frustrated as they send their patients out into communities that are literally making them sick.[7] Recognizing that the illnesses or injuries they were treating could be prevented, clinicians have been effective champions for policies and community changes across a range of community health issues from infant car seats to tobacco control to violence prevention.[8]

CCHH is one approach to bridging the insights and credibility of health care with the community improvement know-how of public health and community partners to achieve improvements in overall population health. The CCHH approach provides a guiding philosophy, a set of capacities and examples practices, and a process that health care organizations can follow to embody and demonstrate their institutional commitment to address community determinants and reach health equity in their communities.

## WHAT IS A CCHH?

A CCHH is a health care organization that acknowledges that factors outside the clinical setting affect patient health outcomes and actively participates in improving them. Thus, the CCHH model adds community-centeredness as a core attribute and functionality of the health home.[9] A CCHH considers the daily living conditions that contribute to injury and illness, interfere with treatment plans, and present obstacles to improving health, and it mobilizes its resources, expertise, and credibility to work in partnership to advocate for change. CCHH practices are grounded in the principles of quality community-level prevention, which honor community wisdom, focus on community determinants of health, take a comprehensive multisector approach, and utilize policy, systems, and organizational practice change as key tools for improving community conditions. Ultimately, being a CCHH reflects an ongoing organizational commitment to advancing health equity by utilizing its influence, expertise, and partnerships to make improvements in health-impacting conditions within the community it serves (Figure 31.1).

Partnerships are critical to the success of the CCHH model, and the intent is not for health care institutions to enact change alone. Health care institutions are credible partners whose assets are valuable for advancing community change. At the same time, public health, community-based organizations, and advocates frequently have more knowledge about community systems and policy processes. Collaboration between health care organizations and local partners—such as local health departments, community-based organizations,

## Figure 31.1 ▼

Structure of a community-centered health home (CCHH).

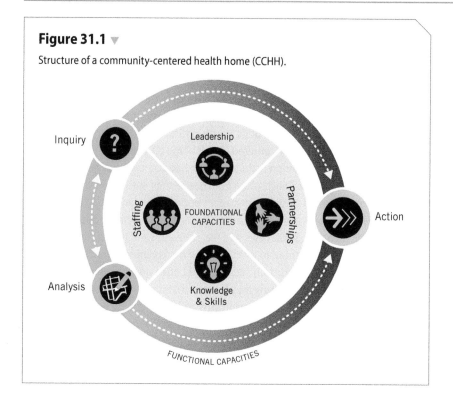

businesses, local government, and schools—presents opportunities for leveraging assets and shared resources, as well as for mutually fulfilling work and engagement in CCHH activities.

The model provides a framework for engaging in policy, systems, and environmental change through a fluid and collaborative process of inquiry, analysis, and action, gathering insights and data about the community context, diagnosing the underlying health issue, and working with community partners to develop a comprehensive action plan. Health care organizations may enter into CCHH efforts anywhere in the cycle, depending on what is going on in their community and the starting place of the organization. To fully engage in the practices of inquiry, analysis, and action, health care organizations will need to invest in strengthening key organizational capacities for developing and sustaining a CCHH approach, including leadership, staffing, knowledge and skills, and partnerships (Box 31.1).

The following sections describe the capacities of the CCHH model and examples practices, which provide a framework for a clinical organization to consider what needs to be in place to apply the model and measure progress in their journey toward becoming a CCHH.

*Adaptive and Engaged Leadership* Executive leadership, senior management, provders, and board members prioritize community-level prevention and healthy equity as part of the organization's vision, mission, and goals, and set the strategic direction for building their CCHH. Structures, systems, and processes are built to support the team with CCHH implementation. Organizational

Foundational capacities *refer to elements that enable a health care organization to fully and strategically integrate a community-centered approach into the fabric of the organization. (Box 31.2).*

## Box 31.1 | Daughters of Charity Services: Gathering Information and Insight to Address Diabetes

The process of inquiry and analysis often go hand-in-hand, as evidenced by Daughters of Charity Services of New Orleans (DCSNO),[11] one of the sites that participated in the CCHH Demonstration Project administered by the Louisiana Public Health Institute (LPHI). When the health center began its community-centered health home (CCHH) work, the staff knew they wanted to focus on diabetes, which had been a major health concern in their community. Clinical data from one of their sites showed rising hemoglobin A1C levels among their patient population; they also had data from a community assessment conducted by Dillard University—one of their partners—that pointed to diabetes as a major health condition in their community. Because they wanted to establish their own relationship with the community (outside of Dillard University), staff began going to community meetings themselves; this is how they learned that the community was aware of the diabetes issue but had other concerns and "did not want another community garden." Those other concerns included food insecurity as well as the lack of safe places for physical activity. The CCHH model allowed the team to think further upstream (than developing a community garden or nutrition classes) and to assess the community's real concerns. In response, they developed and administered their own questions on food resources, physical activity, and safety and added these to their patient registration and adult patient history forms. They had never thought to ask the community or patients these types of questions before. To institutionalize this new focus on community engagement and hear directly from residents (not just their patients), the health center established an advisory council made up of patients as well as other community members to advise them on an ongoing basis.

*Louisiana Public Health Institute. The Community-Centered Health Homes Demonstration Project. New Orleans, LA: Louisiana Public Health Institute; 2017.*

leaders are effective in being stewards of strategic change internally as well as engaging community leaders and stakeholders about common aims.

*Designated and Diverse Staffing* Leadership of the organization identifies internal assets and staff capacities for implementing the CCHH model. Leaders, staff, and clinicians across departments and disciplines understand how community conditions outside the clinical setting shape health and apply that knowledge to their role. Designated CCHH staff, who are proficient in community-level prevention and community engagement, coordinate and implement CCHH initiatives and serve as a bridge between the health care organization and community partners.

*Knowledge and Skills for Advancing Community-Level Prevention* The designated CCHH team is proficient in the models, tools, and competencies needed to advance community prevention. Care teams and frontline staff receive continuing education, tools, and support to identify and address the community

## Box 31.2 | Asian Health Services: Exemplifying the Practices of a CCHH

Ingredients used in popular nail products have been tied to conditions such as cancer, lung diseases, miscarriage, and other illnesses.[12,13] During health outreach trips to local nail salons, clinicians at Asian Health Services (AHS), a Federally Qualified Health Center in Oakland, California, found troubling symptoms amongst the mostly young and female manicurists.

*Inquiry*: Following this disturbing discovery, AHS began work with the Cancer Prevention Institute of California to conduct a health survey of nail salon workers in their county. Other studies followed, collecting both quantitative and qualitative data on the health and experiences of the area's manicurists. Background research confirmed that three chemicals (dubbed the "toxic trio" by advocates and commonly found in nail products) are closely associated with serious health concerns.

*Analysis*: The data collected by AHS and its partners found that nail salon workers were at increased risk for developing gestational diabetes and delivering underweight infants. Interviews with manicurists revealed "epidemic" levels of sickness. Qualitative data collected from individual salon workers included stories of thyroid conditions, breast cancer, asthma, and many other preventable illnesses.

*Action*: AHS initiated the formation of the California Healthy Nail Salon Collaborative, a coalition of more than 40 organizations, including environmental and reproductive justice groups, the salon workforce, nonprofit organizations, researchers, government agencies, and other key stakeholders. AHS serves as its fiscal sponsor and sits on its steering committee. Since its inception, the California Healthy Nail Salon Collaborative has worked to change policies to protect nail salon workers in the county and beyond. Some successes include:

- The passage of legislation in certain California counties and cities that charges local governments to implement a recognition program that confers "Healthy Nail Salon" status on businesses that meet certain criteria that protect the health of their employees and customers.
- Co-sponsorship and the passage of statewide legislation that called for a consumer education program focused on the benefits of patronizing a Healthy Nail Salon and an awareness campaign for local governments on the benefits of implementing recognition programs.
- The launch of a pilot microloan program, housed at AHS, to assist businesses that wish to become Healthy Nail Salons with the up-front costs of ventilation systems that improve air quality.

By engaging with its community, AHS recognized that exposures in nail salons were having a negative impact on health in its service area, and they actively worked to change these conditions through policy, systems, and environmental change—exemplifying the practices of the community-centered health home (CCHH) model.

- Quach T, Gunier R, Tran A, et al. Characterizing Workplace Exposures in Vietnamese Women Working in California Nail Salons. American Journal of Public Health. 2011;101(Suppl 1):S271–S276. doi:10.2105/AJPH.2010.300099.
- About Us. California Healthy Nail Salon Collaborative website. https://cahealthynailsalons.org/about-us/ Accessed September 30, 2018.
- Thu Quach, Asian Health Services, oral conversation, August 28, 2018.
- California Healthy Nail Salon Collaborative website. http://www.cahealthynailsalons.org. Accessed April 2, 2018.

*Functional capacities refer to steps that a health care institution can take to become a CCHH, which include gathering insights and data about the community context, diagnosing the underlying health issue, and working with community partners to develop and play a role in a comprehensive action plan. It is important to note that these steps do not necessarily need to be sequential and that the level of intensity may differ, but that systematic application of these steps is what truly constitutes a CCHH.*

context of their patients as well as to support the CCHH team by lending their knowledge and credibility to CCHH initiatives.

*Authentic Community Partnerships* The health care organization is a credible and trusted partner in the community. It effectively collaborates with multisector stakeholders to leverage collective strengths and enable community-level action to improve conditions that impact health and health equity. It invites and enables patients, community members, and community-based organizations to participate in inquiry, discovery, invention, design, and decision-making related to community prevention strategies.

*Inquiry: Assess and Identify Community Determinants of Health* The health care organization supports the CCHH team to identify, compile, and share internal knowledge and data useful for understanding community health conditions and determinants. The CCHH team is supported in gathering and using internal and external knowledge and data sources that are indicative of the community health conditions. Staff and clinicians have opportunities and venues to contribute their insights into community-level issues, factors, and causation that may be underlying the prevalence of injuries and illnesses in both the clinical and community settings. Patients, community members, and partners participate in the production of knowledge and data regarding community conditions.

*Analysis: Collaborate with the Community on Planning and Priority Setting* The health care organization shares knowledge and data with relevant community partners to support the identification and prioritization of issues and to develop comprehensive intervention strategies. The CCHH team is proficient in presenting and communicating data trends and implications, designing and facilitating collaborative planning processes, and developing action plans in concert with community members and community-based partners.

*Action: Contribute to Improvements in Community Conditions* The health care organization embraces model organizational practices that contribute to community-level prevention. It also participates with partners to improve the community conditions that shape health outcomes and health equity. To achieve this, health care organizations and their partners advocate for community-level changes in policies, systems, practices, and environments.

## EARLY TESTING OF CCHH INITIATIVES

According to Pritesh Gandhi, Associate Chief Medical Officer & Director of Adult Medicine at People's Community Clinic and a participant in the Texas CCHH Initiative,[14] "Clinical interventions alone can't get us to the health outcomes we want without complementary community interventions. At People's Community Clinic, we began to offer ourselves and our clinical expertise as a tool to advance the issue of paid sick leave. We're proud that when community organizations needed a health care advocate, they turned to our clinic to help develop a city-wide policy. In February, Austin became the first city in the South to pass such an ordinance that required paid sick leave."

Shortly after conceptualizing the model, philanthropic investment in three CCHH demonstration projects in the Southeastern United States ensued.

In the Gulf States region, Prevention Institute partnered with the Louisiana Public Health Institute (LPHI) to launch the first CCHH demonstration in the nation. The initiative officially launched in March 2015, with the selection and announcement of five sites (two in Louisiana and one each in Florida, Mississippi, and Alabama) that received grants over 2 years in conjunction with supportive technical assistance. Because it was a 2-year demonstration project, the focus was on developing strategies for how clinics could begin to change their organizational culture, structure, and procedures to support community change as well as the CCHH model, rather than focusing on health outcomes. This included developing the right staffing roles, cultivating leadership, guiding new strategies for collecting and sharing information and data (both internally among clinic patients and staff and externally with community partners), making the case for adoption of this model, and building authentic community partnerships. The project came to a close in April 2017, and LPHI disseminated a final report describing the experience and detailing the program evaluation findings.[10,11] Many of the sites continued some aspect of their CCHH work beyond the program period by growing their relationships and collaborations with partners, participating in local coalitions, advancing internal data collection activities, and changing the way they talk about the clinic's role in the community.

In North Carolina, the Blue Cross and Blue Shield of North Carolina (Blue Cross NC Foundation) developed a strategic priority to increase the capacity of safety net health care organizations and communities to implement practices associated with the CCHH model. The initiative used the CCHH model as a conceptual framework for bringing together health care providers and community-based organizations to work in partnership with community members to advance policy and environmental changes to improve health, but the initiative is not rooted specifically in community health centers. Blue Cross

NC Foundation is currently supporting three grantees who are entering their fourth year of work, and recently selected another six grantees for a planning grant period to be followed by four years of implementation funding. In Texas, Episcopal Health Foundation (EHF), which serves 57 counties in East and South Texas, established the Texas CCHH Initiative in 2016. The foundation is supporting a cohort of 13 community clinics with 18-month or 36-month grants. The goal of the Texas CCHH initiative is to support community clinics in improving the community conditions that contribute to poor health in Texas as a complement to the delivery of healthcare services. This goal is embedded in the foundation's 2018-2022 strategic plan in order to support resource allocation and system reform in the health sector to promote health, not just healthcare. The 13 clinics are focused on a range of issues such as advocating for city paid sick leave policy, addressing food insecurity, and improving community spaces for physical activity.

## CONCLUSION

Work and interest in health care–community integration to improve population health is growing exponentially and will only intensify through increased health system transformation efforts. Focusing on community conditions has the potential to save lives, reduce illnesses and injuries, and facilitate healing. In many cases, this focus also saves resources for health care providers, payers, and patients. CCHH contributes to our nation's journey toward a system of health by highlighting the value of health care in partnering with its surrounding community and offering a systematic approach to partnering with community groups to improve community conditions while continuing to meet the daily priority of delivering high-quality health care.

### REFERENCES

1. Prevention Institute. *Community Centered Health Homes: Bridging the Gap Between Healthcare Services and Community Prevention.* Oakland, CA: Prevention Institute; 2011.

2. Koo D, Michener JL, Castrucci BC, Sprague JB. Why a Practical Playbook for Partnerships Between Public Health and Primary Care? In: Koo D, Michener JL, Castrucci BC, Sprague JB, eds. *The Practical Playbook.* New York: Oxford University Press; 2016:3–12.

3. Magnan S. Social determinants of health 101 for health care: five plus five. NAM Perspectives. Discussion Paper. Washington, DC: National Academy of Medicine; 2017. https://nam.edu/social-determinants-of-health-101-for-health-care-five-plus-five/. Accessed 1/22/2019.

4. Cutts TF, Cochrane JR. *Stakeholder Health: Insights from New Systems of Health.* Winston-Salem, NC: Stakeholder Health Press; 2016.

5. Patient Centered Primary Care Collaborative. Shared principles of primary care. 2018. https://www.pcpcc.org/about/shared-principles. Accessed March 5, 2018.

6. AAFP. Public Statement: Integration of Primary Care and Public Health. 2015. https:www.aafp.org/patient-care.html. Accessed March 1, 2018.

7. Nolen L. Improving population health outcomes by investing in community prevention. *Health Affairs*. November 30, 2017. https://www.healthaffairs.org/do/10.1377/hblog20171130.64591/full/. Accessed March 10, 2018.

8. Cohen L. *Prevention Diaries: The Practice and Pursuit of Health of All.* New York: Oxford University Press; 2017.

9. Mikkelsen L, Pañares R, Anastasoff J, Miller K, Baumgartner E, Mor K, Riccardo J, *Community-Centered Health Homes: Bridging Healthcare Services and Community Prevention.* Oakland, CA: Prevention Institute. Published January 2018.

10. Prevention Institute. *The Community-Centered Health Homes Model: Updates and Learnings*. Oakland, CA: Prevention Institute; January 2016.

11. Louisiana Public Health Institute. The Community-Centered Health Homes Project, 2017 Report. New Orleans, LA. 2017. http://lphi.org/wp-content/uploads/2017/10/CCHHFinalReport.pdf. Accessed 1/22/2019.

12. California Healthy Nail Salon Collaborative website. https://cahealthynailsalons.org/. Accessed March 10, 2018.

13. Itchon NP. How safe is your mani-pedi? *San Francisco Chronicle*. October 22, 2015.

14. Gandhi P. Guest Commentary: Let's address hunger and other community determinants of health. *Modern Healthcare*. http://www.modernhealthcare.com/article/20180310/NEWS/180319995. Published March 10, 2018. Accessed 1/22/2019.

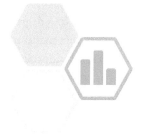

# Chapter 32

# Going Way Upstream: How One Foundation Redefined Its Work to Improve Population Health

PETER LONG AND BRITTANY IMWALLE

In 2016, Blue Shield of California Foundation (BSCF) took the first steps on a journey that would have radical implications for its work and impact. Over the prior 6 years, BSCF had achieved considerable success in its work to expand access to high-quality health care and to end domestic violence in California. (Ending domestic violence has been core to the mission of BSCF since it was significantly expanded in the early 2000s. Today, it is the largest private funder of domestic violence services in California.) Through funding and support, BSCF shaped the creation of health care services that engaged low-income patients[1] and domestic violence services that took into account the experience of survivors.[2] BSCF demonstrated how to integrate disparate health care services, such as primary care and specialty care,[3-5] and behavioral health and primary care,[6] to improve access and quality while potentially lowering costs (visit https://www.blueshieldcafoundation.org/publications/tag/behavioral-health). BSCF created networks of established leaders within the health care and domestic violence safety nets in California[7,8] and influenced safety net systems in California to think and act differently.[9,10]

Despite these notable successes, BSCF struggled to sustain, scale, and spread these innovations to other organizations and systems or to embed them into policy changes. We began to ask ourselves whether there might be new ways to promote the well-being of individual Californians, who in many cases were receiving services from both of the fields BSCF had been working to build and support.

As the strategic planning process began in early 2016, BSCF weighed a number of options, including (1) increasing investments to sustain, scale, and spread previous innovations; (2) choosing different opportunities to impact the health care and domestic violence fields; or (3) fundamentally changing the approach to address the root causes of poor health and violence.

After years of working on improving access to services and the quality of systems serving the safety net, it was clear that something different needed to be done to meet BSCF's goal. A decision was made to shift the focus "upstream," to address root causes. And BSCF did so boldly—not just by a degree or two—in an effort to move closer to the source of the issues that mattered most: improving the health and well-being of the most vulnerable Californians and ending domestic violence. (In the classic public health parable credited to medical sociologist Irving Zola, a witness sees a man caught in a river current. The witness saves the man, only to be drawn to the rescue of more drowning people. After many have been rescued, the witness walks upstream to investigate why so many people have fallen into the river.) BSCF did so with the belief that successful upstream investments can influence outcomes for health and domestic violence and can be sustainable for the long term.

How did one of the largest health grant-making organizations in the state, with a long history of working to improve access to services and the quality of systems serving the California safety net, chart a new path upstream? This journey is described in the pages that follow (Box 32.1).

---

**Box 32.1 | Are You Ready to Move Upstream? Five Questions to Assess Your Organization's Readiness**

- *Are you clear on why upstream work is right for you?* A move upstream is challenging and will be aided by a clear vision of why upstream work to address root causes is important for your organization's future success.
- *Have you embraced complexity?* Upstream work is complex and requires a complex solution set. Consider the diverse and varied perspectives you will draw on to inform new ways of working in the future.
- *Have you assessed how your current strengths can support your future work?* Consider what has made your organization uniquely successful in the past and assess how existing strengths can be utilized to support upstream work in the future.
- *Are you ready for the amount of change required within your organization?* Moving upstream will create change at all levels of the organization. Consider how to consistently engage staff and the board of directors in the process to ensure that they are ready for the magnitude of changes required to be successful addressing upstream factors.
- *What if my organization isn't ready for a full-scale shift in focus?* You can still play a meaningful role in upstream change! Consider engaging other players and partners who are currently working in the upstream space. How can your organizational knowledge and insight contribute to their efforts to create upstream change?

*Adapted from Schroder, SA (2007) We Can Do Better – Improving the Health of the American People. NEJM. 357.1221–8.*

## WHY UPSTREAM?

According to research, 80% of health is determined by factors outside the health care system—things such as access to affordable housing, availability of good schools, level of exposure to violence, and personal health habits (diet, smoking, and exercise), as well as personal and community support networks. This information is not new. For more than two decades, awareness of social determinants of health (SDHs) and the impact that these determinants have on overall health and well-being (Figure 32.1)[11] have been well understood. And yet the preponderance of BSCF's funding remained focused on systems and system solutions.

Simply put, BSCF realized that its work was emphasizing just one side of the supply–demand equation and was focused on improving the services delivered by health care and domestic violence providers to address people's expressed needs (improving supply); BSCF was not focused on how to prevent poor health and domestic violence from occurring in the first place (reducing demand). To reduce demand for services, BSCF would need to focus on prevention.

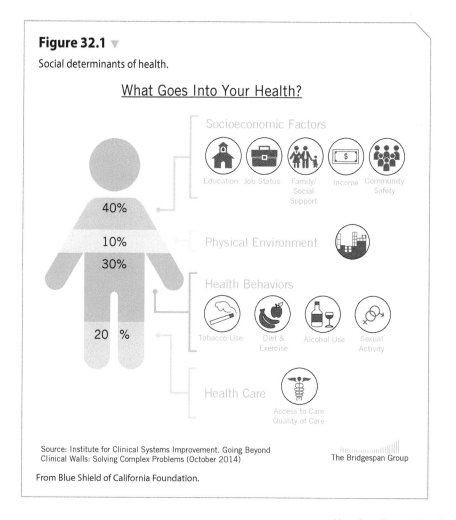

**Figure 32.1** ▼

Social determinants of health.

Source: Institute for Clinical Systems Improvement. Going Beyond Clinical Walls: Solving Complex Problems (October 2014)

The Bridgespan Group

From Blue Shield of California Foundation.

BSCF also realized that improved health and safety are not directly tied to just systems or services—they are also tied to people and community. Although prior investments (such as funding to improve the cultural competence of domestic services providers to better meet the needs of survivors and improve access to health care for low-income Californians) promoted improvements in individual outcomes, systems and organizations were the primary lever for change. To effectively address the root causes of domestic violence and poor health, BSCF needed to ensure that equity, people, and community were at the center of its work.[12] With these revelations in hand, a shift in focus not only felt important, it felt imperative.

## WHERE TO FOCUS

In some ways, defining the challenge ahead was the easy work: it was apparent how the current focus on improving "supply side" services for vulnerable Californians would not directly produce improved health or end domestic violence. Looking ahead, it was apparent how an upstream approach would be a better match to address the complex social problems driving poor health and violence and would hold the potential to significantly impact the lives of all Californians, especially those who struggle the most. The possibility of new, meaningful approaches to address poor health and violence in our communities was energizing. And then the real work began: defining new areas of focus that built on past knowledge and insight yet were radically different from where BSCF had been working in the past.

Utilizing the three-by-three Upstream Medicine Quality Improvement (QI) Project Matrix developed by Manchanda,[13] various pathways to change were explored: via investment in individual change, organizational change, or community-level change, and focusing on the levels of primary, secondary, or tertiary prevention. Recognizing that our final strategy must reflect a unique role and niche for the organization, we used its values (possibility, partnership, integrity, equity, and dignity), organizational characteristics (a California-focused, annual contribution foundation), and an emerging vision for the future to define the upstream approach: informed by past work, BSCF will drive change at the community level to improve outcomes for California's most vulnerable residents. (Blue Shield of California Foundation is classified by the Internal Revenue Service as a private foundation and receives an annual gift from Blue Shield of California. This annual gift is used to fund grant-making and other programmatic investments. Instead of an endowment, a modest reserve fund is maintained by the organization.)

The first upstream investments to improve health and end domestic violence are described in the next sections.

## Breaking the Cycle of Domestic Violence

We know that childhood exposure to domestic violence and trauma leads to increased likelihood of becoming violent and experiencing poor health in early adulthood.[14] That is why BSCF is working to interrupt the cycle of domestic violence with a two-generational approach: healing those who are currently in violent relationships while also promoting prevention by addressing the adverse impacts of exposure to violence. This shifts the focus from domestic violence service delivery to a multigenerational effort to prevent and heal. And it shifts as well from a focus on older survivors of domestic violence to one on children and young adults, whose experiences inevitably create the domestic violence pipeline of the future. By changing gender violence norms through multisector collaboration, public awareness, and policy changes, we will work to shift the frame of domestic violence from that of a private issue between two individuals to recognition of domestic violence as a complex social issue that impacts families and communities. Initial investments are focused on examining domestic violence across the life course and establishing a community-informed design lab. Together, these investments will identify key leverage points and opportunities for impact as BSCF continues to develop our multigenerational approach to prevention and healing.

## Collaborating for Healthy Communities

Analysis has told us that many of today's multisector efforts within communities have been built around service delivery agreements between two organizations and that these collaborative efforts are the result of years—even decades—of hard work across organizations to build trust, understanding, and accountability related to shared outcomes. In the new work, BSCF will shift from testing opportunities for collaboration to work that identifies the fundamental elements that allow collaborations to quickly get off the ground and thrive. The focus is expanded from the effective engagement of service providers within a collaborative to a focus on how collaboratives promote authentic and meaningful engagement of community members. A shift will be implemented from investments in collaborative dyads to investments in integrated collaborations designed to address complex social drivers and explore the optimal role of health care systems within collaborative arrangements. BSCF believes that multisector collaboratives that are truly integrated will be uniquely positioned to improve health and reduce violence in California communities, particularly for our most vulnerable neighbors. Initial stages of work in this area are designed to learn from current collaborative investments (e.g., sites funded through the California Accountable Communities for Health Initiative) as BSCF seeks to identify the elements of collaborative engagement that promote rapid engagement and sustainability.

**Box 32.2 | Our New Work in Action**

Root causes of domestic violence are highly complex and challenging to address. The two projects described here provide examples of how we are drawing in new ideas and engaging new partners to rethink our work in this area.

*Project 1*: A co-design lab, launched in early 2018 with a diverse group of 16 fellows who work both inside and outside the domestic violence field working together to create new solutions.

*Project 2*: We are working with partners to take a hard look at data in order to inform new approaches to promote social change. Through research and analysis, we aim to identify the root causes and predictors of domestic violence, as well as the risk and protective factors that can inform future interventions.

## Designing the Future of Health

As knowledge about what creates health is exploding, we know that current approaches do not match the complexity of the health issues in our communities. BSCF is exploring ecosystem and other system-mapping techniques to learn which trends and frameworks—beyond the current state of health care—might provide breakthrough ideas to achieve long-term gains and generate successful investments in prevention. As we step outside of the health care system and ask fundamental questions about how health is produced within systems and communities, we expect to shift from approaches that address individual drivers of poor health and violence to approaches that consider multiple, complex drivers. We also see promise in the possibility of shifting from exploration of funding for near-term interventions to approaches that reward investment in long-term solutions. The initial investments in this area will move beyond existing frameworks for health and violence prevention to create room for approaches that draw on new ideas, new partners, and new pathways to rapidly accelerate and sustain change over time (Box 32.2).

## CHARTING THE COURSE UPSTREAM

BSCF used a series of new tools and approaches to shift its focus upstream. Initial steps to redefine the work were supported by a simple framing exercise: "From what, to what?" This allowed us to clarify where we wanted to go and what we wanted to achieve (Table 32.1).

## SET A BOLD GOAL AND LEARN

Past practice told us that we were most successful when we were explicit and focused in our work. With this in mind, BSCF developed a bold goal to guide

### Table 32.1 ▼ From what, to what? Blue Shield of California Foundation

| From what? | To what? |
|---|---|
| Investments focused on single-frame issues (access to care, quality of services, etc.) | Recognition that social issues and needs are complex, and our investments must reflect this complexity |
| Focus on addressing health care and domestic violence separately | Recognizing that root causes of poor health and violence are interconnected, and developing integrated approaches for social change |
| Focus on change within systems to improve care for individuals | Focus on change outside systems, creating the conditions for improved health and violence prevention |
| Focus on improving the delivery of services to patients and survivors | Focus on prevention, well-being, and the social determinants of health. |
| Focus on efforts that can create impact within a short-term (2–4 year) timeframe | Focus on efforts that will create impact over a much longer time horizon (10 years or more) |
| Work on issues where steps to attain future state are relatively certain | Work on issues where steps to attain future state are much more uncertain |
| Long-standing relationships with known, trusted partners | New relationships with new groups and voices |
| Multiple, mid-sized, grants ($50k –$250k) made annually to support key organization | Fewer, larger grants ($1 million or more) made over multiple years to support transformative change in communities |
| Emphasis on project-support grants with clearly defined project goals and outcomes | Emphasis on supporting organizational creativity, through large, general operating support grants |

the work upstream: to make California the healthiest state in the country, with the lowest rates of domestic violence and the most empowering community health solutions.

This ambition directs and inspires our progress and underscores the imperative of working differently to create change in the world. It is necessary to innovate and try new things, moving away from resuming old roles, scanning the field for effective practices, creating iterations on those practices to improve performance, and then implementing at scale across the state. We've learned to identify what is working and have devoted significant resources to help teach and coach others.

By contrast, the new goal and the new areas of funding we've identified require moving into the role of explorers: mapping out some early hunches about next steps to take and quickly assessing whether or not we appear to be on the right path. We've moved from work to identify and implement promising practices in areas where pathways to create change were more clear to a world where the pathways forward are unknown, and our job is to be on the lookout for nuggets of insight that can guide us forward—even when things don't proceed exactly as planned.

These insights helped BSCF to recognize that, just as building skills in the area of exploration and innovation was necessary, so was the need to build complementary skills in the area of applied learning: moving from an organization that approached learning as a way to demonstrate progress to an organization that approaches learning as a way to test hypotheses, explore information, invite discussion, reflect on patterns, and adapt as necessary. The notion of applied learning was approached in the following series of steps:

1. *Setting and defining indicators* for the bold goal and anchoring long-term objectives to exploring progress over time.
2. *Developing close-in hypotheses for new initiatives* by deliberately defining key learning questions to track and setting clear points for teams to reflect together on the patterns and results that are emerging. These reflective discussions help us stay on course, whether that means taking the next step forward or circling back a step or two to try an alternative path.
3. *Explicitly defining how we will engage others in our work and thinking,* which may include new community and foundation partners as well as existing nonprofit, government, and public health agencies. We are inviting engagement from communities at the front end of new projects, building in the capacity to share learning with others, and inviting additional reflection and meaning-making from audiences across the state as we attempt to elevate the importance of equity and inclusion in all areas.

These approaches are codified in Figure 32.2.

This multilayered measurement approach is supported by the application of learning loops (Figure 32.3) that help to identify the hypotheses that are being tested, the key pieces of information that will be tracked, and the method that will be employed to gather relevant data. Opportunities to engage communities and partners in the learning process are also shown in Figure 32.3. Whether managed internally or in partnership with others, *learning loops* ensure that there is dedicated time to focus and reflect as well as to maintain a bias toward action as insights are applied to future stages of work.

**Figure 32.2** ▼

Elements of measurement.

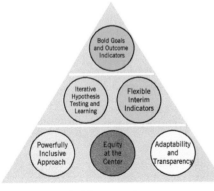

Our Bold Goal: California is the healthiest state in the country, with the lowest rates of domestic violence and the most empowering community health solutions.
Indicators: Comprised of elements of Gallup Well-Being Index

Test and Learn: Iterative tests of change and clear and 3-5 year indicators for each area of investment allow us to track progress over time and learn.

Our Values: Our Foundation values (Equity and Dignity, Partnership, Possibility and Integrity) are reflected in our final set of measurement elements.

From Blue Shield of California Foundation.

The beauty of learning loops is that they have application and use at multiple levels: whether informing board decision-making around strategy or team decision-making around individual work components, learning loops provide a structured process to gather meaningful information and apply what is learned. We have found that it is important to be consistent in the use and application of learning loops—not to employ them only when things don't seem to be proceeding as planned. In fact, the learning loop structure is flexible enough to be applied at several points along a project's life cycle:

- As a body of work is developing
- After a new phase or type of work is completed
- If there are new partners with whom to coordinate measurement and learning
- If data cause a shift in underlying thinking that effectuates new steps

Teams have also utilized the learning loop structure in conjunction with before- and after-action reviews,[15] which provide additional scaffolding for the work of project planning and active reflection, both of which support BSCF's increased focus on applied learning as the work has moved upstream.

**Figure 32.3** ▽

Learning loops.

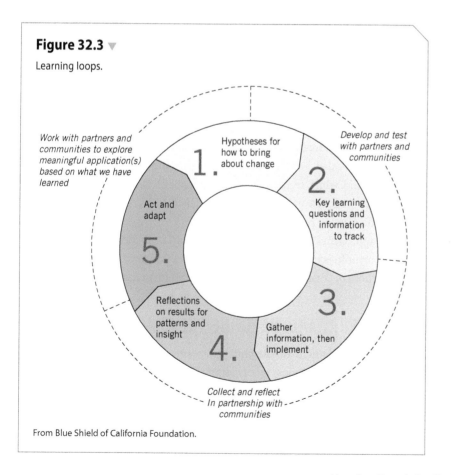

From Blue Shield of California Foundation.

**Box 32.3 | Approaches to Draw in New and Divergent Thinking**

- *Look outside of traditional fields of funding.* For example, we began exploring multisector collaborative efforts that exist outside of health care)
- *Do a deep dive with the data.* For example, we looked across several data sources to draw out new leverage points for the prevention and healing of domestic violence.
- *Engage new partners.* For example, as we seek to redesign the future of health, we've engaged futurist thinkers to help us imagine and build from what can and cannot to be constrained by what we know is true today.
- *Engaging existing partners in new and different ways.* For example, we are exploring new ways of engaging government and public health agencies that focus on how agencies can work together differently to improve the health of communities.
- *Ask for input from your board and staff.* For example, we are deliberately including a broad cross-section of staff and trustees in early work to develop our working hypotheses and explore what we are learning.

## NEW PARTNERS AND NEW APPROACHES

As part of the work to change our organizational focus, we challenged ourselves to hold a "beginner's mind"[16] as we explored new pathways and emphasized the importance of embracing divergent approaches to create change. We were moving *from* an organization that quickly identified and organized around a single path forward *to* an organization that explored possibility and held onto the tension that exists between the risk of taking steps forward based on what we are learning while remaining clear-eyed about what is still not known. Relationships with new partners were undertaken, and groundwork was laid to engage some existing partners in new ways.

These approaches to draw in new thinking and fresh ideas opened up meaningful opportunities to envision new possibilities, and new voices were engaged alongside those of trusted long-term partners to inform future work (Box 32.3).

## FURTHER FORWARD: DEFINING THE BRAND

Another critical element of the shift upstream was a significant investment in strategic communications, recognizing that the strategies require a shift in mindsets. This process began with the rebranding of BSCF.

Not only did we define what we were working toward and got clear about the audiences we intended to engage, but we also developed a complete

**Table 32.2 ▼ Blue Shield of California Foundation brand equation, developed in partnership with Mission Minded)[17]**

| Brand Promise Further forward. | | | |
|---|---|---|---|
| **Brand values** | **Brand value proposition** | **Brand positioning** | **Brand personality** |
| Integrity Partnership Possibility Equity and Dignity | When I partner with Blue Shield of California Foundation, I feel confident and energized, because together we will forge ahead for a healthy California. | The Foundation Willing to think big and do whatever it takes for the well-being of all Californians. | Thoughtful Authentic Collaborative Curious Adaptable Ambitious |

brand equation (Table 32.2) that defines how the new brand promise will be delivered: moving California "Further Forward."

The final brand equation provided important guidance and direction for the look and feel of the new brand image, collateral, templates, and website, and it set expectations for our team as we began to develop and execute against a strategic communications approach that is embedded within all of our upstream work.

For example, the "Further Forward" brand promise formed the backbone for a competitive Request for Applications (RFA) to participate in a co-design lab focused on prevention approaches to break the cycle of domestic violence. The new brand messaging was used to shape descriptions of how the co-design team will lift up voices of underserved Californians, and careful attention was paid to ensure that the value of participating—to spur innovations that can create improved health in California—would be clear. The message distribution strategy was designed to reach new audiences, and the RFA itself reflected the BSCF's new visual identity with white space, bold (yet grounded) colors, and meaningful graphics throughout.

The culmination of the strategy, innovation, measurement, and branding efforts was a refresh of the mission statement of BSCF (Box 32.4), which provides the capstone for the upstream efforts, "To build lasting and equitable solutions that make California the healthiest state and end domestic violence."

---

**Box 32.4 | Sample 1-Minute Message**

- At the Blue Shield of California Foundation, we believe it's possible to improve the lives of *all* Californians.
- That's why, every day, we collaborate with forward-thinking partners who are committed to seeking out the best, most innovative solutions that advance everyone's well-being—especially our most vulnerable neighbors'.
- Because when we work together to improve the lives of those who struggle most, we create a California full of possibility and opportunity for all.

## SUMMARY

We acknowledge that success upstream will take time to demonstrate, but we are optimistic about the chances of success. Clear data exist that define the root causes of the complex social issues we seek to address, tools exist to support a change in focus, and more and more practitioners are working together upstream.

Early takeaways are that a shift upstream requires making a deep commitment across the organization to tackle complex social challenges, having a willingness to develop new approaches that match the complexity of upstream issues and meaningfully engage communities, making an investment in a high-performing learning system that invites reflection and supports action, employing a strategic communications approach designed to draw others into new work as it unfolds, sharing what is being learned, and—finally—having the patience to give new work time to take root in support of lasting social change.

## REFERENCES

1. Blue Shield of California Foundation. On the Cusp of Change: The Health Care Preferences of Low-Income Californians. https://blueshieldcafoundation.org/publications/cusp-change-healthcare-preferences-low-income-californians. Accessed January 2019.

2. Blue Shield of California Foundation. How do Survivors Define Success? A New Project to Address an Overlooked Question. https://www.blueshieldcafoundation.org/sites/default/files/covers/How_Do_Survivors_Define_Success_FFI_Oct_2014_0.pdf. Accessed January 2019.

3. Health Affairs. Los Angeles Safety-Net Program eConsult System Was Rapidly Adopted And Decreased Wait Times To See Specialists. https://www.healthaffairs.org/doi/abs/10.1377/hlthaff.2016.1283. Accessed January 2019.

4. Council of Community Clinics. eConsult in the Safety Net. Workplan for Blue Shield of California Foundation. https://www.blueshieldcafoundation.org/sites/default/files/covers/CCC%20%28SD%29%20eConsult%20Workplan.pdf. Accessed January 2019.

5. Blue Shield of California Foundation. Mission Possible: Implementing eConsult in the Los Angeles County Healthcare System. https://www.blueshieldcafoundation.org/publications/mission-possible-implementing-econsult-los-angeles-county-healthcare-system. Accessed January 2019.

6. Blue Shield of Californai Foundation. Behavioral Health. https://www.blueshieldcafoundation.org/publications/tag/behavioral-health. Accessed January 2019.

7. BTW. Preparing the Clinic Leaders of Tomorrow. The Clinic Leadership Institute Emerging Leaders Program. https://www.blueshieldcafoundation.org/sites/default/files/publications/downloadable/FINAL_CLI-Brief.pdf. Accessed January 2019.

8. Blue Shield of California Foundation. The Legacy of the Strong Field Project. https://www.blueshieldcafoundation.org/sites/default/files/covers/2015%20SFP%20Legacy%20Report%20-%20FINAL_0.pdf. Accessed January 2019.

9. Center for Health Care Strategies, Inc. Advancing Payment Innovation within Federally Qualified Health Centers: Lessons from California. 8 https://www.blueshieldcafoundation.org/sites/default/files/covers/CHCS-CA-FQHC-APM-Brief_052517.pdf. Accessed January 2019.

10. California's 1115 Waiver: An Opportunity to Move from Coverage to Whole-Person Care. https://www.blueshieldcafoundation.org/sites/default/files/covers/1115%20waiver.WPC_.PDF. Accessed January 2019.

11. Institute for Clinical Systems Iprovement, Going Beyond Clinical Walls: Solving Complex Problems. https://www.icsi.org/_asset/w6zn9x/solvcomplexproblems.pdf. Accessed January 2019.

12. The Aspen Institute Health Innovation Project. Accelerating Innovation in Health Care: Five Game-Changing Ideas to Clear the Way. https://www.blueshieldcafoundation.org/sites/default/files/covers/AI_HealthInnovationProject_BigIdeasPaper_0_0.pdf. Accessed January 2019.

13. Moving Healthcare Upstream: Using Quality Improvemetn to Improve Social Determinants of Health and Clinical Care. https://www.sierrahealth.org/assets/HCP/Framework_Improving_Social_Determinants_of_Health.pdf. Accessed January 2019.

14. Centers for Disease Control and Prevention. Morbidity and Mortality Weekly Report. Prevalence and Characteristics of Sexual Violence, Stalking, and Intimate Partner Violence Victimization – National Intimate Partner and Sexual Violence Survey, United States, 2011, Page 14. https://www.cdc.gov/mmwr/pdf/ss/ss6308.pdf. Accessed January 2019.

15. Harvard Business Review. Learning in the Thick of It. https://hbr.org/2005/07/learning-in-the-thick-of-it. Accessed January 2019.

16. Suzuki, Shunryu (1970). Zen Mind, Beginner's Mind. p. 21.

17. Mission Minded is a branding firm that works exclusively with nonprofit organizations. Mission Minded may be contacted by emailing amplify@mission-minded.com.

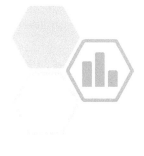

# Chapter 33

# Case Study—Acting (and Funding) Locally: How One Virginia Foundation Is Changing the Way It Supports Communities

PATRICIA N. MATHEWS

N orthern Virginia is among the healthiest places in the United States. Arlington County, Fairfax County, Loudoun County, Prince William County, the City of Alexandria, and the smaller cities they surround, rank among the healthiest areas in the Commonwealth of Virginia. It is a region with a land mass larger than the state of Rhode Island. Northern Virginia is a highly diverse region of more than 2.4 million people, constituting nearly a third of all Virginia residents. And yet more than 500,000 of its residents live below 200% of the federal poverty level (FPL). (A family of four currently living at the FPL has an income of $24,600/year. At 200% FPL, that income is $49,200/year.)

The Northern Virginia Health Foundation (NVHF) was created 12 years ago and charged with a mission that remains in place today: to improve the health and health care of the residents of Northern Virginia, with a particular emphasis on those who are low-income and uninsured. At that time, these individuals and families had limited options when it came to receiving high-quality, affordable health care services. All too often, they sought their health care from very few small health centers, privately funded free clinics, health departments, and hospital emergency rooms, all of which comprised Northern Virginia's health care "safety net." Strengthening and expanding that safety net quickly emerged as a critical grant-making priority for NVHF.

Despite being a small foundation, over the years, NVHF has made significant investments in the health care safety net. Our grant-making approach has been strategic. We fund a range of organizations that, either independently or by coordinating care with other safety net providers, offer low-income residents a patient-centered medical home where they can receive high-quality, well-coordinated care, something every person deserves regardless of ability to pay.

However, low-income residents of Northern Virginia continue to face significant challenges. Roughly 130,000 Northern Virginia residents younger than 64 and who are single, not pregnant, and not disabled live below 100% of the FPL and are uninsured. This is primarily because Virginia has one of the country's most stringent Medicaid policies, and legislators are only now discussing the possibility of expanding Medicaid, something that was not done under the Patient Protection and Affordable Care Act (ACA).[2] It became increasingly clear that just focusing on improving and expanding safety net services was not the answer to improving the health of residents of Northern Virginia.

## SYSTEMS CHANGE: UPSTREAM INTERVENTIONS

Continuing to be true to the mission, NVHF expanded its grant-making to include a focus on system change. This was certainly not an unusual idea; across the country, conversations were taking place about health equity and social determinants of health (SDOH)—those factors that affect health beyond health care, such as income, housing, education, ethnicity, race, gender, transportation, and access to healthy foods. Indeed, for several years, staff had been actively participating in cross-sector partnerships and coalitions and had come to understand the importance of working upstream—of recognizing that most of what makes us sick has less to do with health care than where we live, work, play, and pray. And we knew that one sector couldn't address these issues on its own.

This is the reason that, a little more than 2 years ago, NVHF issued a Request for Proposal (RFP) for "upstream interventions"; we asked that applicants be coalitions comprised of at least one nonprofit organization, one nonprofit health care provider, and one local government agency. Staff held an informational webinar for prospective applicants and stressed the importance of submitting letters of intent that focused on factors that caused poor health outcomes that could be prevented. Although more than 70 organizations participated in the webinar, far fewer submitted a letter of intent, and even fewer were asked to submit a full proposal.

After careful review, NVHF awarded $125,000 in planning grants to each of five local coalitions that proposed to work on an issue that addressed one of the social factors that contributed to poor health outcomes in Northern Virginia. Each of these coalitions included a mix of local government agencies, community organizations, and health care providers who used their planning grants to develop collaborative strategies to enhance their work.

## LOUDOUN COUNTY: ADDRESSING CHILD ABUSE AND NEGLECT

Of particular note is a coalition led by Stop Child Abuse Now (SCAN) of Northern Virginia, which is working to shed light on child abuse in Loudoun County. Loudoun County, declared by *Forbes Magazine* to be the nation's wealthiest county in 2016, has a median household income of $134,464,[3] double the national median. Moreover, 76% of the population own their own homes, 60% are families with children, and the labor force participation rate is 75%. In the past few years, the county has grown quite rapidly, with a population that now exceeds 312,000.

But there is a flip side to this positive picture. In 2014, 1,462 children were involved in 1,205 valid reports of child abuse in Loudoun County. More than 1 in 5 of these reports involves a child exposed to domestic violence. Because social services positions have not increased at the rate of the children's population growth in the county, staff are stretched thin. Although the Child Welfare League of America's standards recommend no more than 12 cases per child protective services investigator, and nearby Fairfax County has a maximum of 9 cases per worker, Loudoun County child protective services investigators typically have more than 20 cases each.

A substantial body of research has shown that child maltreatment is arguably a causal factor for many of the most pressing health status concerns, having an adverse impact on physical health, behavioral health, and well-being. Child maltreatment has been shown to disrupt and impair brain development.[4] The stress of childhood adversity and trauma have a negative impact on emotional regulation and is a risk factor for persistent psychological issues (e.g., low self-esteem, depression, and antisocial, including violent, behavior). These children also demonstrate delays in cognitive capacity and language development, and their academic achievement is lower than that of their nonabused/neglected peers.[5]

To address this issue, SCAN of Northern Virginia brought together a group that included Loudoun Citizens for Social Justice, the county's Department of Family Services, and HealthWorks for Northern Virginia (one of only three Federally Qualified Health Centers in Northern Virginia). The group determined that it would form a steering committee and add other organizations to the collaboration as its work progressed.

Its first piece of work was to gather data drawn from structured interviews, group interviews, health center data, and data from county government agencies, which was an important step. Once the group had collected data, it could work on recommendations to address the issues identified and create and disseminate a report that could educate the residents of Loudon. As a result of their efforts, the steering committee grew to 10 active organizations, and plans were made for publication of "Resilient Children, Resilient Loudoun!—A Collaborative Report on the Needs of Children and Recommendations to Best

Support Loudoun County's Most Vulnerable Children & Families" (the full report can be downloaded at www.scanva.org/loudoun.)

With subsequent funding from the NVHF, the steering committee continued dissemination of its report, targeted opportunities for advocacy, and offered training to local providers on key topics related to the recommendations. Community leaders and elected officials participated in meetings with steering committee members. And there was some system change: the Board of Supervisors of Loudoun County agreed to fund two new positions for child protective services. New county regulations also took effect in July 2017, which require Child Protective Services to make a priority response (i.e., within 24 hours) to reports of an infant at risk, although there was some confusion about how that response should be handled.

In 2018, the steering committee will focus on just one of the adverse childhood experiences: growing up with a parent who has a substance abuse issue. One of the best practices in addressing this growing epidemic and reducing the negative consequences to children is universal screening of all prenatal patients, at both public clinics and by private obstetricians. A number of other communities have found universal screenings to help reduce stigma, enhance the system's ability to assess the scope of the problem, and facilitate more and earlier referrals to treatment. This is the logical next step for the steering committee. Also, studies show that one-third to two-thirds of child maltreatment cases involved some degree of substance abuse.[6] Nonetheless, this will be a challenge.

## LESSONS LEARNED

The NVHF and its "upstream" grantees have already learned a number of lessons from this work:

1. *Genuine partnerships are difficult.* Our "upstream interventions" require all of the participants to engage in the work and to have a specific role in achieving the objectives that were put forth in the proposal's logic model. All too often, organizations agree to lend their support as "partners" but have no intention of being an active participant, and they leave it to the applicant to call the organization when or if they're needed. These grants required the active engagement of *all* partners.

2. *Nonprofit organizations often don't see themselves as "peers" of government agencies.* Nonprofit organizations—particularly smaller ones—often find it difficult to question, challenge, or disagree with government agencies, particularly if they are receiving funds or other support from the government. Although many funders, private or public, are aware of this "power dynamic," they are often not sensitive to it. Yet it is essential that nonprofits see themselves as peers to lead an effective partnership.

3. *Disruption happens.* Changes in staffing, whether in the applicant organization or among partner participants, may require renegotiating the nature of the partnership.

4. *Genuine partnerships take time to develop.* This new way of working together doesn't just happen; time is required to develop the relationships necessary to move the work forward. Expecting things to move quickly, although understandable, can lead to frustration and delay, which can result in more delay. And time is needed at various points to ensure that consensus is built and maintained as the work proceeds to its next level.

5. *Systems change is very difficult.* While recognizing the need for systems change, it is easy to focus on undertaking a project or starting a new program. If something isn't working, the usual reaction is to say "Okay, let's just create something that does work." This is completely understandable; seeing systems change is a relatively rare occurrence. Unfortunately, starting something new means that whatever has been created is on top of that which doesn't work. The original problem is still there; staff is still working the same way and funds are still being expended. Yet, when that new project stops, the underlying problem remains. Changing systems requires a different way of thinking, but it is the only path to lasting change.

6. *Data are essential.* All of us have had occasion to drive through a community and know that vulnerable residents live there. But what do we actually know? Having data, rather than anecdotes, assumptions, or beliefs, is a key ingredient to any advocacy strategy, and it is essential to systems change.

In light of these lessons, the NVHF took several steps that we thought would be helpful.

1. *We commissioned data.* In 2016, the NVHF engaged the Center on Society and Health at Virginia Commonwealth University to provide census tract data on five indicators: life expectancy; median household income; percentage of residents with a bachelor's degree or higher; percentage of residents who are black, non-Hispanic; and percentage of Hispanic residents. Each of these indicators was mapped for each census tract, and a companion report, "A Study in Contrasts: Why Life Expectancy Varies in Northern Virginia," was also prepared (https://novahealthfdn.org/wp-content/uploads/csh-nova-report-v10.pdf). NVHF staff knew that data on a countywide or citywide basis would mask the disparities in the jurisdictions, as would zip code data. It was important to provide granular data to ensure that the disparities were highlighted. And they were highlighted: among the facts that were revealed is that life expectancy at birth (i.e., the number of years an average newborn can expect to live) varies by as much as 13 years across Northern Virginia.

   Last year, we deepened that work. We again commissioned the Center on Society and Health to update and provide additional indicators for the census tract maps, this time looking at 13 indicators in the areas of education, economic distress, housing, and health care. As had been the case previously, a companion report. "Getting Ahead: The Uneven Opportunity Landscape in Northern Virginia," https://novahealthfdn.org/getting-ahead-report/ was prepared by the VCU team, led by Steven H. Woolf, MD, MPH. The report detailed 15 "islands of disadvantage" interspersed among the affluent communities of Northern Virginia, where residents face multiple challenges, including poverty, poor education, unaffordable housing, and lack of health insurance. People of color, who represent a disproportionate share of residents in these neighborhoods, face greater challenges getting ahead. Some of the neighborhoods are, literally, directly across the street from affluent census tracts. As an example, in Fairfax County, one census tract has a median household income of $192,750, and the census tract on its border has a median household income of $47,214. And in Loudoun County, there are 12 census tracts where people have a median household income of less than $50,000.

Both of these reports are being used by local government agencies and numerous nonprofit organizations to begin to delve more deeply into the challenges faced by vulnerable residents in Northern Virginia.

2. *We provided additional technical assistance.* Another step that NVHF took was to require each of the upstream grant recipients to attend training on effective partnerships. Each had to bring a representative from every collaborative participant, thereby ensuring that the information learned and shared was received by all who would be engaged. The facilitator who led each session (without NVHF staff present) prompted discussions about roles and responsibilities of partnership participants, expectations of each partner, and clarification of the work to be achieved. Feedback on these sessions was quite positive, and future sessions are being envisioned as the NVHF continues to explore its role in upstream interventions.

## CONCLUSION

Cross-sector collaboration is difficult and, in many instances, expensive. But the return on investment is potentially strong. Creative and focused efforts to change systems can reverse economic decline and help mitigate the fragile living conditions that fuel social discord, drug abuse, crime, and gang violence. Such efforts could also boost economic productivity by cultivating a more educated, healthy, and competitive workforce, which would be attractive to the business community.

Of course, this work also gives rise to the question, "What if?" What if the Centers for Disease Control and Prevention were to require states to report at the census-tract level? What if the data that are already available was communicated in such a way that those hearing it didn't have to be epidemiologists to understand it? What if hospitals in our region were more receptive to getting engaged in upstream interventions, as have some other hospitals and health systems around the country? What if the business community understood the actual economic benefit to addressing social determinants of health? What if local government agencies that weren't health departments understood the effects that their programs, plans, and systems have on the health of individuals? What if "cross-sector collaboration" wasn't something that was all too frequently done to acquire a grant, but became instead a way of thinking about strategic problem-solving? What if the issues of race and class were not so sensitive and so politicized that they could be discussed in ways that contributed to the solutions that are sorely needed?

The "what if?" possibilities are continuing challenges that all of us, philanthropic, nonprofit, for-profit, government, and, most especially, health sectors, need to continue to address, however small the individual step. At the end of the day, we are not just looking for systems change in the macro sense; we also are looking for behavior change in each and every one of us.

Poverty in the suburbs is a growing problem throughout the nation. Economic and demographic trends indicate that the problem will worsen without action. As Dr. Martin Luther King, Jr., observed, "Injustice anywhere is a threat to justice everywhere." This is certainly true for Northern Virginia. The NVHF is looking forward to continuing to work on these issues for improvement of the health and well-being of the region.

## REFERENCES

1. Robert Wood Johnson Foundation. County Health Rankings and Roadmaps-Virginia. http://www/countyhealthrankings.org/app/virginia/2018/overview. Accessed 1/22/2018.

2. Balch, B. (2018, October 18). Medicaid expansion enrollment to begin Nov. 1. *Richmond Times Dispatch*. Retrived from www.richmond.com

3. Loudoun County Facts and Figures. https://www.loudoun.gov/173/Facts-Figures. Accessed 1/22/2019.

4. Child Welfare Information Gateway. *Long-Term Consequences of Child Abuse and Neglect*.Washington, DC: US Department of Health and Human Services, Children's Bureau; 2013.

5. Romano E, Babchishin L, Marquis R, Fréchette S. Childhood maltreatment and educational outcomes. *Trauma Violence Abuse*. 2015;16(4):418–37. https://doi.org/10.1177/1524838014537908

6. Child Welfare Information Gateway. *Long-Term Consequences of Child Abuse and Neglect*. Washington, DC: US Department of Health and Human Services, Children's Bureau; 2013.

# Sustainability and Finance: Supporting Partnerships over Time

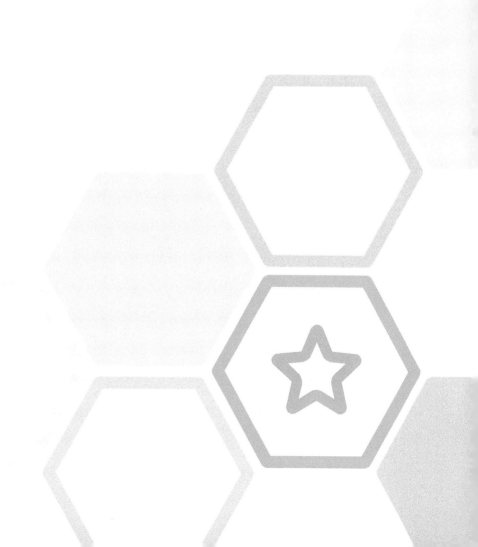

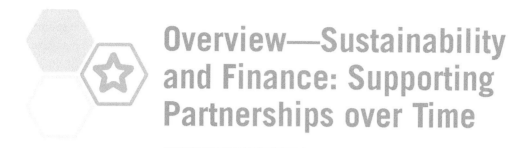

# Overview—Sustainability and Finance: Supporting Partnerships over Time

CRAIG W. THOMAS AND BRIAN C. CASTRUCCI

Disclaimer text: *The opinions expressed by authors contributing to this publication do not necessarily reflect the opinions of the U.S. Department of Health and Human Services, the Public Health Service, the Centers for Disease Control and Prevention, or the authors' affiliated institutions.*

Across the country, cross-sector collaboratives to improve population health are under way to accelerate the movement toward value-based health systems. Key to these efforts is a focus on prevention strategies to address social determinants of heath as well as collective efforts to improve population health outcomes. Furthermore, if the growing number of health disparities across the country are to be eliminated, dedicated and innovative strategies are needed to close the gaps and reduce the need for health care services.

Effectively acquiring, managing, and sustaining financial investments in health is fundamental to the success of multisector and community-led health improvement initiatives. Catalyzed by grant dollars in response to acute and long-standing community health problems or by enterprising institutions seeking to promote their healthy community mission, these partnerships are rapidly developing between health care, social services, public health, and organizations that support, among others, housing, public safety, and transportation.

Sustainability and financing are essential to ensuring the success of population health improvement initiatives throughout the life cycle (i.e., initiation, maintenance, adaptation, and continual improvement) and for achieving and expanding its impact. For example, support for sustainable community health initiatives can be achieved in partnerships with hospitals and health systems through alignment of diverse funding sources for health improvement interventions and by reinvestment of a portion of the savings from interventions back into the community.

Cross-sector partnerships play a critical role in ensuring the sustainability and financing of population health initiatives. By combining assets, services, and investments, these partnerships will have a wider impact than would spending by a single organization alone. Commitment to shared resources, flexible funding practices, and investment strategies are reflected in many current national guidelines and model practices for health improvement, including the Community Health Improvement Navigator Program from the Centers for Disease Control and Prevention (CDC), the Foundational Public Health Services framework from the Robert Wood Johnson Foundation, and the Public Health 3.0 framework from the US Department of Health and Human Services.

This section highlights the importance of developing and maintaining diverse partnerships and innovative resource strategies. The chapters in this section illustrate a range of new and evolving financial strategies that are currently under way to support partnerships for improved population health outcomes.

In Chapter 35, Jutte introduces readers to the community development sector, an extensive network of financially skilled institutions and members that work collectively to reduce poverty in underserved and underresourced communities by addressing social and structural determinants of health. Offering innovative and sizeable financial opportunities to invest in and improve vulnerable communities, this sector shares a common mission to improve health, generates economic growth, and catalyzes and sustains multisector partnerships for population health improvements. Also in this chapter, Gillman adds her expertise as a funder at the Robert Wood Johnson Foundation and describes how it has become involved with community development financial institutions.

Clary and Riley, in Chapter 36, present innovative funding strategies to help state Medicaid and public health decision-makers plan for possible changes to the structure and levels of federal funding for public health. Four scenarios are presented that represent a range of responses to possible changes and reductions in federal funding. Creating greater flexibility in funding is a central component of their strategy to support and sustain cross-agency work. Blended, braided, and block grant strategies are discussed, as are state-based examples of these strategies that have been adopted to safeguard and promote the health of their communities.

Also in Chapter 36, Deloso discusses a rural case study on sustainability of a mental health initiative to strengthen social support and leadership development. Led by a Federal Qualified Health Center, this multisector partnership includes public health, health care, and community support partners. Through this collaborative, partners share ideas, pool resources, share meeting space, and provide peer-to-peer training to develop a sustainable workforce capable of providing social support services and needed job skills to youth and veterans.

In Chapter 37, Zuckerman, Ansell, and Davis describe a new and compelling role for hospitals and health systems as anchor institutions. Representing significant economic and human capital resources, anchor institutions are grounded, sound business practices, and, in the realities of the local communities they serve, they are well placed to effectively align, leverage, and invest resources to improve the health of their communities. An important and highly effective partner for health, examples of successful institutions that have adopted this approach are described, as is a national network to help hospitals and other institutions adopt and advance an anchor mission within their organizations and communities.

Bellow, Brewster, Chennisi, and Oestman, in Chapter 38, provide a case study on how building ties with the business community has sustained and expanded local efforts to improve community health and wellness in Pasadena, Texas. This example highlights how businesses can be a powerful partner in promoting economic development and creating community health as well as in sustaining and expanding health improvement initiatives through funding, strategic partnership, and implementation support.

The chapters in this section underscore the value and benefits of developing strategic partnerships with institutions that represent sizeable economic and human capital resources and share a commitment to making investment strategies that promote economic development, address determinants of health and inequity, and drive population health improvement within the communities they serve.

Despite the number of successful examples of sustainability and innovative financing presented here, we do need to understand which organizational and financing strategies work best and under which circumstances. In particular, we need to identify which sustainability strategies are most effective in underserved and underresourced communities. In certain geographic areas and in specific populations, institutions, funding, and resources are lacking.

Tribal and rural communities are particularly affected by geography as well as by lack of programs, community organizations, and partnerships to improve health and wellness. For example, tribal chapter communities often have no community wellness centers for youth. The isolation of rural tribal communities also contributes to food deserts and problems accessing fresh fruits and vegetables (well-stocked grocery stores may be 30–50 miles away).

In rural America, Shaping Our Appalachian Region (SOAR) is a nonpartisan economic development agency serving 54 counties tasked to expand job creation; enhance regional opportunity, innovation, and identity; improve the quality of life; and support all those working to achieve these goals in Eastern Kentucky. Through collaboration and innovation, and with local leadership, SOAR has created the Healthy Communities Initiative, which is focused on maximizing collaboration and education to reduce the physical and economic impact of obesity, diabetes, and substance abuse. The Community Health Action Team (CHAT) is working to help create sustainable economic infrastructure and healthy communities.

It is important to note that funding, although indistinguishable from sustainability, is only one piece of the sustainability puzzle. Other sustainability practices include sustainability planning, conducting annual reviews, continuing action plans, maintaining partnerships, and tracking and monitoring progress.

These practices emphasize the importance of working sustainability into the planning, resourcing, implementation, and evaluation of population health initiatives, and they ultimately support the success and impact of multisector partnerships.

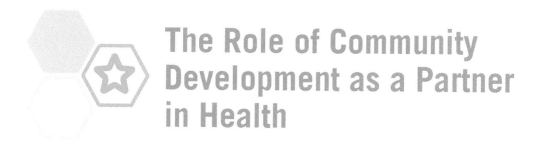

# Chapter 35

# The Role of Community Development as a Partner in Health

DOUGLAS JUTTE

More jumbles of letters: LIHTC, NMTC, CRA, AMI, TOD, HFFI, HFAs, CDFIs, CDCs (no, not that CDC). What do any of them have to do with health?

In this chapter, we describe the work—and the jargon—of the community development sector, a vast, financially savvy, mission-driven industry that tackles poverty in our most under-resourced neighborhoods (Box 35.1). In doing so, this sector also improves the health of vulnerable communities through interventions addressing important social determinants that underlie the enormous health inequities we see across cities, regions, and the country as a whole.

The importance of this potential collaboration cannot be overstated. In the United States, we currently spend at least $3.5 trillion per year on health care.[1] More than 85% of those resources are spent on chronic disease, and we know that a substantial portion of chronic disease is preventable, linked to poverty, and concentrated in low-income communities.[2] This translates to at least *$1 trillion* spent annually on avoidable chronic disease among residents of low-income neighborhoods. These are precisely the places where community development invests its time, resources, and expertise tackling many of the determinants of poor health.

Despite being relatively unfamiliar to clinicians and public health practitioners, the community development sector has been around for decades and now invests nearly $200 billion annually into low- and moderate-income neighborhoods across the country.[3] This sector is comprised of several thousand organizations that finance and build affordable housing for families, develop supportive housing for the homeless and elderly, place grocery stores in

### Box 35.1 | Community Development Acronym Buster

AMI: area median income
CRA: community reinvestment act
CDC: community development corporation
CDFI: community development financial institution
ELI: extremely low income
HFA: housing finance agency
HFFI: healthy food financing initiative
LIHTC: low income housing tax credit
NACEDA: National Alliance of Community Economic Development
    Associations
NALCAB: National Association of Latino Community Asset Builders
National CAPACD: National Coalition for Asian Pacific American Community
    Development
NMTC: new markets tax credit
NOAH: naturally occurring affordable housing
OFN: Opportunity Finance Network
SAHF: Stewards for Affordable Housing for the Future
TOD: transit oriented development

For detailed definitions, visit the Build Healthy Places Network's Jargon Buster at www.buildhealthyplaces.org/jargon-buster/.

food deserts, and construct charter schools, preschools, child development centers, community clinics, and other neighborhood infrastructure while also investing in locally owned small businesses. Driven by a mix of public and private resources—federal and state grants and tax incentives as well as federally mandated investments by for-profit banks—the community development sector intervenes to address many of the social determinants of health (SDHs) and inequity that clinicians and public health practitioners hold dear: housing, education, child care, transportation, access to healthy foods, recreation, and jobs (Box 35.2).

Too often, public health, primary care, and community development are working in the same neighborhoods, often with the same people, but don't know one another. By joining forces and harnessing each other's strengths and resources, these sectors together can have a more powerful impact on improving population health and addressing long-standing, persistent health inequities. The Build Healthy Places Network (the Network) where I am executive director, is the national center at the intersection of community development and health working to bridge these fields and advance a common vision: equitable communities where all people can live healthy and productive lives.

## Box 35.2 | Robert Wood Johnson Foundation Funding in CDFI Work

*Amy Gillman*

For more than 40 years, the Robert Wood Johnson Foundation (RWJF) has worked to improve health. What we've learned is that focusing on health *care* alone is not sufficient because most of what shapes our health happens outside the doctor's office. Our strategic vision is to build a national Culture of Health that enables all people to lead a long, healthy life—regardless of where they live or the social or economic challenges they may face. Community development financial institutions (CDFIs) and other community developers play a critical role in improving health because of their ability to improve conditions in low-income neighborhoods where it can be more difficult to be healthy—places without safe, affordable housing or places to walk or play, or access to good jobs or high-quality schools. They are important partners in our work, and in the work of all public- and private-sector funders including national, regional, and local philanthropies whose mission is to improve health and well-being.

Funders of all sizes can play a variety of roles to foster community investment that improves the health and vitality of neighborhoods; effective partnerships between the community development and health sectors can make this possible. Note the following examples:

- *Flexible project capital.* Funders can provide flexible capital—grants, loans, or guarantees—for projects such as safe housing, grocery stores, early childhood centers, and other physical infrastructure that makes communities healthier. Philanthropic dollars can support projects at an early stage and help reduce the cost of funds or risks seen by lenders who may hesitate to invest in lower income neighborhoods. Funders such as RWJF and the Kresge Foundation have collaborated to catalyze new financing models, such as the Healthy Neighborhoods Equity Fund, which is a transit-oriented development investment pool that looks at community, environmental, and health impacts in addition to financial returns. Smaller philanthropies and community foundations can contribute to this type of local or regional fund or support proven models in their geography.
- *Data and measurement.* As CDFIs increasingly turn their attention to health, they face the challenge of assessing the health impacts of their activities and investments. Philanthropy can play a role in making data and measurement tools available and easier for practitioners to understand and use, both to build the evidence base and engage a broader circle of partners, including the health sector. That's why we're supporting the 500 Cities Project and City Health Dashboard to provide neighborhood- and census tract–level data on health and the factors that drive health in communities. These data allow leaders from the health, community development, and other sectors to better identify the most pressing health issues, dig deeper into how to address those challenges, and target strategies more effectively.

- *Cross-sector learning and collaboration.* CDFIs have only recently begun to recognize the health benefits of community development and often have limited understanding of health indicators or the culture and operations of health institutions. At the same time, many health actors are unfamiliar with community investment or how to engage with CDFIs to support healthy communities. Funders can help by convening partners and identifying and communicating about promising models and practices. The Build Healthy Places Network is an example of an important RWJF investment in promoting work at the intersection of community development and health by having a place to connect and learn about each sector and how sectors can work together. RWJF also participates in the Convergence Partnership, a network of more than 80 local and regional funders that are making investments in food systems, resilient economic development, and prevention and health systems, all of which provide opportunities for partnership between the community development and health sectors.

## WHAT IS COMMUNITY DEVELOPMENT?

### Brief History

The modern community development sector has its roots in the War on Poverty of the 1960s. Importantly, however, community development today is not the centralized urban renewal of that era, an approach that too often resulted in the industrial-scale public housing projects we associate with the urban core of many American cities. Those sorts of Department of Housing and Urban Development (HUD)-funded efforts fell out of favor under President Nixon and were slashed under President Reagan. In their place gradually arose a network of community-based, local and national, largely nonprofit organizations that responded to the unabated need for affordable housing. There are now thousands of these organizations across the country, representing communities large and small. Partnering with one another and using new sources of federal and private capital, these more nimble, mission-driven institutions were better able to incorporate resident voices and build the housing and other neighborhood infrastructure that best responded to the community's needs.

### How Much Money? And Where Does It Come From?

As a result of multiple funding streams of different types, sources, and definitions, estimates of the total investments made annually through community development are difficult to come by. But adding together the main categories brings us to approximately *$200 billion per year* invested expressly into low-income neighborhoods.

### Low-Income Housing Tax Credit

The workhorse of community development funding is the Low-Income Housing Tax credit (LIHTC, pronounced "LieTeck" by those in the industry). Created as part of the Tax Reform Act of 1986 to encourage private investment in affordable housing, LIHTC vouchers are distributed by the states and amounted to nearly $9 billion in 2017 alone.[4] In a somewhat complicated dance, organizations allocated tax credits by their state housing finance agencies (HFAs) sell them to corporations for cash that they can then use for their work. The corporations then use the credits they've purchased as payment for future taxes, saving money in the process. Interestingly, there is substantial bipartisan political support for this program. Conservatives see it as a way to provide tax credits to corporations and engage the private market in the development of affordable housing. Meanwhile, liberals see LIHTC as a way to get substantial resources into the hands of community-based organizations through the tax code and thus avoid risky annual budget fights.

The LIHTC funds must be spent on the production or preservation of affordable rental housing. "Affordability" is defined as economical for residents earning 60% of area median income (AMI), with rents capped at 30% of their income, less utilities. Notably, nearly half of residents living in LIHTC-subsidized apartments make less than 30% AMI, or are extremely low income (ELI).[4] Housing can be in the form of fully affordable or mixed-income housing and can include multi-family or, less often, single-family homes; special-needs housing for the elderly or disabled; and supportive housing for homeless families and individuals. Remarkably, fully 30% of the 10 million units of affordable housing in the country have been developed through the LIHTC program. That represents more apartments than all the federally funded housing built prior to 1987, effectively making it "the most successful social program that nobody has heard of."[5]

### New Markets Tax Credit and Healthy Food Financing Initiative

Another important tax credit program, the New Markets Tax Credit (NMTC),[6] is managed by the Treasury Department and, since 2001, has provided nearly $55 billion targeted at job creation in low-income neighborhoods ($3.4B in 2017 alone).[7] These dollars can be invested directly in small businesses or into other job-creating community facilities. In recent years, community clinics have been seen as important job creators in low-income neighborhoods and thus are increasingly being built using NMTC funding. In addition, since 2010, through a parallel mechanism jointly run through the US Treasury, the US Department of Agriculture (USDA), and US Department of Health and Human Services (HHS), the federal government has provided hundreds of millions of dollars via the Healthy Food Financing Initiative (HFFI).[8] HFFI provides grants, loans, and financial assistance to community development organizations to put grocery stores into food deserts and undertakes other efforts to increase the availability of fresh, healthy food in low-income neighborhoods.

### Community Reinvestment Act

But as important as the aforementioned funding streams are for driving resources into low-income neighborhoods, they pale in comparison to the impact of the Community Reinvestment Act (CRA). Passed in 1977, the CRA is often called an "anti-redlining" law because it responded to decades of disinvestment in predominantly African American neighborhoods across the country's cities driven by discriminatory lending practices. The term *redlining* arose from the red color used to shade neighborhoods considered high risk due to the "detrimental influences" of, among other things, residents of non-white minority groups.

The CRA requires for-profit banks to invest by providing loans and mortgages to the low-income neighborhoods where they take deposits. The results of the CRA have been staggering. In 2016 alone,[9] banks made CRA investments totaling more than $255 billion. Even considering only larger loans over $100,000 that are more likely to represent true community development investments, the total adds up to more than $150 billion in just that 1 year.

## Who Does the Work?

Having described the sources of the hundreds of billions of dollars going into community development, it's important to highlight the types of organizations that do the hard work of investing the money in the communities that need it. Broadly, one can break down the major players into three groups: (1) community development corporations (CDCs), (2) affordable housing developers, and (3) community development financial institutions (CDFIs).

### Community Development Corporations

With the help of Robert Kennedy, the first CDC was founded in 1967, in New York City—the Bedford Stuyvesant Restoration Corporation—to serve the impoverished, predominantly African American, Brooklyn neighborhood of the same name. These CDCs, nonprofit organizations incorporated to support and promote community development efforts in struggling neighborhoods, now number more than 4,000 across the country. They are in almost every urban neighborhood as well as in many smaller cities and rural areas. Prominent examples include Chicanos por La Causa, a statewide CDC serving Arizona; East Bay Asian Local Development Corporation (EBALDC) in Oakland, California; and Hill Community Development Corporation serving Pittsburgh's Hill District.

EBALDC, for example, arose in 1975, with a group of activists and community leaders initially working to serve the Chinatown neighborhood of Oakland. Subsequently, the organization expanded its focus to respond to the large-scale destruction of affordable housing by freeway development and other forms of urban renewal prevalent in that era. And, more recently, EBALDC has been one of the most innovative and forward thinking CDCs nationally in its explicit incorporation of health into its work.[10] EBALDC now owns and manages 30 residential developments and commercial space serving childcare and health centers, nonprofits, a resident-owned market, and popular locally owned restaurants. And they have developed and preserved 2,200 affordable homes, helping Oakland resist the effects of intense local gentrification and displacement pressures.[11] (You can find case studies and articles featuring the recent work of EBALDC and other CDCs on our website, www.buildhealthyplaces.org.)

### Affordable Housing Developers

More narrowly focused on housing and more often regional or national in scope than CDCs are the nonprofit and for-profit affordable housing developers. A national organization, Stewards for Affordable Housing for the Future (SAHF), represents the 13 largest nonprofit affordable housing developers in the country, with members including Mercy Housing Inc., National Church Residences, Retirement Housing Foundation, and the Community Builders. Together SAHF members own and operate more than 130,000 rental apartments serving low-income residents across the country. In addition, dozens of for-profit developers also provide affordable and mixed-income housing across the country, with just the 10 largest constructing more than 11,000 affordable homes in 2016 alone.[12] Both nonprofit and for-profit affordable housing developers rely heavily on LIHTC resources and investments from CRA-motivated banks to do their work.

### Community Development Financial Institutions

CDFIs make up a third important category of community development organizations. At root, CDFIs are nonprofit banks with the mission to provide lending and financial resources to low-income neighborhoods underserved by the for-profit banking sector.

The origins of CDFIs can be traced back to the early 1970s and the mission-focused loan funds started by religious orders of nuns to provide low-interest loans to economically disadvantaged residents in their communities.[13] At the same time, the first community development bank in the country, ShoreBank in Chicago, was founded by young, banking activists in 1973 to fight against the growing tide of racist lending practices.[14] Inspired by these earlier efforts, in 1994, President Bill Clinton championed the creation of the CDFI Fund within the US Treasury Department to support and spread the work of CDFIs nationally.[15] The field has grown substantially over the past 20 years, with the CDFI Fund now certifying more than 1,000 CDFIs across the country (https://ofn.org/cdfi-coverage-map). The CDFI Fund itself has distributed more than $2 billion since its inception and, in 2017 alone, financed more than 14,700 small business and microenterprise loans, nearly 28,000 affordable housing units, and served more than 470,000 individuals with financial literacy or other training.[16]

One of the most important roles for CDFIs is to coordinate the complex financial transactions required of modern community development. Most community development investments require the blending and braiding of multiple streams of capital: philanthropic dollars, tax credits (LIHTC and/or NMTC), CRA-motivated investments, and market-rate loans. Though more successful in getting resources directly into the hands of communities than the previous centralized, HUD-based model, this more complex, networked approach to obtaining necessary resources also demands a level of financial expertise that exceeds the capabilities of all but the most sophisticated CDCs or affordable housing developers. CDFIs are, thus, important partners for increasing the capacity and capability of community developers and for driving investments that address local needs.

### National Umbrella Organizations

As noted earlier, the large, nonprofit affordable housing developers utilize SAHF as a shared organization advocating for the importance of their work at the national and regional level. Similarly, the CDFI industry has a national membership body called the Opportunity Finance Network (OFN) that provides support, training, and a national forum for gathering and guiding the field. At this time, CDCs lack a national institution, but a pair of organizations fills part of that gap. The federally funded NeighborWorks America supports more than 240 CDCs that meet its rigorous membership criteria, and the National Alliance of Community Economic Development Associations (NACEDA) provides a forum for the many state and regional CDC associations.

Importantly, all four of these national organizations—SAHF, OFN, NeighborWorks America, and NACEDA—have dramatically increased their focus on SDHs in recent years. Thus, they are important associations to recognize because they represent excellent partners for collaborative work with health care and public health and because they can help identify member organizations working in your own neighborhood, city, or region.

## THE ZIP CODE IMPROVEMENT BUSINESS

It is often said that your zip code is more important than your genetic code in determining your lifelong health. It could also be said, then, that community development is in the zip code improvement business.

Much as state and county public health departments can provide on-the-ground interventions to address public health threats, I believe that the community development sector is well positioned to serve *population health* as a similar action arm for intervention. Simply studying the consequences of poverty or specifying in greater and greater detail the negative health effects of important SDHs is not enough. But actually intervening to reduce levels of poverty or improve neighborhood-level factors tied to poor health has seemed beyond the reach of health practitioners. The community development sector is at its root an anti-poverty movement. Thus, by joining forces, health and community development can together have a greater positive influence on SDHs and advancing health equity.

A pair of recent speeches drives home this point. In a plenary session before a national audience of CRA-regulated banks in 2016, then-president and CEO of the Robert Wood Johnson Foundation, Risa Lavizzo-Mourey stated, "We are likely to look back at this time and wonder why community development and health were ever separate sectors."[17] But perhaps even more surprising than the CEO of one of the world's largest health foundation speaking to a ballroom full of bankers was Ben Bernanke, Chair of the Federal Reserve Board of Governors, saying in a speech in 2013, "Perhaps one of the most promising new partners in community development is the health-care sector." He pointed out that neighborhood factors such as safety, income, educational success, and access to healthy food are correlated with both economic health and physical health and concluded by saying that "health-care professionals and community development organizations are seeing new opportunities for cooperation in low-income communities."[18] The time is now to act on their forward thinking.

## A Health ROI and Opportunities for Research and Partnership

Because the work of community development brings financial resources to low-income communities to improve important SDHs, they are creating a health return on investment (ROI). However, that health ROI is only beginning to be adequately acknowledged, it is still not being routinely measured, and it is almost never paid for by the health care system. This, then, is a critical role for public health and clinical researchers: to measure and document the health benefits that arise from community development investments.

Though research has demonstrated positive effects of housing affordability on child well-being,[19] most work focuses on the negative consequences of exposures like parental debt on child socioemotional well-being,[20] unstable housing on physical and mental health[21] and home foreclosure on hospital admissions for child abuse.[22] A particularly robust literature exists on the consequences of food deserts.[23] And the well-known Moving to Opportunity study found mixed health impacts on families randomized to receive vouchers allowing them to move out of public housing to potentially higher opportunity neighborhoods.[24-28]

But studies on the health effects of moving people *out* of neighborhoods are not equivalent to studies on the health benefits of investments made *into* neighborhoods. Furthermore, much of the existing research has not attempted to put a price tag on the value of health improvements. Research demonstrating the social and health care cost savings resulting from interventions that improve neighborhoods—as well as calculating the positive value of healthier and more productive residents—is critical to making the case for more robust upstream investments. Without this evidence of both savings and value, we risk simply continuing to treat, at great expense, the downstream health consequences of inaction.

An intriguing new pilot study now under way in Ohio is an example of this type of intervention research that addresses health ROI. Led by the Ohio Housing Finance Agency, the project will examine whether providing affordable housing to homeless or unstably housed pregnant women can reduce the high infant mortality rate in this population.[29] This is just one example of the substantial but usually unstudied investments made into low-income neighborhoods every year. There is great potential for public health and clinical researchers to systematically explore the health benefits of community investment interventions.

## Growing Interest Across Sectors

A number of recent developments provide evidence of growing interest in the community development sector around health. For example, two of the national organizations mentioned earlier, SAHF and NeighborWorks America, now have full-time health staff, including SAHF's new senior vice president for health who is a board-certified pediatrician. And the Federal Reserve Bank of San Francisco's community development division recently hired a public health PhD as a member of their research team. Enterprise Community Partners, by far the largest of the CDFIs, has hired a vice president for health, has a physician on their Board of Trustees, and has created a Health Advisory Council, on which the Network sits, to guide their strategic planning in this area. Similarly, the Local Initiative Support Corporation (LISC), the second largest CDFI, recently hired a new health team, announced a pledge to invest $10 billion over 10 years to fight neighborhood-level disparities in life expectancy,[30] and has committed to a $45 million partnership with ProMedica, an Ohio-based integrated health system.[31] The president and CEO, Maurice Jones, stated, "our entire organization is a health organization" (Jutte D: Personal communication, 2017).

This excitement and activity is not limited to the community development sector. In late 2016, with the Network's guidance, the American Public Health Association published the first ever national policy statement on community development that stressed the importance of partnership with public health in tackling important SDHs and provided recommendations for next steps.[32] The Association for Community Health Improvement, a nonprofit arm of the American Hospital Association, has had a community development track at its annual meeting since 2015. The national health care system Kaiser Permanente has a new C-suite executive with the title Chief Community Health Officer. And, at the request of the new Surgeon General, Dr. Jerome Adams, the Network recently provided a community development briefing and organized a tour of the Villages of East Lake in Atlanta, one of the earliest examples of a comprehensive community development investment.[33] A growing number of hospitals and health care systems are also using community development financial tools or investing directly into the creation of neighborhood infrastructure serving low-income communities, a few of which are described in Box 35.3.

## Box 35.3 | Kaiser Permanente's Thriving Communities Fund

*John Vu*

In May 2018, Kaiser Permanente launched the Thriving Communities Fund, an impact investment commitment of $200 million focused on addressing housing stability and homelessness prevention, among other community needs. Initial investments will focus on preventing displacement or homelessness of lower and middle income households in rapidly changing communities, reducing homelessness by ensuring access to supportive housing, and making affordable homes healthier and more environmentally sound.

Many of the communities that Kaiser Permanente serves are grappling with some of the highest costs of housing and highest rates of homelessness in the United States, leading to significant challenges for the health of our members and residents. Across America, homelessness affects 550,000 people[1] and more than 12 million renter and homeowner households are considered "cost-burdened," paying more than 50% of their annual incomes for housing, indicating they may have difficulty affording necessities such as clothing, transportation, and medical care[2]

Alongside the investment commitment, Kaiser Permanente joined the Mayors and CEOs for US Housing Investment, a first-of-its-kind bipartisan coalition comprised of 17 mayors (and growing) and five CEO business leaders who have publicly committed to advancing public–private partnerships and key federal housing priorities. The coalition positions affordable housing as a critical infrastructure investment and recommends policy changes related to (1) maximizing funding for existing federal programs that work; (2) issuing new innovation, investment, and reform grants; (3) building on successful HUD-Veterans Affairs Supportive Housing model; and (4) creating a housing stabilization fund to provide short-term emergency housing assistance to households in need.

"Affordable housing will be a significant focus of Kaiser Permanente's impact investing portfolio to generate housing stability and improve health outcomes," said Bernard J. Tyson, chairman and CEO of Kaiser Permanente, of the commitment. "We hope our commitment creates a broader national conversation on homelessness, and encourages other companies to join with us to advance economic, social, and environmental conditions for health."

These dual commitments reflect Kaiser Permanente's long-standing mission to support member and community health, its preventative care model, and a growing understanding that health is much more expansive than health care. The quality of where and how people live, work, learn, and play has a big impact on their health. Specifically, we know that only 20% of health outcomes are attributable to medical care. The other 80% are controlled by nonmedical, socioeconomic, and environmental determinants of health.

Poor quality and/or unstable housing has specifically been associated with a wide array of health complications, including lead exposure and toxic effects, asthma, and depression.

Kaiser Permanente's commitment reflects their belief that better health outcomes begin where health starts: in communities.

### References

1. Kinciad E. *Health System Invests $200M in Programs To Reduce Homelessness.* Forbes. May 18, 2018. https://www.forbes.com/sites/elliekincaid/2018/05/18/health-system-invests-200m-in-programs-to-reduce-homelessness/#68d09c881446. Accessed 1/18/19.
2. U.S. Department of Housing and Urban Development. *Affordable Housing.* https://www.hud.gov/program_offices/comm_planning/affordablehousing/. Accessed 1/18/19.

## Challenges and Barriers

### Scale and Alignment

Despite community development's substantial scale, it's simply not enough. To put it in perspective, the $200 billion invested yearly by the community development sector represents less than 6% of annual expenditures on health care. Second, poor health and poverty are the result of complex, interwoven systems; but to date, community development efforts have not been coordinated or aligned to achieve their full impact. Rather, investments are generally driven by financial considerations that produce one-off transactions responding to the simultaneous availability of real estate and financial resources. This results in an apartment building here, a grocery store there, and a new clinic across town. Although the total investments add up, an individual, family, or neighborhood may not experience the combined impact needed to meaningfully improve health or eliminate poverty. The solution is more partnerships across sectors and holistic community investment strategies like those described in the following text.

### Measurement

Despite growing recognition of the potential health benefits of the work of community development, it remains primarily a field of practitioners, not evaluators or researchers. Historically, success has been measured by what health researchers would consider *outputs* rather than *outcomes* (e.g., the number of units of housing built, jobs created, child care slots opened, or loans repaid on time). What has not been measured is whether a family's or individual's life improved as a result of that apartment, childcare slot, or job. Those in community development tend to come from real estate or finance backgrounds, so they are simply not well positioned to measure impacts on health and well-being.

Although some might argue that public health and medicine measure disease more effectively than health, this shortfall in meaningful and practical metrics of success in the work of community development represents a huge opportunity for partnership and collaboration.

### Gentrification and Displacement

Investments into previously disinvested neighborhoods raise important concerns of gentrification. The National Alliance for Latino Community Asset Builders' (NALCAB's) *Guide to Equitable Neighborhood Development* describes gentrification as "a type of neighborhood change in which real estate price appreciation leads to involuntary displacement and significant cultural change."[34] Unfortunately, what begins as valuable and necessary neighborhood revitalization in communities that have experienced periods of stagnation can lead to unintended gentrification and resulting displacement.

The Prevention Institute's 2017 report, *Healthy Development Without Gentrification*, notes that the critical component for preventing displacement is available affordable housing.[35] The report highlights a lengthy list of risk factors for displacement, including being near gentrifying or high-value areas, existing transit infrastructure, low property values, a high proportion of renters, and little subsidized housing. Fortunately, increasing affordable housing is a primary goal of the community development sector, and it is in the very conditions that draw speculative real estate developers that community development organizations should have their greatest role. In fact, nonprofit affordable housing developers actively seek out what's known as *naturally occurring affordable housing* (NOAH). In an approach known as "produce, protect, and preserve," they build and rehabilitate housing—produce and protect—while also purchasing NOAH properties to permanently preserve their affordability in the face of rising rents and real estate prices. The Voorhees Center for Neighborhood and Community Improvement at the University of Illinois at Chicago has published a comprehensive guide, *Gentrification and Neighborhood Change: Helpful Tools for Communities*, that suggests additional steps to prevent displacement. These include community land trusts and policies such as inclusionary zoning, tax abatement policies, and strengthened renter protections.[36]

### Innovations in Financing, Investment, and Health

A number of recent innovations have linked community development finance and health. These include different types of loan and equity funds, partnerships with hospitals to use real estate and community benefit dollars, and more comprehensive approaches using multiple tools to tackle several SDHs at once.

### Loan Funds and Equity Funds

The simplest finance tools are loan funds. These are pools of capital that provide private investment dollars in the form of low-interest loans for community development efforts. The innovation is either in the criteria that must be met to gain access to those dollars or in the source of the funding.

For example, the Healthy Futures Fund (HFF) is a $200 million loan fund developed jointly by LISC, Kresge Foundation, and Morgan Stanley, the for-profit investment bank. HFF incentivizes a particular type of investment by requiring that its resources only go toward the development of community clinics that are built in conjunction with or adjacent to affordable housing.[37] The only example of its type for a number of years, the HFF has been joined by the AIM Healthy fund (https://nff.org/learn/AIM-healthy) launched in December 2017 by the Nonprofit Finance Fund, another national CDFI, and a pair of funds now in the works by Enterprise Community Partners.

At least two hospital systems have also created similar community development loan funds. Dignity Health, a large Catholic health care system, has made a small fraction of its investment portfolio available as a $140 million loan fund. Overseen by a Community Economic Investment subcommittee of its national board of trustees, on which the Network sits, Dignity provides below-market rate loans to community development projects in low-income neighborhoods served by its member hospitals. One innovative example is a $1.5 million loan made to support the opening a new children's museum in Phoenix, Arizona that has helped serve as an anchor to turn around what had been one of the roughest neighborhoods of the city.[38] Another large Catholic system, Trinity Health, based in Michigan, has a similar loan fund of $75 million.

A more complex investment tool, and to date the only one of its type, is the Boston-based Healthy Neighborhoods Equity Fund (HNEF). Focused on transit-oriented development (TOD), HNEF makes equity investments into mixed-use and residential developments in low-income neighborhoods, near transit, that are vulnerable to gentrification. HNEF's goal is to create health promoting neighborhoods using an aggressive real estate investing strategy that ensures every neighborhood has key characteristics that promote upstream social determinants.[39]

HNEF blends government tax credits, philanthropic dollars, bank capital, and other private investor dollars, including investments from two area hospitals, Boston Medical Center and Boston Children's Hospital. Unlike a loan fund that provides assured repayment with interest using the development as collateral, HNEF participants are at-risk equity investors in the neighborhood, with no guaranteed return. Rather, they earn revenue from rents—a portion of which are maintained as affordable to those making 30–80% AMI—and from the increasing value of the property they partly own. The return is then obtained when the investor later sells their higher value share of the ownership to either the owners of the building or a new investor. This process, in effect, harnesses gentrification to provide part of the return while preserving commercial space and homes for low-income residents.

## Hospital Partnerships in Community Development

While such cases are still rare, a handful of recent innovative examples have been seen of hospitals directly partnering with community development organizations to improve low-income neighborhoods. For example, in Stamford, Connecticut, the Stamford Hospital partnered with the local housing authority, Charter Oak Communities, and, through a land swap and use of community benefit dollars, replaced a large, dilapidated public housing project adjacent to their campus with six small townhome communities nearby. This allowed the hospital to build a new high-rise tower without displacement of residents or loss of a single unit of affordable housing. And in the center of the new communities now sits Fairgate Farm, an agricultural oasis and teaching facility available to all of the local residents (Figure 35.1).[40]

In Columbus, Ohio, Nationwide Children's Hospital partnered with a local CDC, Church and Community Development for All People, in a Healthy Homes Initiative (HHI) for its impoverished south side neighborhood. Providing $8 million of $18 million in total resources, the hospital has built on vacant lots or has rehabbed 58 abandoned homes for sale to low-income residents, has rehabbed or built 73 affordable townhomes and apartments, and has provided 65 home-improvement grants of $15,000 each to local residents. And, working with the City of Columbus and JPMorgan Chase bank, the hospital just recently opened the Residences at Career Gateway: 58 townhomes and apartments reserved for low-income residents and an onsite career

**Figure 35.1** ▽

Vita Health & Wellness District: The image is of one of several small communities of public housing developed by Charter Oak Communities (the Stamford, Connecticut housing authority), in partnership with Stamford Hospital, to replace a large, dilapidated public housing complex.

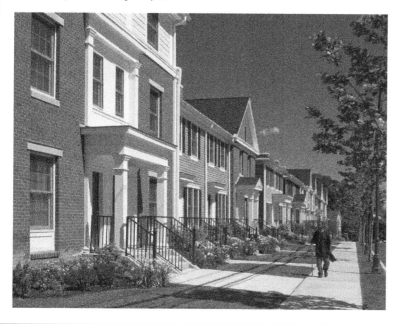

**Figure 35.2** ▼

South Philadelphia Community Health and Literacy Center developed in partnership with the Children's Hospital of Philadelphia and using New Markets Tax Credits.

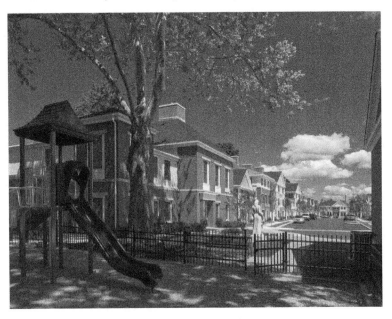

development and workforce training center as a pipeline for well-paying jobs at the hospital.[41] In another children's hospital example, the Children's Hospital of Philadelphia partnered with the city and the Free Library of Philadelphia to use city-owned land and $40 million in NMTC resources to build the South Philadelphia Community Health and Literacy Center. The new center includes a city-run Community health center, playground and recreation center, community library, and pediatric clinic (Figure 35.2).[42]

## Community Development Efforts Addressing Multiple SDHs

As noted previously, a challenge for the community development industry has been aligning investments in a way that tackles multiple social determinants at once to increase the likelihood of meaningful positive impact on the health and well-being of the families and individuals being served. But one great example of doing just that is the Conway Center, now being completed in Washington, DC.

Initiated by a faith-based organization called So Others Might Eat (SOME) and located in distressed northeast Washington, DC, the Conway Center is a $90 million investment that received $34 million of its financing from the Healthy Futures Fund described earlier in this chapter. Comprising 200 units of affordable housing, half for low-income families and half for homeless single adults, a community clinic that will serve 15,000 local residents annually, a job training center run by SOME, and retail and office space, the Conway Center also has a park and playground on its roof and is located across the street from a DC Metro station. So not only is it addressing multiple needs for the neighborhood at once, its easy access to green space, clinical care, and transit provides important additional ingredients for good health for its residents who are already benefiting from the affordable housing.[43]

Even larger scale, comprehensive, neighborhood-level community development investments exist. In San Francisco, for example, the multibillion dollar HOPE SF effort is tackling the four largest remaining public housing projects in the city while also countering several negative aspects of the controversial, federally funded Homeownership Opportunities for People Everywhere (HOPE VI) program that preceded it.[44,45] Like HOPE VI, the goal is to transform decrepit public housing projects into mixed-income, service-rich, healthy communities that are integrated into their larger neighborhoods. But, in sharp contrast to HOPE VI, the HOPE SF program will not lose a single unit of affordable housing and aims to avoid any displacement of existing residents during the redevelopment.

Another prominent example of holistic community development is the Purpose Built Communities network. Purpose Built Communities, based in Atlanta, provides free technical assistance and nonfinancial support to 22 communities nationally that are working to implement its model. Based on its work in the East Lake neighborhood of Atlanta, their place-based approach focuses on three pillars within a geographically defined neighborhood: high-quality mixed-income housing, a cradle-to-college educational pipeline, and community wellness.[46,47] Their "secret sauce" (personal communication, Carol Naughton, President of Purpose Built Communities, 2.1.18), as they call it, is the community quarterback: a small, usually newly created nonprofit whose sole purpose is to align local partners, sources of financing, social services, programs, and other resources to maximally support the health and success of every resident in the neighborhood.

## WHAT IS THE ROLE FOR CLINICIANS AND PUBLIC HEALTH PRACTITIONERS?

Although understanding community development generally, not to mention considering partnership opportunities, can feel huge and overwhelming, there are a number of ways that clinicians and public health practitioners can participate in that sector's efforts to address poverty and improve important SDHs.

### Learn

The Build Healthy Places Network has developed a number of resources to help make navigating the community development sector easier: Community Close-Ups provide detailed case studies on community development investments that address multiple SDHs at once; *Crosswalk Magazine* includes easy-to-read essays describing innovative partnerships and exploring complex topics such as gentrification, aging in place, and rural development; and the Jargon Buster demystifies the acronyms and language of community development. Review the report developed by NACEDA and Community Catalyst to learn the similarities between CRA banking and hospital community benefit requirements. And Prevention Institute's report on Healthy Development without Displacement teaches you the signs of an at-risk or resilient community in the face of gentrification and displacement.[35]

### Identify

Locate high-poverty neighborhoods within your hospital's or public health department's geographic footprint to identify where CDCs and CDFIs are likely to be active. The Network's MeasureUP metrics portal has consolidated a number of mapping tools that allow users to find or create maps with data available at the census tract level. These include the Child Opportunity Index, HealthLandscape, PolicyMap, Community Commons, Opportunity 360 (https://www.buildhealthyplaces.org/measureup/measurement-tools/#opportunity360), and more.

Use the Build Healthy Places Network's Partner Finder to identify which community development organizations work in your community, city, county, or metro area. Collected in one place are membership directories for several important community development umbrella groups including NACEDA, OFN, NeighborWorks America, NALCAB, and the National Coalition for Asian Pacific American Community Development (National CAPACD).

### Engage

Once you've identified which community development organizations are in your area, engage. Reach out to local or regional CDCs, CDFIs, affordable housing developers, or members of the associations just listed. Remember that community development is not only an activity. It is also an industry with leaders who are excited about health and well-being as an outcome of their work and are interested in the potential for new partnerships with health care and public health. Meet with these community development leaders in your area to learn more about their work and the nature of their local investments. Tell them about your organization's populations and neighborhoods of concern and the work you're doing there, and identify common ground for collaboration.

Invite community development organizations to participate in the development of community health assessments (CHAs) and community health needs assessments (CHNAs). Join the board of a CDFI or CDC. You might be surprised by their excitement in having an interested professional from the public health or health care field join. I'm a pediatrician and sit on the National Board of Trustees for Mercy Housing, the nation's largest nonprofit affordable housing developer. I don't understand the nuances of every financial transaction, but I bring a different and valuable perspective to their work. Likewise, if you work for a clinic, hospital, or health care system, invite a leader from community development to join your board. Their insights and perspectives will similarly enrich your board.

## Align

Consider ways to align the resources and expenditures of your hospital or public health department with those of local or regional community development organizations. What are your common goals? Which are your shared neighborhoods of concern? The anchor institution model promoted by the Democracy Collaborative suggests ways that a hospital's hiring and purchasing practices, as well as their investment strategies, community benefit expenditures, and real estate holdings, can be aligned with the needs of the local neighborhood or used to accelerate the work of community development.[48] Are there ways that local community development organizations can help your public health department or hospital address needs identified in the CHA or CHNA? Has your public health department or hospital identified a "hot spot," a cluster of high-risk patients in a neighborhood, building, or complex that could be the focus of future community development investments or partnerships?[49]

Community development organizations want successful investments that provide the greatest possible impact. Importantly, they also are more likely to receive funding for projects that demonstrate community buy-in and partnership with important local institutions such as hospitals and public health departments. Help them build a "pipeline" of future projects ready for investment that also address your needs. Those billions of dollars in annual community development resources are going to go somewhere, with or without your help. Use your clinical or public health experience to guide where and how those investments are made. Where are the neighborhoods of greatest need; what types of investment are needed (e.g., housing, food, childcare, education), and which population will benefit most (e.g., the elderly, veterans, families, the disabled)?

## CONCLUSION

The community development sector is in for the long game. They may not be able to provide for the patient or family sitting in front of you right now, but over time, they are able to make investments that improve neighborhoods and help break the cycle of intergenerational poverty. By joining forces, public health, primary care, and community development together can have a more powerful impact on improving the lives of our most vulnerable populations. A trillion dollars a year spent on avoidable chronic disease in low-income communities is at stake. So consider where, how, and with whom you can partner, and use the tools, resources, and acronyms provided in this chapter to take your first steps.

## REFERENCES

1. Keehan SP, Stone DA, Poisal JA, Cuckler GA, Sisko AM, et al. National Health Expenditure Projections, 2016–25: Price increases, aging push sector to 20 percent of economy. *Health Affairs.* 2017;36(3):553–63.

2. Gerteis J, Izrael D, Deitz D, LeRoy L, Ricciardi R, Miller T, Basu J. *Multiple Chronic Conditions Chartbook.* AHRQ Publications No. Q14-0038. Rockville, MD: Agency for Healthcare Research and Quality; 2014.

3. Jutte DP, Miller JL, Erickson DE. Neighborhood adversity, child health, and the role for community development. *Pediatrics*. 2015;135(Suppl 2):S48–57.

4. Gramlich E from the National Low Income Housing Coalition (NIHLC). http://nlihc.org/sites/default/files/AG-2018/Ch05-S09_LIHTC_2018.pdf. Accessed May 3, 2018.

5. Dougherty C. Tax overhaul is a blow to affordable housing efforts. *New York Times*. January 18, 2018. https://www.nytimes.com/2018/01/18/business/economy/tax-housing.html. Accessed May 3, 2018.

6. January 2018 Summary sheet: https://www.cdfifund.gov/Documents/NMTC%20Fact%20Sheet_Jan2018.pdf. Accessed May 3, 2018.

7. CDFI Fund. Fiscal Year 2017 Summary. https://www.cdfifund.gov/Documents/Final%202017%20NMTC%20Award%20Book%20v4%20021218.pdf. Accessed May 3, 2018.

8. Office of Community Services, U.S. Department of Health and Human Services. https://www.acf.hhs.gov/ocs/programs/community-economic-development/healthy-food-financing. Accessed May 3, 2018.

9. Federal Financial Institutions Examination Council. https://www.ffiec.gov/CraAdWeb/pdf/2016/N1.PDF. Accessed May 3, 2018.

10. Miller J. *San Pablo Avenue Corridor, Oakland, California: Community Development 2.0—Collective Impact Focuses a Neighborhood Strategy for Health*. San Francisco, CA: Build Healthy Places Network; 2017. https://buildhealthyplaces.org/whats-new/san-pablo-avenue-corridor-oakland-california/ Accessed May 3, 2018.

11. East Bay Asian Local Development Corporation. *Our History*. http://ebaldc.org/about-us/our-history/.Copyright 2019. Accessed 1/16/2019.

12. Affordable Housing Finance. Top 50 affordable housing developers of 2016. April 11, 2017. http://www.housingfinance.com/management-operations/top-50-affordable-housing-developers-of-2016_o. Accessed May 3, 2018.

13. Walsh D. Nun funds: The original impact investors. *Shelterforce*. January 24, 2018. https://shelterforce.org/2018/01/24/nun-funds-original-impact-investors/. Accessed May 3, 2018.

14. Douthwaite R. Short circuit: Strengthening local economies for security in an unstable world. June 1996. Feasta. http://www.feasta.org/documents/shortcircuit/index.html?sc4/shorebank.html. Accessed May 3, 2018.

15. CDFI Coalition website information. http://cdfi.org/about-cdfi-coalition/history/. Accessed May 3, 2018.

16. Community Development Financial Institutions Fund, U.S. Department of the Treasury. *Build Your Community-Based Financial Institution with Capital from from the CDFI Fund*. https://www.cdfifund.gov/Documents/CDFI7205_FS_CDFI_updatedDec2017.pdf. Accessed May 3, 2018.

17. 2016 Federal Reserve Bank of San Fransciso. *National Interagency Community Reinvestment Conference*. https://www.frbsf.org/community-development/events/2016/february/2016-national-interagency-community-reinvestment-conference/. Accessed 1/16/2019.

18. Bernanke BS. *Creating Resilient Communities*. April 12, 2016. https://www.federalreserve.gov/newsevents/speech/bernanke20130412a.htm. Accessed 1/16/2019.

19. Harkness J, Newman S. Housing affordability and children's well-being: Evidence from the National Survey of America's families. *Housing Policy Debate*. 2005;16:223–55.

20. Berger LM, Houle, JN. Parental debt and children's socioemotional well-being. *Pediatrics*. 2016;137:2.

21. Sandel M, Sheward R, Ettinger de Cuba S, et al. Unstable housing and caregiver and child health in renter families. *Pediatrics*. 2018;141:2017–2199.

22. Wood JN, Medina SP, Feudtner C, Luan X, Localio R, Fieldston ES, Rubin DM. Local macroeconomic trends and hospital admissions for child abuse, 2000–2009. Pediatrics. 2012;130:2. https://www.ncbi.nlm.nih.gov/pubmed/22802600. Accessed 1/18/19.

23. Walker RE, Keane CR, Burke JG. Disparities and access to healthy food in the United States: A review of food deserts literature. *Health Place*. 2010;16(5):876–84.

24. Kling JR, Liebman JB, Katz LF. Experimental analysis of neighborhood effects. *Econometrica*. 2007;75:83–119.

25. Leventhal T, Dupéré V. Moving to Opportunity: Does long-term exposure to low-poverty neighborhoods make a difference for adolescents? *Soc Sci Med*. 2011;73:737–43.

26. Ludwig J, Sanbonmatsu L, Gennetian L, et al. Neighborhoods, obesity, and diabetes—a randomized social experiment. *N Engl J Med*. 2011;365:1509.

27. Ludwig J, Duncan GJ, Gennetian LA, Katz LF, Kessler RC, Kling JR, Sanbonmatsu L. Neighborhood effects on the long-term well-being of low-income adults. *Science*. 2012;337(2):1505–10.

28. Schmidt NM, Lincoln AK, Nguyen QC, Acevedo-Garcia D, Osypuk TL. Examining mediators of housing mobility on adolescent asthma: Results from a housing voucher experiment. *Soc Sci Med*. 2014;107:136–44.

29. Viviano J. Can housing help prevent infant mortality? Ohio will find out. Tribune News Service. January 3, 2018. http://www.governing.com/topics/health-human-services/tns-infant-mortality-ohio-rent.html.Accessed 1/16/2019.

30. Jones, MA. *LISC New Commitment to Health*. LISC. December 13, 2017. http://www.lisc.org/our-stories/story/lisc-pledges-new-commitment-health.

31. LISC and Promedica. *A Bold New $45 Million Partnership Takes Aim at the Health Gap*. LISC. March 13, 2018. *http://www.lisc.org/our-stories/story/bold-new-45-million-partnership-takes-aim-health-gap*.

32. APHA. Opportunities for health collaboration: Leveraging community development investments to improve health in low-income neighborhoods. November 1, 2016. https://www.apha.org/policies-and-advocacy/public-health-policy-statements/policy-database/2017/01/17/opportunities-for-health-collaboration. Accessed May 4, 2018.

33. Adams, J. U.S. Surgeon General. February 1, 2018. https://twitter.com/surgeon_general/status/959117095668731905.

34. DeManche P, Buitrago C, Esparza, A, Lopez, S, martin L, Medina M, Poyo N, Reyes, M. et al. *Guide to Equitable Neighborhood Development*. National Association of Latino Community Asset Builders (NALCAB) 2018: 5–6. https://www.nalcab.org/wp-content/uploads/2018/02/NALCAB_GuideToEquitableNeighborhoodDevelopment_Final.pdf. Accessed May 4, 2018.

35. Aboelata MJ, Bennett R, Yañez E, Bonilla A, Akhavan N. *Healthy Development Without Displacement: Realizing the Vision of Healthy Communities for All*. Oakland, CA: Prevention Institute; 2017. https://www.preventioninstitute.org/sites/default/files/publications/Healthy%20Development%20without%20Displacement%20-%20realizing%20the%20vision%20of%20healthy%20communities%20for%20all.pdf. Accessed May 4, 2018.

36. Nathalie P. Voorhees Center for Neighborhood and Community Improvement. Gentrification and neighborhood change: Helpful tools for communities. Chicago, IL: University of Illinois at Chicago; 2015. http://voorheescenter.red.uic.edu/wp-content/uploads/sites/122/2017/10/Gentrification-and-Neighborhood-Change-Toolkit.pdf. Accessed May 4, 2018.

37. LISC. *Healthy Futures Fund.* LISC. http://www.healthyfuturesfund.org/section/aboutus/overview.Accessed 1/16/2019.

38. Duffrin L. Building on tradition, catholic hospitals invest in community to improve health. San Francisco, CA: Build Healthy Places Network; 2017. https://medium.com/bhpn-crosswalk/building-on-tradition-catholic-hospitals-invest-in-community-to-improve-health-2b0d9238edd1. Accessed May 4, 2018.

39. Costanza K. *Investing with Health in Mind.* San Francisco, CA: Build Healthy Places Network; 2015. https://medium.com/bhpn-crosswalk/investing-with-health-in-mind-f9a07416d7f1. Accessed May 4, 2018.

40. Miller J. Vita Health & Wellness District, Stamford, Connecticut: Hospital partners with housing authority to put health at the center of a neighborhood transformation. San Francisco, CA: Build Healthy Places Network; 2017. https://www.buildhealthyplaces.org/whats-new/vita-health-wellness-district-stamford-connecticut/. Accessed May 4, 2018.

41. Ray B. A new responsibility for children's hospitals: The health of neighborhoods. San Francisco, CA: Build Healthy Places Network; 2017. https://medium.com/bhpn-crosswalk/a-new-responsibility-for-childrens-hospitals-the-health-of-neighborhoods-257107d6051f. Accessed May 4, 2018.

42. Miller J. Community Health and Literacy Center, Philadelphia, Pennsylvania: A hospital partners with a city to develop a health, literacy and recreation hub. San Francisco, CA: Build Healthy Places Network; 2017. https://www.buildhealthyplaces.org/whats-new/community-health-and-literacy-center-south-philadelphia-pa/. Accessed May 4, 2018.

43. LISC. $34 million into D.C. development that addresses housing, health, employment needs. July 29, 2015. https://www.prnewswire.com/news-releases/healthy-futures-fund-pours-34-million-into-dc-development-that-addresses-housing-health-employment-needs-300120545.html. Accessed May 5, 2018.

44. Orenstein N, Ray B. Hope—and healing—go into massive redevelopment effort. San Francisco. Build Healthy Places Network; 2017. https://medium.com/bhpn-crosswalk/hope-and-healing-go-into-massive-redevelopment-effort-99e4e82aef44. Accessed May 4, 2018.

45. Howard K, Blackwell F. Bringing Together Collective Impact and Pay for Performance: A New Approach to Breaking the Cycle of Poverty. In Bartlett V, Bugg-Levine A, Erickson D, Galloway I, Genser J. Talansky J, eds. *What Matters: Investing in Results to Build Strong, Vibrant Communities.* San Francisco, CA: Federal Reserve Bank of San Francisco; 2017. https://www.investinresults.org/chapter/bringing-together-collective-impact-and-pay-performance. Accessed May 4, 2018.

46. Miller J. The Villages of East Lake, Atlanta, Georgia: Tipping point: Deep, neighborhood-scale transformation creates lasting change. San Francisco, CA: Build Healthy Places Network; 2017. https://buildhealthyplaces.org/whats-new/the-villages-of-east-lake-atlanta-georgia/. Accessed May 4, 2018.

47. Miller J. Columbia Parc at the Bayou District: Holistic redevelopment to bring lasting change to a distressed neighborhood. San Francisco, CA: Build Healthy Places; 2017. https://www.buildhealthyplaces.org/whats-new/columbia-parc-at-the-bayou-district-new-orleans-la/. Accessed May 4, 2018.

48. Howard T, Norris T. *Can Hospitals Heal America's Communities: "All in for Mission" Is the Emerging Model for Impact.* Washington, DC: The Democracy Collaborative; 2015. https://democracycollaborative.org/content/can-hospitals-heal-americas-communities. Accessed May 5, 2018.

49. Gawande A. The hot spotters: Can we lower medical costs by giving the neediest patients better care? New York: The New Yorker; 2011. https://www.newyorker.com/magazine/2011/01/24/the-hot-spotters. Accessed 1/18/19.

# Chapter 36

# Braiding, Blending, or Block Granting?: How to Sustainably Fund Public Health and Prevention in States

AMY CLARY AND TRISH RILEY

State health officials nationwide know that many factors outside the clinical care system, such as nutritious food and safe housing, are important to achieving and maintaining health. Yet state public health agencies have historically relied on narrowly focused federal funding streams that target only one disease or condition. The tension between tightly targeted funding and broader, cross-sector approaches to health exists in a context of recurring federal proposals to reconfigure and curtail public health funding.

State innovation, such as transforming Medicaid to address a broader range of prevention and social factors that affect health, is taking place against a backdrop of federal funding uncertainty. There is an urgent need for state health policymakers to plan for changes that could ensue should federal decision-makers block grant Medicaid or public health funding, combine public health programs, or enact other sweeping changes.

This chapter draws on insights from state public health and Medicaid policymakers to help federal and state leaders think strategically about possible responses to potential policy and funding changes, such as recent federal proposals to blend, braid, or block grant funds for public health and prevention (Box 36.1). It is intended to help chart a way forward for states interested in maximizing their ability to sustainably finance their priorities by coordinating work and resources across programs (Box 36.2).

## Box 36.1 | Advancing Mental Well-Being in Rural South Carolina Through Collaborative Funding Strategies

*Katrina Deloso*

In rural communities, while close interpersonal relationships and camaraderie may be plentiful, social isolation is still problematic. Despite the closeness and strong sense of community among small, rural communities, the experiences of social isolation are hard to combat and are often exacerbated by physical isolation, limited resources, and the lack of community awareness of mental health challenges. Veterans and men and boys of color are two groups disproportionately impacted by mental health challenges. Veterans often struggle in transitioning back to civilian life, whereas men and boys of color frequently experience the impacts of cultural bias, stigma, and racism. These experiences can decrease mental wellness and increase risk-taking behaviors, substance misuse, and suicide. To help remedy this, and to provide social support to these populations, HopeHealth, a Federally Qualified Health Center, leads a coalition of public health, health care, and community support partners in the rural Pee Dee Region of South Carolina.

Because rural communities at times have fewer resources or organizations, HopeHealth provides a critical role by convening partners and encouraging them to collaborate in innovative ways that leverage what is available. "Having different partners at the table has provided another level of thinking," said Shawn Maxwell, Project Coordinator at HopeHealth, Inc., and Making Connections Project Lead. "The partners are more creative in how they consider collaboration, which helps with sustainability." An example of this is the development of a shared-use-of-space agreement among partners that expands opportunities for social support. The Boys and Girls Club, which is mostly unused during the school day, offered space to SC Thrive for peer-to-peer veteran mentoring sessions. As a result, SC Thrive now operates a day session in addition to those that take place in the evenings in other locales. The Boys and Girls Club benefits by reaching veterans—many of whom are parents, caregivers, or family members of the children who attend their programming—and both organizations can easily share knowledge and learning. In a small town like Hemingway, where the Boys and Girls Club center is located, this shared-use agreement is particularly valuable; there are few gathering spaces other than churches, so this presents an alternative safe and comfortable space for veterans.

HopeHealth's Making Connections collaborative emphasizes peoples' compassion and skills in supporting one another. One of the partnership's core strategies is peer-to-peer mentoring, which not only has an impact on those mentored, but also enhances the worth, esteem, and transferable job skills of the helpers. As part of this, SC Thrive, a veteran-serving organization, cross-trains veterans in skills including Mental Health First Aid, suicide prevention, and SC Thrive's own Benefit Bank of South

Carolina online application tool, which provides trained counselors the ability to help individuals apply for multiple social support resources at once. Similarly, the Boys and Girls Club and Alpha Phi Alpha are engaged in training to further develop and support peer-led programming within youth programs "We've heard very eloquent responses about what youth want and need," said Maxwell. "They don't always have to be handheld. They can take the lead—we can give them some parameters and then watch them develop."

Strengthening social supports and leadership development programming, particularly in rural communities, are significant achievements, and they open the door to even more promising implications for the future. Continuously building these collaborations between health and community is essential to promoting social connectedness, an essential component of long-term sustainability of mental well-being that, once built and maintained, lasts well beyond any funding mechanism.

*HopeHealth is one of 16 sites for Making Connections for Mental Health and Well-Being Among Men and Boys, a national initiative to transform community conditions that influence mental well-being. Making Connections is funded by the Movember Foundation, coordinated by Prevention Institute, and evaluated by the University of South Florida.*

*For further information on Making Connections, please contact Sheila@preventioninstitute.org*

## Box 36.2 | Saving Lives and Money During the Opioid Crisis: Creative Funding Mechanisms in Minnesota

An innovative state approach to improving population health is helping to combat the opioid crisis in Minnesota. In Morrison County, the Unity Accountable Community for Health (ACH) reports is saving Medicaid $3.8 million through reduced prescription opioid and related drug claims, due in part to providers prescribing 540,000 fewer doses and safely reducing or stopping drug use for more than 450 patients. The percentage of Medicaid beneficiaries with eight or more opioid claims declined from 14.8% to 12.8% in 1 year.

The Unity ACH model includes local health care providers, pharmacies, insurers, local public health and social services agencies, and local law enforcement. The ACH's lead agency, Catholic Health Initiatives' St. Gabriel's Health, uses a controlled substance care team that works closely with providers and patients to coordinate patient care and help patients safely manage their medications. The care team also identifies the health-related social needs of patients and connects them with services for housing, transportation, insurance, and mental health.

The ACH implemented medication-assisted treatment (MAT) in May 2016 to treat heroin and opioid addiction and expanded MAT into the Morrison County Jail. This initiative—the first of its kind in Minnesota—shows promising results. Before using MAT, 36 people surveyed reported serving an average of 17 days in jail. After participating in MAT, they reported less than 1 day in jail on average. This suggests the potential for significant cost savings to county jail systems.

Each ACH in Minnesota received federal start-up funding through Minnesota's State Innovation Model grant, and the Unity ACH and five others received additional SIM funding. One of the priorities of the additional funding was to support the ability of the accountable care organizations (ACOs) that partner with the ACHs to collect, analyze, and report utilization and quality data for the populations served by both the ACH and its partnering ACO. ACOs are the only entities with whom ACHs are required by the state to partner. This partnership also enables ACHs, such as the Unity ACH, to develop sustainability models and gain access to crucial health care information, such as utilization and cost data.

The Unity ACH model has also led to local-level policy change. Providers are standardizing their screening processes and increasingly accessing the Minnesota Prescription Monitoring Program database, an information-sharing system that helps providers track patients' prescriptions to inform their prescribing practices.

In 2017, the Minnesota General Assembly appropriated $1 million for accountable community opioid abuse prevention projects, which will allow eight other communities to replicate the Unity ACH model. The ACH's reach will spread further through the Echo Hub program, supported through SAMHSA's State Targeted Response to the Opioid Crisis. The grants will support weekly eLearning sessions for providers on opioid care and case management. More broadly, the Unity ACH, in partnership with the state, is considering how savings might be reinvested to support health-related social needs such as transitional housing and healthy food. By incorporating a focus on the opioid crisis and community health within its health care delivery reform, Minnesota may provide a model for other states seeking to build community capacity to improve health and lower costs.

## EXISTING FLEXIBILITIES IN MEDICAID AND PUBLIC HEALTH FUNDING

Historically, block granting public health and social services funding has provided states with flexibility while reducing overall funding available to states. For example, the passage of the 1981 Omnibus Budget Reconciliation Act (OBRA) combined more than 50 existing funding streams into nine block grants (Table 36.1), which were funded at lower levels than the programs they replaced. According to a 1984 Government Accountability Office (GAO) report, "It was often difficult for individuals to separate the block grants—the funding mechanism—from block grants—the budget-cutting mechanism."[1]

| Table 36.1 ▼ Nine block grants created in 1981 by the 1981 Omnibus Budget Reconciliation Act (OBRA) |
| --- |
| Alcohol, drug abuse, and mental health services |
| Community development (Small Cities Program) |
| Community services |
| Education |
| Low-Income Home Energy Assistance Program |
| Maternal and child health services |
| Preventive health and health services |
| Primary care |
| Social services |

Such budget cuts make it difficult for states to assess the impact of the flexibility provided by block grants.

Despite the creation of the Reagan-era OBRA block grants, states still rely on Centers for Disease Control and Prevention (CDC) categorical funding streams, many of which address specific conditions and risk factors, such as tobacco use and different types of cancer. Many states rely on the categorical funding streams to support staff and programs with the focused expertise necessary to produce the deliverables required by each grant. "We created silos for functional reasons," said one state official.

In turn, federal officials acknowledge that many states operate separate programs for conditions such as diabetes and hypertension because of the categorical nature of CDC funding requirements. In an effort to enhance flexibility available under current funding streams, federal policymakers combined some funding streams to states through CDC programs such as the Coordinated Chronic Disease Prevention program and the State Public Health Actions to Prevent and Control Diabetes, Obesity, and Associated Risk Factors, and Promote School Health (DP13-1305) program. Some state leaders are making the most of these opportunities by fashioning their own flexible solutions while working within the defined parameters of CDC's categorical funding streams.

## MEDICAID

Roughly one in five people in the United States—69 million individuals—are covered by Medicaid, a program designed to cover low-income people, including children, senior citizens, pregnant women, some adults, and people with disabilities.[2] People who qualify for Medicaid under their state's eligibility requirements are entitled to guaranteed coverage, whether or not they live in a state that expanded Medicaid. The fact that Medicaid is guaranteed to those eligible sets it apart from non-entitlement programs, such as affordable housing programs that serve fewer than one-third of eligible recipients.

Medicaid is a partnership between states and the federal government, with both parties bearing a portion of cost. In return for the federal funds, state Medicaid programs must follow federal requirements to cover certain populations and provide them with certain services. Within these federal requirements, states have the flexibility to tailor their Medicaid programs. States can use Medicaid State Plan Amendments to make a range of permanent changes to their programs and waive some federal requirements. States can also use waiver authorities such as Section 1115 demonstrations to, for example, test the effectiveness of changes to Medicaid eligibility requirements, benefit packages, or service delivery methods.

### State Example: Washington

States are increasingly using the flexibility available through Medicaid waiver authorities to support efforts to address nonclinical health needs. For example, Accountable Communities of Health (ACH) are an important component of Washington's Medicaid Section 1115 waiver program. The ACHs are permitted to pay for services not ordinarily reimbursed by Medicaid, such as those associated with supportive housing and supportive employment. ACHs are required to include at least one local public health jurisdiction on their decision-making body, which can help ACHs take a regional approach to developing health improvement projects. The state public health agency is also alert to the opportunity to align the priorities of Medicaid, public health, and community partners through the work of ACHs.

## FOUR TYPES OF STATE RESPONSES TO POSSIBLE FEDERAL FUNDING CUTS OR CHANGES

Some federal proposals have advocated reducing the current constellation of federal block grants and categorical funding sources to fewer, and potentially smaller, block grants in exchange for greater administrative flexibility. States may respond by keeping their operations status quo, albeit on a smaller scale. Alternatively, federal changes could spur greater inter- and intra-agency alignment because state leaders could use flexible funding to break down categorical silos and maximize efficiencies in administration.

The following four scenarios contain concrete examples of state innovations that represent a range of responses to possible funding changes. The scenarios and examples are intended to help state policymakers craft their own strategic responses. Although the scenarios appear to represent a continuum of approaches, from more siloed to less, the situation on the ground may not be so clear or linear, and states' responses to federal changes are not necessarily either/or reactions. The degree of difficulty and change inherent in each of the four scenarios may also not follow a straight-line trajectory. The four scenarios highlight the pros and cons of hypothetical state responses, designed to help state officials consider responses to changing federal funding for public and population health. The first three scenarios respond to this fictional funding situation.

As described in the preceding paragraph, some states try to keep their public health programs as close to status quo as possible in the face of budget cuts by absorbing cuts evenly. Alternatively, states could prioritize some programs and cut others. Either way, significant reductions in federal funding eventually result in states discontinuing or scaling back public health programs due to lack of funds, as happened in the aftermath of the 2008 recession. When their diminished resources are overwhelmed, states may lean more heavily on federal assistance to respond to emergencies, such as natural disasters or emerging infectious disease outbreaks—if such funding is available.

Maintaining the status quo sidesteps the need for organizational restructuring and the upheaval that often ensues. However, diminished funding will nevertheless force leaders to make difficult decisions about which programs to prioritize and sustain. In the meantime, staff and infrastructure are likely to be overwhelmed and stretched past capacity. "Trying to stay status quo with reduced funding leads to disaster," noted one state official. However, continuity avoids fracturing coalitions of public health advocates who may have invested considerable resources into building relationships and expertise and even reduced programs provide a framework that can be rebuilt if the fiscal environment changes.

Some states braid, blend, and/or align funding streams to maximize available resources in support of public health priorities. In this scenario, states identify areas in which their health department's work was previously siloed by separate federal funding streams and make strategic decisions to combine and/or more closely align their work in those areas. States also look for other efficiencies by coordinating and possibly braiding funds across programs within a state's public health department.

*A new block grant has replaced existing public health block grants and many CDC categorical formula grants. States now have greater flexibility to apply federal public health dollars to their state-specific needs. However, net public health funding to states is cut significantly. This would be the latest in a lengthy series of state public health funding cuts.*

Scenario 1: Status Quo: A State Maintains Its Health Department's Structure, but Scales Back in Response to Budget Cuts
*A state's health department continues its work and programs as usual. However, it lays off some staff in response to budget cuts and leaves some vacant positions unfilled. These losses are spread fairly evenly across programs, and the surviving staff try valiantly to maintain the same level of service and productivity that existed before the budget cuts. As federal funds dwindle, staff and resources are spread so thin that it becomes difficult to achieve desired outcomes in any program area. Legislators and stakeholders point to the ineffectiveness of the resource-starved department as justification for further cuts. Public and population health suffers.*

Scenario 2: Department-wide Change
*With support from executive leadership, a state health department decides to invest time and resources to reorganize. After spending a year speaking with stakeholders, reviewing funding sources and accountability requirements, and identifying department-wide goals and priorities, the department rolls out its plan. Some programs and functions are cut or transferred to community partners. Remaining programs are integrated, with a focus on aligning initiatives, metrics, and data collection. Some staff leave, and those who stay take time to adapt to their new roles. Eventually, after the planning and adjustment period, the department ramps up its new integrated programs and is on track for measurable success. The new block grants reduce staff time spent on reporting and administration, but it is not clear whether that time saved compensates for the overall loss of funding.*

## State Example: Oregon

Between 2008 and 2012, the Oregon Health Authority's Public Health Division reorganized its siloed Health Promotion and Chronic Disease Prevention Section into a more integrated model. The goal was to integrate programs funded by more than 20 categorical grants to better address the factors underlying a range of chronic diseases. It also sought to ensure that staff and partners worked collaboratively toward that common mission. Oregon did not require a waiver from federal officials in order to braid together its categorical funding. Instead, officials aligned their grant objectives before submitting applications. As a result, they were able to bring together more than 20 different categorical funding streams to support their integrated model. Although this approach did not require a federal waiver, it also did not reduce Oregon's reporting burden. State officials had to show federal funders that they were meeting the expectations of the categorical programs while simultaneously proving to federal leaders that their new strategy was moving toward systemic change in the state.

To accomplish this department-wide breaking down of silos, the division reorganized its staff according to function (e.g., disease surveillance, communications, or policy) instead of segregating them by disease condition or topic area as had been done previously. As a result, their tobacco staff person could be simultaneously working on cancer objectives, or vice versa. Instead of having staff funded by categorical tobacco and cancer grants, each analyzing data from the Behavioral Risk Factor Surveillance System (BRFSS) separately for use in their respective programs, dedicated staff perform one BRFSS analysis and share it across the department.

Attention to upstream prevention and the social determinants of health (SDHs) does not stop at the doors of state public health and Medicaid agencies. In addition to aligning priorities and funding within health departments and across state agencies, states might consider whether they would benefit from a new waiver idea that would bestow flexibility—similar to Medicaid waiver authority—on public health, housing, or other state agencies to address public and population health and upstream prevention. This approach would build on strategies currently employed in some states to marshal the resources of a host of agencies— such as public health, Medicaid, housing, education, social services, transportation, and criminal justice agencies—and devise innovative funding structures to support the cross-agency work.

Scenario 3: Cross-Sector Integration

*After working for years with private philanthropy groups and state Medicaid, housing, and education agencies, the state's public health agency asks federal officials for permission to pool its newly block granted—and reduced—federal public health funds with federal funds that support the state's housing authority or education department. Those pooled funds would be used to address upstream prevention, such as tobacco-free housing for homeless children with asthma or diabetes and their families, with access to safe recreational spaces and healthy food choices. To administer the pooled funds at the state level, executive staff would create a governance structure composed of leadership from all the state agencies involved and task them with establishing shared goals and priorities for the funds. State staff from those agencies would be required to work together on shared terminology, eligibility requirements, and data and reporting systems. For the pool to be successful, all constituencies and their advocates need to support the shared goals and believe that their interests were served. This may be challenging to accomplish with the reduced levels of federal funding.*

## State Example: Virginia

Virginia's Children's Services Act blends state juvenile justice, behavioral health, education, and social services funds to provide flexible funding to address the health and social needs and goals of at-risk youth and families. The program's child-centered approach and pooled funding system gives it the flexibility to provide unorthodox services to support children and families, such as building an addition on a grandmother's house to keep her grandchildren out of foster care. Child-serving state agencies collaborate on the administration of this state-supervised, locally administered program. Medicaid funds are braided with pooled state funds to support an overall plan of services and supports.

## State Example: Vermont

Vermont's Blueprint for Health similarly braids funding from private partners to support initiatives such as the Support and Services at Home (SASH) program. SASH braids funds from a number of state agencies and programs, as well as a Medicaid Section 1115 demonstration waiver, a Multi-Payer Advanced Primary Care Practice initiative from Centers for Medicare and Medicaid Services (CMS), the Million Hearts initiative from CMS and CDC, and private sources. The program seeks to lower costs and improve health outcomes for elderly residents of affordable housing by providing individualized nurse coaching, care coordination, and health and wellness education, and by linking participants to community resources. An independent evaluation of the program found that Medicare expenditures grew more slowly for SASH participants than for a comparison group. Going forward, SASH will be funded by Medicare through the Vermont All-Payer model via the Medicare Next Generation Accountable Care Organization (ACO) Risk Program.

## State Example: South Carolina

South Carolina couples the flexibility available through Medicaid waivers with private philanthropic donations and pay-for-success investments in support of population health goals. The South Carolina Department of Health and Human Services (DHHS) leads a Nurse-Family Partnership Pay-for-Success Program that braids Medicaid funding through a 1915(b) waiver with pooled philanthropic funds. DHHS entered into a contract to conduct an evidence-based program in which public health nurses visit low-income new mothers in their homes to reduce preterm births and improve health outcomes. If the program is successful, as determined by an outside evaluator, the state will make "success payments" to its funders.

The program blends funds into several braids. It blends funds from several private investors and philanthropic organizations together, and then braids them with Medicaid funds pursuant to a Medicaid Section 1115 demonstration waiver. The braided funds are all collected and held in escrow by an outside trustee who disburses the success payments and protects the funds from shifts in political leadership. The state was able to successfully leverage its public health and Medicaid infrastructure to attract outside investors.

Scenario 4: No Federal Change
*State health policymakers have heard federal officials promise more flexibility to design and administer public health programs and to modify Medicaid design and eligibility standards. They have also heard that federal funding for their health programs might be reduced. Faced with this federal uncertainly, state officials take matters into their own hands.*

*First, they take an inventory of what program flexibility is currently available to them. They note all the existing types of Medicaid waivers and state plan amendments that could enable innovation. Next, officials examine the ways in which public health agencies in other states have aligned categorical programs to achieve a common goal without requiring federal approval. After completing their research, they develop an internal work plan that helps them maximize existing resources and flexibilities—including actions that don't require federal approval.*

Within state public health agencies, some leaders are managing work plans, staff, and resources to align their disparate categorical funding streams. These changes allow some states to break down silos created by categorical funding and maximize the efficient use of staff and resources to achieve data-driven goals.

## State Example: Rhode Island

The Rhode Island Department of Health (DOH) determined that the categorical approach to chronic disease and health promotion was not maximizing its effectiveness at meeting the needs of local communities. DOH officials first tested collaboration through integrated projects, such as bringing together staff from diabetes, obesity, and maternal and child health programs and community partners to work on a shared initiative. They then took stock of their funding sources and looked for opportunities to divest from categorical funding and invest in place-based funding. They ultimately designed a method to braid funds within DOH and issued a request for proposals aligned with their emphasis on health equity and local health priorities. The work initially focused on cross-cutting interventions, such as needs assessments and infrastructure-building.

The state DOH did not need federal authorization for its braiding model because each funding source maintained its own identity. That placed the burden on the DOH to create a system that aligned the work done in the communities with the work plans and deliverables attached to each funding stream. Developing a database that linked grant-specific requirements with the work plans and timelines of staff in the field helped the DOH track categorical grant requirements in a way that was invisible to staff in the field. State leaders organized staff into policy teams that met weekly to discuss progress toward collaborative goals.

## State Example: Louisiana

As part of its permanent supportive housing program, Louisiana Medicaid covers some supportive housing services, such as assisting beneficiaries to find and apply for housing and help them communicate with landlords and neighbors. Research shows the program reduced unnecessary emergency department (ED) visits and lowered Medicaid costs. The close working relationship between Medicaid and the Louisiana housing agency has contributed to the success of the program. In Louisiana, the public health and Medicaid agencies both sit within the Louisiana Department of Health, which may facilitate the cross-agency focus on common goals.

The tenancy supports provided by the program are included in the state's Medicaid Section 1915(c) Home and Community-Based Services waivers for people with disabilities, as well as in its mental health rehabilitation state plan amendment. Louisiana enhances these Medicaid flexibilities by braiding Medicaid funds with the Community Development Block Grant and a range of affordable housing programs to house people with disabilities who need support to live in the community. This braiding lends a measure of resilience, so that services can continue even if there is temporary disruption to one of the funding sources.

## POTENTIAL STRATEGIES FOR POLICYMAKERS

The scenarios in the previous paragraphs illustrate the current and potential challenges for state policymakers who seek to improve health in the context of diminishing, siloed, and uncertain funding. They also demonstrate the innovations happening at the state level. Looking beyond the four scenarios, an ad hoc group of state officials suggested that the following strategies, properly funded and implemented, might have potential for maximizing the effectiveness of state health programs. These ideas reflect key issues of concern to state leaders and may help inform important conversations among federal and state health policymakers.

- Develop a pathway to enable states to pilot large-scale cross-agency federal demonstration waiver projects that braid, blend, and align public health and Medicaid funding beyond what is permitted under current law. Such waiver projects could include funding from agencies such as CMS, CDC, Department of Housing and Urban Development (HUD), Health Resources and Services Administration (HRSA), Substance Abuse and Mental Health Services Administration (SAMHSA), and the US Department of Agriculture (USDA) in order to efficiently address health-related needs for food, shelter, and other supports. States can also work within existing waiver authorities to reinvest Medicaid savings from addressing nonclinical health needs and prevention.
- Pilot an optional, well-funded, public health block grant of at least 5 years' duration to test the collective impact of state public health and Medicaid agencies working together to address factors outside of the health care system that influence health. Such a public health block grant could help states define and clarify the changing roles of public health and Medicaid in an era of transforming payment and delivery systems. The test could start with a small number of self-selected states that choose to participate.
- Consider what states can do without new federal action. Using existing federal waiver authorities or state-level actions, states can make policy

decisions to address health-related social needs and prioritize prevention. States could develop a cross-agency systems approach to state
health strategy that views health as affected by things outside of the clinical context. State agencies steward a range of resources that affect these
things and are well-positioned to align those resources for maximum
impact. States can also work within existing waiver authorities to reinvest Medicaid savings from addressing nonclinical health needs and
prevention.

- Align funding cycles, eligibility requirements, application processes, and
reporting obligations across existing federal grant programs. Medicaid
and safety net programs currently have different eligibility thresholds.
Some states are already working to align these programs to maximize
their impact, such as Louisiana's enrollment of residents into expanded
Medicaid using Supplemental Nutrition Assistance Program (SNAP) eligibility data (Box 36.2).

## CONCLUSION

Proposals to create block grants and cut public health funding to states require focused attention from state public health officials. Assiduously tracking,
preparing for, and responding to such proposals may also help state Medicaid
and public health agencies clarify their shared goals and roles and identify actionable steps they can take even without any additional federal flexibility.

When asked about the prospect of increased flexibility and reduced funding
for public health, many state officials were wary:

- "My fear is that a block grant would just be less money and less accountability, which would make it hard to demonstrate our programs' effectiveness, which would lead to even greater funding reductions."
- "Block grants would make my life much easier by eliminating some complicated and unnecessary reporting and accountability systems. Flexibility
would be much easier, but I would be concerned with the level of funding
cuts. I would keep the reporting burden to keep the funding. Our level of
funding already isn't what it needs to be. It's a dangerous zone."

The possibility of changes to the structure and level of funding for public health
represents an opportunity for state leaders to articulate their visions for the future and to determine the funding levels and mechanisms that will help them
achieve their goals. At a time when much attention is focused on changes flowing
from Washington, DC, strategic state leaders can navigate this uncharted territory to safeguard and promote the health of communities nationwide.

### REFERENCES
1. Bowsher CA. States use added flexibility offered by the Preventive Health and
Health Services block grant. *Report to the Congress by the Comptroller General of*

*the United States* (GAO/HRD-84-41). Washington, DC: Government Accounting Office; 1984:75. http://www.gao.gov/assets/150/141487.pdf. See also GAO, *Block Grants: Characteristics, Experience, and Lessons Learned* (GAO/HEHS-95-74). Washington, DC: Government Accounting Office; 1995. http://www.gao.gov/assets/230/220911.pdf.

2. Medicaid. As of the May 2017 enrollment report: https://www.medicaid.gov/medicaid/program-information/medicaid-and-chip-enrollment-data/reporthighlights/index.html. http://www.kff.org/medicaid/issue-brief/10-things-to-know-about-medicaid-setting-the-facts-straight/.

# Chapter 37

# Rethinking the Mission of Health Systems: Improving Community Health as Anchor Institutions

DAVID ZUCKERMAN, DAVID ANSELL, AND MICHELLENE DAVIS

## ADVANCING THE ANCHOR MISSION OF HEALTH CARE

Despite the position of the United States as the wealthiest nation in the history of the world, a staggering 43 million Americans and 1 in 6 children live in poverty—a level greater than that of its peers. Four in 10 Americans could not sustain living at the poverty level for just 3 months if their main source of income disappeared tomorrow. White family wealth remains seven times greater than African American family wealth and five times greater than Hispanic family wealth, as of 2016.[1]

These significant economic inequities, amplified by a long legacy of racial exclusion, create an impossible headwind in our nation to improving health and well-being if not addressed intentionally and systematically. Today, the difference in lifespan after age 50 years between the richest and the poorest has more than doubled—to 14 years—since the 1970s,[1] and communities a few miles apart experience life expectancy differences of more than 20 years. According to Philip Alston, United Nations US Special Rapporteur to the United States, "Americans can expect to live shorter and sicker lives, compared to people living in any other rich democracy, and the 'health gap' between the United States and its peer countries continues to grow."[2]

We must apply a health equity—as well as a racial equity—lens to our strategies, acknowledging both historical and systemic inequities as identifiable root causes of poor health that need to be explicitly named. Furthermore, and equally important, our communities and their leading institutions must therefore reevaluate the toolbox of solutions we bring to address these named systemic problems. Despite these staggering challenges, locked in our communities are unbelievable resources that we could align, leverage, and deploy in more thoughtful and creative ways to lay the foundation for a more equitable and healthy society.

These resources are anchor institutions, or nonprofit or public enterprises that are rooted locally because of their mission, physical investment, and/or the communities they serve and that have emerged as notable economic engines. Their ownership status creates greater accountability to the public and community and creates an opportunity for them to orient long-term in a way that benefits both their institution and their community's most in-need residents. Among the largest employers and purchasers, anchor institutions represent "sticky capital" that can be more effectively channeled to strengthen the local economy and address economic inequities. Health systems and universities are the most common anchors, but this group may also include local government, public schools, place-based philanthropy, public utilities, and other community-owned institutions.

Health systems and universities alone have expenditures of more than $1 trillion annually, have nearly $1 trillion in investment assets, and have more than 9 million employees. Their scale is enormous, and the potential for impact on these systemic problems is equally great. If a thriving and healthy community requires a focus on equity, then the challenge becomes to discover how these institutions can more effectively align their business operations with their missions of health care and education to tackle these structural and economic drivers of poor health. That approach is an "anchor mission." It requires going beyond traditional notions of corporate social responsibility and rethinking the very foundation of the institution's role and how it deploys its economic and social assets in the community.

## The Anchor Mission

An anchor mission is a commitment to intentionally apply an institution's long-term, place-based economic power and human capital in partnership with its community to mutually benefit the long-term well-being of both.

Without embedding a core set of principles to guide its approach, an anchor institution is likely to perpetuate the same inequities we currently face. It is important to consider how the policies and practices implemented take into consideration the following factors with a systems-approach: (1) health, racial, and economic equity; (2) community connectivity; (3) individual agency; and (4) place-based impact.

The degree of current inequities previously outlined creates a sufficient moral imperative to act. Still, defining this imperative by community and context is often step one. It is critical to helping activate a new coalition needed to tackle these problems and lay the foundation for collaboration through new practices, such as reorienting everyday purchasing, hiring, and investment practices to disinvested zip codes and disconnected residents.

Although the urgency of this work is readily apparent, anchor strategies are ultimately insufficient tools if they are not grounded in rebuilding social bonds that have splintered as the resource gap has widened in our communities. Momentum for an anchor mission will be driven by the small wins that can come through changes in practices and policies, but also through the depth of empathy between institutional actors and community members. Relationship building, building trust, and cultivating power-sharing are all essential elements of this process. Achieving these elements cannot be rushed and may frustrate actors hoping to move more quickly, but avoiding this process will derail the impact of this approach. Naming and nurturing this process is an important early step.

As anchor institutions around the country have grown as notable local actors, they find themselves in close proximity to communities that have been pummeled by poverty and racism. Although not exclusively the same story everywhere, the result is that the social distance between senior leaders of these institutions and those living in these communities is immense. As institutions secure senior leadership buy-in and move toward implementation, staff biases—both implicit and intrinsic—and their beliefs regarding innate negative business consequences from a new approach focused on social impact can conspire to keep individual projects from being successful.

Many of our senior leaders have participated in events in high-hardship anchor communities, allowing them to experience first-hand the neighborhood conditions that lead to poor health outcomes. Normalizing these community experiences for senior leaders along with employees from the same neighborhood allows leaders to connect strategy with personal day-to-day experiences.

Anchor institutions also have an economic imperative to act. The role of repairing local economic ecosystems so that well-being outcomes are more equitable, sustainable, and healthy can be an amorphous proposition. Why should we reorient our business practices and take on more responsibility for society's ills, especially with shrinking margins?

Articulating this long-term value proposition is an essential foundational step in the process of achieving an anchor mission. We as a society and our communities cannot move forward and prosper while leaving more people behind. This fact is only reinforced by the gaps in life expectancy outlined earlier in the chapter as well as the fact that we as a nation spend more per capita on health care than any other country in the world. The long-term return on investment from these strategies on investment lies in a healthier population—living in equitable, civically engaged, diverse, safe, and economically strong communities.

In advancing an anchor mission, short-term actions must be nested within longer term strategies and within a new institutional culture that more effectively aligns organizational assets and connects with other community partners. This requires new roles and responsibilities internally and more formal structure to encourage collaboration and alignment across large institutions—especially among their business units (e.g., procurement, human resources, treasury, facilities and real estate, and government and community relations).

The following sections highlight examples of how two institutions—Rush University Medical Center in Chicago and RWJBarnabas Health, at various locations in New Jersey—are beginning to operationalize this approach, both within their institutions and in partnership with their communities. In addition, leading health systems nationally are coming together to embed this strategy within health care more broadly through the Healthcare Anchor Network (healthcareanchor.network), a national collaboration of more than 30 health systems seeking to improve health and well-being by building more inclusive and sustainable local economies.

## RUSH UNIVERSITY MEDICAL CENTER

Rush has been a health care fixture in Chicago for 181 years, tracing its incorporation as the area's first medical school to 3 days before the city of Chicago itself was incorporated in 1837. Rush is a regional integrated academic health system with multiple sites across the Chicago region. The flagship medical center, Rush University Medical Center, sits on the Near West Side of the city. Quality of care is a hallmark of Rush, which is a four-time Magnet Nursing designated hospital, a multiple recipient of the Leapfrog A safety designation, consistently in the top 10 hospitals in the United States in the Vizient Quality and Accountability Study, and the only Centers for Medicare and Medicaid Services five-star hospital in Chicago.

The mission of Rush is to improve the health of the individuals and the communities it serves.

Yet neighborhoods just a mile away from the medical center have health outcomes and life expectancies similar to those of Iraq or Bangladesh, rather than those of a developed nation. It was the recognition of these large life-expectancy gaps that led Rush to reconsider its strategy and obligation to the residents in these neighborhoods. These nine West Side neighborhoods, largely segregated communities of concentrated poverty, high unemployment, and poor educational outcomes, are home to almost 500,000 residents (larger than Miami or Cleveland.) In July 2016, the Board of Trustees at Rush endorsed a broad-based health equity strategy that aimed to have Rush lever its size and success as the largest private employer on Chicago's West Side to be a "catalyst for community health and economic vitality" there. Rush's Community Health Needs Assessment named structural racism and economic deprivation as two root causes of the health gaps in these neighborhoods and also acknowledged that its many community-focused programs had not "moved the needle" quickly enough to narrow these gaps. There was also an acknowledgment among the senior leadership team that because the life expectancy gaps were driven by inequity, there was an urgency to act. A new senior vice president role was created on the senior leadership team to coordinate Rush's health equity agenda.

In addition to identifying Chicago's West Side as a geographic focus, Rush named its low-wage employees as its "first community." Applying analytics and performing focus groups, Rush could begin to understand the financial and other struggles of its low-wage employees (many of whom lived in the neighborhoods surrounding Rush). The leadership was able to identify how well-meaning institutional policies and a lack of a career ladder program may have contributed to these difficulties. As a result of this analysis, Rush has developed programs to create opportunities for career growth and to promote financial literacy and reduce hardship among these low-wage employees. One unexpected consequence of this effort was the degree to which our employees were ambassadors for their neighborhoods within Rush. They transmitted their enthusiasm and pride for their communities, often depicted negatively in the media, to senior leaders, most of whom had never ventured into them.

Rush partnered with the Civic Consulting Alliance, a pro bono arm of the Commercial Club of the City of Chicago, to build an anchor mission strategy, to hire locally, to develop wealth-creating career pathways, to purchase locally and stimulate new business development on Chicago's West Side, to invest locally, and to volunteer locally. These efforts were documented in *The Anchor Mission Playbook*, which was co-edited by The Democracy Collaborative.[3] Rush also convened 100 community-based organizations and six other anchor health care institutions into a health-equity focused collaborative called West Side United to develop a place-based, multisector, private–public partnership to address health and economic well-being on the West Side. The ultimate aim is to reduce the life expectancy gap between Chicago's Gold Coast and the West Side neighborhoods by 50% by 2030 by addressing population and community health, educational outcomes, economic development, and the built environment. Nine health care anchor institutions have joined the West Side Anchor Committee under the West Side United umbrella. Collectively, these institutions have almost 45,000 employees and 6,000 new hires yearly, and they have enormous purchasing power. These institutions have committed to directing a portion of their economic and job engines to the economic vitality of Chicago's West Side.

The Rush health equity strategy is an inside-out, outside-in strategy. While West Side United is building high-value external partnerships to address the structural root causes of poor health outcomes on Chicago's West Side, inside Rush, a reorganization of the quality infrastructure was initiated to address health care inequities. Partnered with the Institute for Health Care Improvement, Pursuing Equity project, Rush began a project to screen and refer patients who experience negative social determinants of health (e.g., transportation, food and housing insecurity). Rush has also assembled its health care quality data to better understand by race, gender, age, insurance status, language, gender and sexual identity, and geography who among its patients were not thriving. The quality plan for Rush now includes specific goals related to health care equity with an infrastructure to lead equity projects. The work to improve the lives of our low-wage employees, while reorganizing Rush business units to the anchor mission, also reflects the impact of the new equity strategy. Finally, a new 5-year Diversity and Inclusion plan for Rush includes community health equity as a pillar, as well as a goal to achieve demographic parity to better reflect the voice of the community in all leadership roles across the organization.

All of this work is organized under a senior vice president for community health equity and a department of community engagement and health equity. An anchor mission manager was hired to manage the business unit activities. Staff were added to Human Resources and Quality to manage new programs. The health equity mission needed specific ongoing investments to succeed. The Civic Consulting Alliance in 2017 provided almost $4 million in pro bono consulting services in addition to the in-kind time of business unit leaders across Rush. The work is painstaking and requires a high degree of organizational focus. Yet the Rush leadership is convinced that, in addition to the moral imperative to repair historical injustices, there will be a longer term return on investment when the population of the surrounding neighborhoods experiences improved health and economic vitality.

## RWJBARNABAS HEALTH

RWJBarnabas Health (RWJBH), the state's largest integrated health care delivery system, treats and serves more than 5 million patients each year. This system reaches from northern New Jersey to the state's ocean shores and serves diverse populations, cities and townships, and urban, suburban, and rural areas. System leaders are committed to providing the highest quality of patient care and health education to the community and the region.

Beyond addressing health care through the provision of patient care within the walls of its hospitals, clinics, and home-care facilities, RWJBH leaders are driven to make a unique impact in local communities throughout the state. The ultimate aim is to make communities healthier. RWJBarnabas Health's leadership believes that the system has a responsibility to meaningfully serve its communities; to be an anchor institution that fosters health and well-being by playing its part in addressing the social determinants of health. In order to realize that belief, RWJBH has established its social impact and community investment practice, a system-wide professional operation aimed at helping to advance the organization's vision of improving the health, quality of life, and vitality of New Jersey communities.

The RWJBH social impact and community investment practice leverages the system's range of assets to advance a culture of health and lift the quality of life in New Jersey communities. With a programmatic emphasis on ensuring health equity, the practice spearheads innovative social-impact and external affairs initiatives that address the social, economic, and environmental conditions that have a significant impact on health outcomes. The policy arm leads the practice as it seeks to change systems, structures, and policies through the equity lens to create a more equitable future for all New Jerseyans.

Despite the aspirational desired outcome of a more equitable future for all, large-scale organizations struggle with the naturally occurring strategic tensions that present themselves during an organization's attempt to alter missions and cultures. At RWJBH, the constant in the battle is not of good versus evil, but of traditional bottom-line focus versus community health and wealth-building focus. One such tension presents itself in the departure from traditional community benefit project planning, which often occurred behind institutional ivory walls by hospital executives and then resulted in new projects erected in communities in a "if-you-build-it-they will come" manner. Rather, RWJBH's adoption of an anchor mission required both the formalization of a corporate office-led Anchor Roundtable and an enhanced understanding that while community health needs, county health rankings, and state department of health data utilization have their place, a community solution needs to be led by the community.

To transform an organization into a true community change agent requires an entity to adopt the humble position of active listener. The challenge remains ripe as we further embed the social impact practice throughout the system and adopt a position of co-learning and co-leading with community-based organizations and residents in order to fulfill the mandate of assisting our communities to build community wealth. This work moves only at the speed of humility. As such, since adopting this understanding, we have witnessed a welcome into community-based organizations that have existed for years but that have never opened themselves up to the hospital that has been in their neighborhood for 119 years. They now do so after witnessing the appreciation of the community members' daily living experience and expertise.

To embed this practice into the institution's operations side, we created a Corporate Anchor Roundtable (CAR). The CAR is co-chaired by the system CEO and the Executive Vice President who are charged with driving this work across the system. The composition of the CAR includes the system's asset leaders, including supply-chain, Human Resources, construction, and facilities management; information technology and services; and treasury. The CAR members convene quarterly to update the system CEO on the progress of the use of local diverse suppliers, the hiring rate of local residents, and investment into community building. Moreover, the Social Impact and Community Investment practice adaptation into system operations is the sixth pillar of the system's strategic plan. As such, it is measured and tracked just as every other strategic initiative is within the business' strategic plan. Furthermore, a one and half full time equivalent (FTE) (.75 to be exact) is required to drive this work across the system as staffers need to work with each facility to coordinate and align the identification of local purchasing and local hiring target goals.

An important element of our local hiring initiative is our Hire Newark program, conducted in partnership with our local municipality, the City of Newark, as well as with the Hire Newark program and the Mayor's local hire program, Newark2020. Hire Newark trains and places participants in businesses in Newark to help close the gap between Newark's unemployment rate and that of the state of New Jersey.

## CASE EXAMPLE

One of our participants actually had a dream to work for herself as a commercial wedding cake baker but had enrolled in our program out of necessity. The married mother of five showed such promise that she was placed in a job with the hospital's dining vendor in order to secure the 300 hours of baking in a commercial kitchen needed to satisfy her small business certificate. She continues to thrive on her own as a bona fide minority- and woman-owned diverse local supplier of professional baked goods. As a result of this opportunity, she recently announced the purchase of her first home. The work is equity-focused with the constant of creating opportunity in order to help build community wealth and to push back the tide of generational poverty.

## SCALING FOR IMPACT: A NATIONAL COLLABORATION IS FORMED

The challenges facing our communities are systemic. Our solutions for addressing them and meaningfully achieving health equity must be equally bold. We need this approach to take root in each of our communities. All of our institutions must rise to the occasion.

An example of this is the Healthcare Anchor Network. Formed in early 2017, it is a growing collaboration of more than 35 leading health systems, representing more than 600 hospitals, that are committed to deepening their understanding and implementation of strategies that leverage their business operations (e.g., hiring, purchasing, and investment) to benefit the communities they serve and to address economic and health disparities. The purpose of the Healthcare Anchor Network is to help institutions more effectively advance an anchor mission in their institutions, in partnership with their communities and across the health care sector.

Any health system committed to these goals can join the Healthcare Anchor Network. Together, we can help collectively to forge a new narrative in health care related to practical—but perhaps not initially intuitive—strategies that health systems and partner anchor institutions can take to meaningfully address the systemic inequities that have contributed to the current disparities we continue to confront in the United States.

Anchor institutions represent significant economic resources. If reoriented with an equity lens toward broader impact and leveraged along with other local resources in our communities, we could finally bring to the equation the resources needed to ensure that all in our country can live healthy lives with dignity.

## REFERENCES

1. Tavernise S. Disparity in life spans of the rich and the poor is growing. *New York Times*, February 12, 2016. https://www.nytimes.com/2016/02/13/health/disparity-in-life-spans-of-the-rich-and-the-poor-is-growing.html. Accessed 1/18/19.

2. Philip, A. *Statement on Visit to the USA, by Professor Philip Alston, United Nations Special Rapporteur on extreme poverty and human rights.* United Nations, Human Rights. Office of the High Commissioner. December, 15, 2017. http://www.ohchr.org/EN/NewsEvents/Pages/DisplayNews.aspx?NewsID=22533. Accessed 1/18/2019.

3. Rush University Medical Center. *The Anchor Mission Playbook.* Chicago, IL: The Democracy Collaborative; 2017.

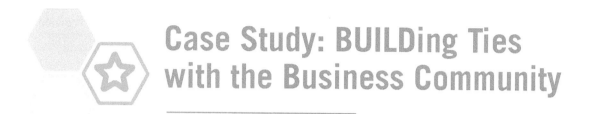

# Case Study: BUILDing Ties with the Business Community

KATHERINE OESTMAN, ROSALIND BELLO, CATHERINE CHENNISI, AND ANNA BREWSTER

## OVERVIEW OF PASADENA, TEXAS

About 20 miles southeast of downtown Houston is Pasadena, Texas, the second largest city in Harris County with just over 150,000 people. It is a strong, cohesive community with a unique local history and culture, connected through bonds of common industry (petrochemical) and geography (proximity to bayous and the Houston Ship Channel). In 1970, the City of Pasadena created an industrial district that contains more than 60 chemical plants.[1] Local business volume for the industrial district-related enterprises exceeds $829 million annually with 11,000 jobs directly attributable to the complex.[1] The city's commitment to economic development is evident through outcomes such as earning the 2013 Community Economic Development Award from the Texas Economic Development Council, and the city's slogan is: "New opportunities and old-fashioned values. You can have them both in Pasadena."

Although Pasadena defines itself in terms of economic opportunity, many Pasadena residents face economic challenges that impact health. At the time of publication of this case study, the most recent publicly available data (from The University of Texas School of Public Health, Health of Houston Survey[2]) was 8 years old, illustrating the dearth of locally available and timely community health data on children's weight status. According to the 2010 Health of Houston Survey, 65% of children aged 12–17 years in the Pasadena/South Houston area are at an unhealthy weight, the highest rate in Harris County. The survey also showed that the greater Pasadena area has a high proportion of residents in only fair or poor health and contending with social and economic disadvantage. Other local data sources show few health-supporting policies and systems in Pasadena to build a culture of health; namely, there are few fitness facilities, no public urban agriculture, no farmers' markets, and several food deserts (areas where residents live more than 1 mile from the nearest supermarket) (Table 38.1).

| Table 38.1 ▼ Pasadena, Texas, by the numbers | |
|---|---|
| **Total Population, 153,256** | |
| Race/ethnicity | Most residents living in Pasadena are Hispanic (67%) or white (28%). |
| Income | The median household income is $48,607 (compared to Harris County, with a median income of $55,584). |
| Education | 29% of the population older than 25 years does not have a high school diploma. |
| Poverty | 20% of the population lives below the federal poverty level. |

From American Community Survey (ACS) Demographic and Housing Estimates, 2012–2016 5-year estimates, 2018. Washington, DC, US Census Bureau, 2018.

Concurrent to these challenges, Pasadena has many community assets, including an engaged school district and active civic clubs, which form a strong foundation for community health collaboration and programming. Pasadena Independent School District (ISD) is the largest employer in Pasadena and is among the 30 largest school districts in Texas, with 54,000 students. Pasadena ISD has built a strong foundation of learning that educates today's students for tomorrow's workforce. Through postsecondary, specialized, and technical opportunities, many students are prepared for jobs in Pasadena's industrial complex. The district has championed innovative educational learning as well as health initiatives that foster student and community health, including an award-winning School Health Advisory Council.

## Building a Foundation for Collaboration with Businesses in Pasadena

Harris County Public Health (HCPH) was one of the first public health–focused organizations to begin building ties with the business community in Pasadena. In 2011, HCPH launched Healthy Living Matters (HLM), a collective-impact initiative aimed at curbing childhood obesity. After an extensive needs and assets review, HLM released a Community Action Plan (CAP) outlining policy priorities. HLM also selected three priority communities in Harris County, one of which was the City of Pasadena. In 2014, HLM established a community health coalition of Pasadena-area stakeholders and community members, known as the HLM-Pasadena Community Task Force. This community health coalition, inclusive of multiple sectors that have an interest in the health and wellness of the community, has led to collective action supportive of obesity prevention activities in Pasadena. Stakeholders from area businesses regularly engage with the community health coalition in collaboration with representatives from local government, Pasadena ISD, health care providers, and resident participants. Local business owners provide a unique perspective on the health priorities addressed by the community health coalition. In addition, local businesses offer in-kind benefits to the community, such as hosting health fairs and donating space for health-related activities and events.

The community health coalition has not only acted as a convener but also as a catalyst, proactively bringing funding, additional support, and capacity-building resources to Pasadena. In 2015, the coalition received a BUILD Health Challenge award ($250,000) to address the nutrition-focused CAP priorities and food insecurity in Pasadena. The BUILD Health Challenge is a national awards program supporting "bold, upstream, integrated, local, and data driven" (BUILD) community health interventions in low-income urban neighborhoods. The BUILD Health Challenge was founded by the Advisory Board Company, the de Beaumont Foundation, the Colorado Health Foundation, the Kresge Foundation, and the Robert Wood Johnson Foundation. Locally, the BUILD Health Challenge award helped strengthen partnerships between local non-profit organizations, hospitals and health systems, and Harris County Public Health to improve the health and well-being of Pasadena. In 2016, Pasadena was selected for the Pasadena Vibrant Community initiative, which brought an influx of corporate funding to the community, which is further detailed in the following section.

## Strengthening Ties with Businesses in Pasadena: Businesses Serving as Funders, Strategic Partners, and Implementation Partners

The public health stakeholders in Pasadena engaged the Boston College's Center for Corporate Citizenship to refine a strategy for strengthening ties with businesses. The Center for Corporate Strategy defines community involvement as "in-kind and financial donations, employee volunteer days, or enduring partnerships that have the power to bring positive, measurable change to both your company and the communities in which you operate." As such, public health organizations in Pasadena have categorized business partnerships as funders, implementation partners, and strategic partnerships.

### Funders

Businesses that as serve funders provide necessary financing for programming and infrastructure support as aligned with key social investment strategies. Within the social investment framework, funds and resources can be leveraged to impact to both the businesses themselves and the communities where they operate. To that end, businesses also bring a unique partnership perspective. Businesses play a critical role in supporting health and wellness programming in Pasadena through philanthropic funding and partnership support. Two key examples are described here.

The Pasadena Vibrant Community is an initiative of the University of Texas MD Anderson Cancer Center (MD Anderson) made possible by an investment from and collaboration with Shell Oil Company (Shell), a large employer in the area. The initiative is a program of the Cancer Prevention and Control Platform within the Moon Shots Program at MD Anderson. The Pasadena Vibrant Community brought critical funding to Pasadena to further mobilize the community to promote health and wellness. Leveraging the foundational work of HLM, MD Anderson and Shell chose Pasadena for this initiative after a community selection process, based on community need and community capacity, for the execution of objectives related to improving dietary behaviors and increasing physical activity. Shell chose to make this investment because the company believes in investing in the communities where it operates and where employees live. Shell operates a number of facilitates in and around Pasadena, including Shell Deer Park, which is a 2,300-acre manufacturing site with 1,500 employees and 1,200 contractors. Shell promotes its own culture of health with its employees. Key learning gleaned from the Pasadena Vibrant Community initiative is serving to inform MD Anderson's Be Well Communities program, which is mobilizing communities to promote wellness. Be Well Communities unites individuals, schools, workplaces, government agencies, health care providers, and policymakers to plan and carry out community-led solutions that will make positive, long-lasting changes in people's health.

General Electric (GE) is another key funder and collaborator for the Pasadena community in terms of community health capacity-building. A part of GE's healthymagination commitment, GE developed the HealthyCities Leadership Academy. The HealthyCities Leadership Academy mentors and supports leaders in communities to develop and support new strategies to tackle population health challenges. The goal of the initiative is for community and business leaders to work together to help the cities, towns, and communities in which they live and work to address significant health challenges. The community health coalition in Pasadena was selected as part of the inaugural cohort of the HealthyCities Leadership Academy. The GE funding helped augment existing programming in support of expanding a local network of healthy food suppliers and distributors.

### Implementation Partners

Businesses that are implementation partners work with public health stakeholders to integrate programs that support health and wellness as a part of their core business. In Pasadena, through the Healthy Corner Store Initiative and Healthy Dining Matters, HCPH partners with businesses to create healthier food environments. Initial funding was provided to corner stores and restaurants to implement changes in the food retail environment. Once the changes were implemented, the businesses have been able to sustain the changes with little or no additional funding.

The Healthy Corner Store Initiative was launched in 2014, with CAN DO Houston. The program was implemented in Pasadena with initial funding from the Centers for Disease Control and Prevention (CDC) and expanded through BUILD Health Challenge funding. This program retrofits local "mom-and-pop" grocery and convenience stores to provide healthy alternatives to traditional store snacks. To help engage the corner stores in Pasadena, the community health coalition relied on the Greater Houston Area Retailers Collaborative Association, which is aimed at supporting independently owned and operated convenience stores in the greater Houston area. This group helped spread the word about the Pasadena efforts and helped with the recruitment of some of the participating corner stores. There are now three corner stores participating in Pasadena, and, every other Friday, an HLM representative conducts food demonstrations using the fresh foods now available in the store.

Similar efforts are being made to help owners of small, nonfranchise restaurants in Pasadena develop and offer healthy options on their daily menus through the Healthy Dining Matters Program. The goals of the program are to help restaurants make healthier options, create a healthy dining environment, and promote healthy choices to customers who are dining out. Currently, two restaurants in Pasadena are fully engaged in the program and are preparing meals with healthier ingredients, promoting healthier options, and adding new meal options designed by a registered dietitian. These businesses view engagement as an opportunity to further their investment in the community. For example, the head chef at one of the participating restaurants was already supporting nutrition services at Pasadena ISD when he was approached to become involved with the Healthy Dining Matters Program. The chef thought that the program strengthened the restaurant's connection with the community. Furthermore, he wanted to provide healthy options to the older adults who frequent his establishment. However, the program does encounter some barriers to restaurant participation, including staffing and different conceptions regarding the connection between the food environment and health.

To facilitate the implementation of both programs, the community health coalition worked to form relationships with local restaurants, corner stores, and grocers to help improve access to healthy food in the community. The business case was initially presented to the food retailers, but their involvement was mostly dependent on their dedication and commitment to the community. Most businesses did not want to take the risk of making changes to their food retail environment that might not be profitable. The retailers that did join the efforts in Pasadena saw the value in the demand that the overall programming was creating for the new food offered. The community health coalition assisted with promoting the participating businesses through several channels (e.g., at health fairs, within the Healthy Dining Guide, inclusion in the city water bill inserts, via social media and newsletters, and in a public service announcement developed by the city, discussed in the next paragraph).

Beyond the Healthy Corner Store Network and Health Dining Matters, the community health coalition partnered with John Manlove Marketing and Communications to create and disseminate a public service announcement (PSA) in English and Spanish augmented by pro bono services. The PSA featured the mayor of Pasadena and was developed to make Pasadena residents aware of the healthy options available at participating corner stores, restaurants, schools, and food pantries. The PSA encouraged residents to "buy local" by purchasing affordable produce from retail locations.

### Strategic Partnerships

Businesses or business networks also work with public health stakeholders through strategic partnerships. Businesses networks that serve as strategic partners may not necessarily fund or implement specific programming but are aligned around a common goal or complementary strategies. A business network such as a chamber of commerce furthers the interests of business and can support public health priorities in a unique way. In addition, an economic development corporation, usually a 501(c)(3) nonprofit, can complement the work of a chamber of commerce in planning for the longer term economic growth of a community, including city planning efforts that can impact health.

The Pasadena Economic Development Corporation (EDC), also known as the Second Century Corp., was created "for benefitting and accomplishing public purposes on behalf of the City by promoting, assisting and enhancing economic development activities as provided by the Development Act of 1979." The EDC is supportive of the community health coalition and the coalition's efforts to develop the city-owned flood plain lots into a physical activity corridor. At the time of publication of this case study, the City of Pasadena Parks and Recreation Department is developing a plan for the corridor on behalf of the community health coalition.

The Pasadena Chamber of Commerce serves as a stakeholder on the community health coalition in Pasadena and supports programming where appropriate. The mission of the Pasadena Chamber of Commerce is to "promote economic development and community growth to ensure the prosperity of Pasadena's businesses and citizens." The Chamber leads, serves, and grows the community. The signature health initiative of the Chamber is coordinating the Annual Rugged Race, a fundraiser for playgrounds and tracks for Pasadena ISD schools. The Chamber also hosts a yearly event focused on highlighting Pasadena area restaurants, including the Healthy Dining Matters locations. Additional areas of strategic alignment between the Chamber and the community health coalition are currently being explored, such as promoting resources for healthier workplaces.

## CONCLUSION

Businesses play a significant role in community health improvement, and public health stakeholders in Pasadena have identified several mechanisms for engaging businesses as funders, implementation partners, and strategic partners. Businesses that serve as funders in Pasadena provide necessary financing for programming, while implementation partners actually play a central role in program execution. Additionally, businesses that function as strategic partners in Pasadena work to support community health in unique and complementary ways. Looking to the future, public health stakeholders in Pasadena will need to continue to build ties with the business community and identify additional ways to engage businesses in community health improvement.

### REFERENCES

1. City of Pasadena Economic Development Corporation. Major employers in Pasadena. 2018. http://www.pasadenaedc.com/. Accessed 1/16/2019.

2. The University of Texas School of Public Health. Health of Houston survey. 2011. https://sph.uth.edu/research/centers/ihp/health-of-houston-survey-2010/. Accessed 1/16/2019.

# Policy: Achieving Sustained Impact

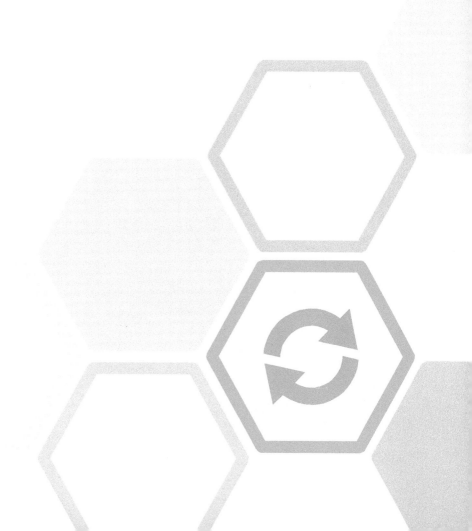

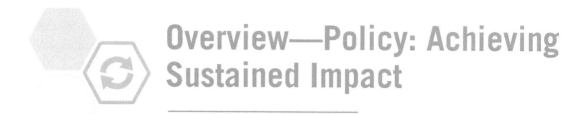

# Chapter 39

# Overview—Policy: Achieving Sustained Impact

## EDWARD L. HUNTER AND DON W. BRADLEY

Policy approaches were included the first edition of this book (*The Practical Playbook: Public Health and Primary Care Together*[1]), but the editors of this new edition felt it was important to provide more prominence to successful examples of policy partnerships being pursued across the United States. This new emphasis stems from a number of important realities.

First, there is growing recognition of the role that policy plays in the pursuit of community health goals. Public health leaders have articulated the importance of policy as a public health approach (Public Health 3.0[2]); similarly, wide experimentation is taking place regarding the use of policies on health care reimbursement to reshape the contribution that delivery systems can make to community health objectives. Though historically "health policy" has been dominated by consideration of strategies related to insurance and access to care, these discussions increasingly include how policies in housing, education, transportation, and other sectors help shape a community's health.

Second, policy is a prime example of the importance of cross-sector collaboration. Policy can affect all sectors, and it is rarely developed, implemented, and sustained without the active engagement of a broad coalition of interests. Policy is an art as well as a science—relying often on judgments and strategies more commonly familiar to those *outside* the public health and medical communities. This makes it all the more important for *The Practical Playbook 2: Accelerating Multisector Partnerships for Health* to highlight positive examples of success as well as to suggest ways that multisector coalitions can access both the science and the strategies needed to successfully pursue policy.

"Policy" is a term that is applied in multiple ways. Institutions can set policies to govern their own practices (e.g., how hospitals control infections, manage protection, or share patient data). Employers and health plans can establish policies that affect the working conditions and benefits of their employees and covered populations. Health systems (including those managed by governments) can implement policies that affect all of their member institutions, with wider impact. At the broadest level, laws, regulations, entitlements, and other measures adopted by governments—public policies—can have broad, sustainable impact and set a context for the actions of others in the community.

Public policy, the primary focus of this section, is responsible for many of the most important advances in health in the past century. Health-specific policies have included the removal of lead from paint and gasoline, control of second-hand exposure to tobacco, near elimination of many childhood diseases by financing and mandating vaccines, and regulating exposure to environmental toxins. More broadly, governments have sought to tackle poverty and other underlying social determinants of health—with varying degrees of success—through the tax code (e.g., the Earned Income Tax Credit), housing ordinances, and direct assistance programs (e.g., Supplemental Nutrition Assistance Program [SNAP] and Women, Infants, and Children [WIC]).

Collaboration related to policy takes multiple forms and involves multiple parties. Evidence arises from experimentation and evaluation of initiatives often undertaken by institutions, systems, philanthropy, or local governments. Advocacy helps to distill this evidence and to translate it to other jurisdictions for broader population impact. Engaged stakeholders keep public officials accountable through implementation and encourage evaluation and revision.

This section reviews examples of successful pursuit of policy strategies at multiple levels of government, often the result of active partnerships between public, private, and philanthropic interests. These examples highlight the diversity of topics addressed as well as the strategies and geographic focus. Importantly, the authors demonstrate that leadership on policy comes from many quarters and that successful approaches frequently involve nontraditional partnerships.

The chapters in this section highlight important steps in the policy process.

Vernick and Schneider (Chapter 40) provide an example of focused work at the local level to achieve policy goals related to food and nutrition and discuss the role of philanthropy in leading a multisector partnership. This theme is echoed elsewhere in the *Playbook*, specifically in a contribution from the Aetna Foundation in the Innovation section (Chapter 30) that amplifies the constructive role philanthropies can play in policy.

Skillen and Hearne (Chapter 41) discuss the importance of evidence and describe their work in the Centers for Disease Control and Prevention's (CDC) HI-5 Initiative and CityHealth program (a joint inititiative of the de Beaumont Foundation and Kaiser Permanente), which distill the broad range of evidence on effective policies into a form more readily actionable at state and local levels.

Fraser, Butler, and Tucker (Chapter 42) outline the central role of state health officials in the policy process, illustrated by the collaborative approach to the complex opioids epidemic.

Archer and Hall (Chapter 43) demonstrate the power of nontraditional partnerships to achieve policy change at the local level. Their review of the work of the Kansas City Chamber of Commerce and the KCMO Health Department to motivate adoption of Tobacco 21 initiatives in multiple jurisdictions highlights the importance of business and public health working together.

As in the first edition of *The Practical Playbook*, policy is woven into other sections of this text.[1] Of particular note are the following:

- In Chapter 7, Hall provides insight into what motivates businesses to enage in efforts to improve community health, including engagement in the policy process.
- In Chapter 14, Hunter provides insight into working with elected officials and their multiple influences on decision-making, which is often the key to achieving policy goals.
- In Chapter 37, Zuckerman, Ansell, and Davis discuss the role of hospitals as "anchor institutions," a role that in many communities extends to engagement in the policy process.

Policy remains an emerging tool in communities struggling to make improvements in health and the conditions that lead to poor health. Many in the public health community seek to improve the capacity of public health officials to address these and other strategic challenges.[3] Taken together, these chapters are designed to help readers get a jump-start on engaging in the policy process in their communities, with the guidance of practical examples of how partnerships lead to success.

## REFERENCES

1. Michener JL, Koo D, Castrucci BC, Sprague JB (eds). *The Practical Playbook: Public Health and Primary Care Together* (1st ed.). New York: Oxford University Press; 2016.

2. US Department of Health and Human Services. Public Health 3.0. A call to action to create a 21st century public health infrastructure. https://www.healthypeople. gov/sites/default/files/Public-Health-3.0-White-Paper.pdf. Accessed 1/17/2019.

3. de Beaumont Foundation and the National Consortium for Workforce Development. *Building Skills for a More Strategic Public health Workforce: A Call to Action.* Published by the de Beaumont Foundation. July 18, 2017. https://www. debeaumont.org/wp-content/uploads/Building-Skills-for-a-More-Strategic-Public-Health-Workforce.pdf. Accessed 1/17/2019.

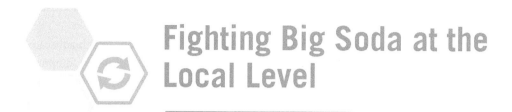

# Chapter 40

# Fighting Big Soda at the Local Level

NIKKI HIGHSMITH VERNICK AND GLENN E. SCHNEIDER

Big Soda is the new tobacco. Research has identified products made by multibillion dollar companies that are harmful to health, especially for children. Communities across the United States that are advancing the health of children and families are going up against beverage companies with vastly more marketing prowess, money, and lobbying power. But public health advocates are taking public policy plays from the successful anti-tobacco playbook, updating them for the 21st century social media environment, and winning. As a public health foundation in central Maryland, the Horizon Foundation has taken on Big Soda, the purveyor of high-sugar, heart disease–causing drinks, by effectively engaging a broad coalition of community partners, managing an aggressive marketing and media campaign, advocating for state and local policy change, and measuring our success along the way.

## LOCAL POLICY OPTIONS TO REDUCE SUGARY DRINK CONSUMPTION

Sugary drinks are the largest single source of daily calories and sugar in a child's diet.[1] Compelling research exists linking drink products with added sugar to obesity, type 2 diabetes, and cardiovascular disease.[2, 3] A third of all children and teens are overweight or obese, "causing a range of health problems not previously seen until adulthood."[4] As a result, the United States "may see the first generation of children that will be less healthy and have a shorter life expectancy than their parents."[5]

The Institute of Medicine report on *Strategies for Reducing the Consumption of Sugar-Sweetened Beverages* recommends that communities adopt policies to reduce the consumption of sugary drinks to prevent childhood obesity.[6] As decades of public health research have shown using the social ecological model of change, comprehensive strategies that promote change at the interpersonal level, the organizational level, the community level, *and the policy level* have been successful in achieving better health outcomes, such as increasing use of seat belts, reducing second-hand smoke exposure, or increasing vaccination rates in children.[7]

Taking lessons from these public health victories, public health advocates have outlined policy changes that could reduce sugary drink consumption, particularly in children. For example, Change Lab Solutions has outlined 10 policy strategies that would collectively reduce sugary drink consumption and move the public health needle (Table 40.1).[8] These strategies include a host of local and state policy interventions to reduce sugary drink consumption, such as making healthier drinks more widely available on public property, making healthy drinks the default offering on restaurant children's menus, and imposing taxes on sugary drinks.

The Horizon Foundation launched a comprehensive, multifaceted campaign in 2012 to reduce sugary drink consumption in Howard County, Maryland.[9] Over the course of several years, the Horizon Foundation convened, organized, and funded a broad and diverse coalition of local and state partners, supported in part by the American Heart Association through the Robert Wood Johnson Foundation's Voices for Healthy Kids program.[10] The coalition assessed these public policy opportunities within our local and state political and community environments and developed several successful policy campaigns that led to the passage of the following policies to reduce sugary drink consumption:

- *A local school wellness policy* in 2013 that removed student-accessible vending machines from middle schools and required that all food and beverages offered or sold on school property meet Institute of Medicine Nutrition Standards

## Table 40.1 ▾ Sugar-sweetened beverages playbook

**The 10-Strategy Path to Reduce Sugary Drink Consumption (strategies pursued in Howard County, Maryland are in boldface type)**

1. **Launch public awareness campaign**
2. **Make healthy drinks more widely available on government property**
3. Make healthy drinks more widely available in workplaces
4. **Restrict sales of sugary drinks on and near school grounds**
5. **Make healthier drinks the default in childcare and after-school programs**
6. **Restrict sugary drinks marketing in schools**
7. Make healthier drinks the default offering on restaurant children's menus
8. License sugary drinks retailers
9. Tax sugary drinks
10. Limit sugary drink portion sizes

*From Sugar-Sweetened Beverages Playbook. ChangeLab Solutions, 2013. (https://changelabsolutions.org/sites/default/files/SSB_Playbook_FINAL-20131004.pdf). Funded by the Robert Wood Johnson Foundation.*

- *Statewide childcare legislation* in 2014 that required all licensed childcare centers in Maryland to support breastfeeding mothers, limit screen time, and only serve healthy beverages
- *Local healthy vending legislation* in 2015 that created healthier drink and snack options in vending machines on government property and in government-sponsored youth-oriented programs (e.g., after-school programs and summer camps)

These public policy strategies each had (1) a strong rationale for creating heathier community environments, especially for children; (2) a significant evidence-base related to their effectiveness; and (3) a growing number of communities where they have been successfully enacted.[11,12,13] These communities represent a patchwork of progress, but they are collectively tilling the soil for others. Critically understanding what led to these public health victories is essential to creating a national movement.

## CAMPAIGN COMPONENTS

The Horizon Foundation is the largest independent health philanthropic foundation in Maryland. With total assets of $95 million and annual spending of approximately $5 million, the Foundation's mission is to lead community change so that everyone in Howard County can live a longer, healthier life. We are a local health foundation working locally, regionally, and statewide to influence better health outcomes for our residents. Howard County is geographically situated between Baltimore and Washington, DC. It is predominantly a suburban community of approximately 317,000 residents, but includes urban and rural areas as well. Finally, Howard County is a relatively affluent community, with high levels of both education and wealth. Despite these positive social determinants of health, the county still experiences high rates of chronic disease and obesity that are similar to those of the rest of the country.

In 2012, the Horizon Foundation embarked on a new, 5-year strategic plan, which included an ambitious goal for *all* children in Howard County to achieve a healthy weight by kindergarten and maintain a healthy weight through at least ninth grade. The Foundation chose to work on sugary drinks after an assessment of the data and on the recommendations of national experts, given that these drinks represent the largest single source of added sugar in children's diets and that research has clearly linked daily consumption to childhood obesity and chronic disease epidemics.[14,15] The Foundation measures long-term success (i.e., over a 5- to 10-year time frame) by evaluating changes in body mass index in children and assessing short-term behavioral changes in both children and adults by measuring sugary drink consumption patterns, sugary drink availability in homes, and objective sugary drink grocery sales. Recently, a research team led by the Rudd Center for Food Policy and Obesity at the University of Connecticut published a study in *JAMA Internal Medicine* showing that our multifaceted Howard County Unsweetened campaign lowered the sales of soda in Howard County by 20% and fruit drinks by 15% over a 3-year period.[16] So what did we do?

The Foundation's work was guided by the 4Ps of philanthropy—People, Programs, Policy, and Proof—which map back to the social ecological model of change.

- We engage *people* to make healthier decisions by providing nutritional tools and resources to assist them in finding healthier beverages, by engaging residents in broad community collaboration building, and by conducting an effective marketing and media campaign to engage the public.
- We help community organizations, such as the local hospital, sports leagues, and Head Start *programs*, often through grant funds, to help change their organizational beverage offerings and educate their members, clients, and visitors about the dangers of sugary drink consumption.
- We advance *public policy* that will change community consumption patterns and create lasting change.
- We offer *proof* of our work by steadfastly evaluating our work and showing progress along the way.

These 4Ps guided our work and allowed our board of trustees to be more comfortable investing in public policy and advocacy as one tool in our philanthropic tool box. Advocacy is one of the most important and most challenging aspects of philanthropy, particularly in the early stages. Moving our board from a philanthropy that made investments in individual programs to a catalytic organization that invested in public health advocacy movements took education, early wins that showed progress, and a broad culture of risk-taking fostered over several years. This shifting belief that philanthropy has a role in public advocacy that could create transformative and lasting social change has been elevated across the sector and across the county.

## WHAT REALLY WORKED

Taking on Big Soda at the local level requires more than just good evidence and a framework for change; it requires carefully selecting the right policy levers, building a broad and deep coalition, anticipating opposition responses, framing and reframing messages, being omnipresent on traditional and social media, and having funding to execute successful campaigns that can win.

### Pulling the Right Policy Lever

Even though public policy strategies related to sugary drinks were emerging from national organizations and other communities that offered a pathway forward, our coalition needed to strategically assess the political and community landscape and choose policies that resonated at the state and local levels.

The coalition knew it would need ground-softening campaigns at the local level that could make a tangible difference and pave the way for bigger statewide changes. The Horizon Foundation and another local nonprofit had developed a voluntary healthy child care certification program in Howard County. Licensed childcare centers that served healthy beverages, supported breastfeeding mothers, and limited screen time were certified as healthy child care centers and publicly recognized. This program, in which the child care centers implemented evidenced-based changes and showed financial viability, allowed us to test a county "pilot" and develop statewide legislation that could embed these voluntary standards into state licensure requirements. The bill, the Maryland Healthy Eating and Physical Activity Act of 2014, gained bipartisan support for enactment.[17]

At the county level, many individual council members had a good track record on public health issues, particularly working on anti-tobacco legislation, such as smoke-free air, and creating a health insurance program for the uninsured (prior to the Patient Protection and Affordable Care Act). These council members understood the need for creating healthy environments, particularly in public spaces and particularly for children. After extensive engagement, the county council supported healthy vending machines on government property and in government-sponsored, youth-oriented programs as a first step toward obesity prevention in Howard County.[18] Subsequently, state coalition efforts led to the passage of health vending policies in five neighboring jurisdictions. (Healthy vending policies were passed in Baltimore City, and in Montgomery, Prince George's, and Charles counties, as well as by the Maryland-National Capital Park and Planning Commission, which oversees park and recreation programs in the Washington, DC area.)

An assessment of the community landscape also provided opportunities. Because of the county's high affluence and adult educational achievement, residents and elected officials place a high value on quality K–12 education and on having one of the best school districts in the nation. In 2013, the Rudd Center assessed the Howard County School System's wellness policy using its evidence-based Wellness School Assessment Tool (WellSAT) and found that it ranked in the bottom third of the country. This gave the coalition a strong case to put forth a new school wellness policy that built on community values and stoked a desire to protect deep-seated community pride.

Finally, the coalition worked with a well-respected pollster in Maryland to poll eligible voters to better understand voter knowledge related to sugary drinks and voter sentiment related to a range of policy options. This data helped drive our policy selections in tandem with our qualitative assessment of the policy and community environment.

## Engaging Broad, Multisector Coalition Partners

As most public health advocacy organizations know, partnership building takes lots of time, intentional effort, and patience. The coalition targeted organizations whose missions aligned with children's health, brought credibility and authenticity to the campaigns, represented the diversity of our community, and brought community assets (mostly time and people) to the partnership. The coalition was purposefully built with "grasstops" organizations that had political influence with policymakers and elected officials, as well as grassroots organizations with sizeable memberships that could be activated. Locally, this broad and diverse partnership included the following:

- Faith partners, including People Acting Together in Howard County, a power-building organization of 13 faith organizations and more than 500 faith leaders
- Health care providers, including the local hospital, pediatricians, and hygienists
- Childcare providers, including home care providers and childcare centers
- Organizations representing communities of color, such as the African American Community Roundtable and the local chapter of the National Association of the Advancement of Colored People (NAACP)
- The Local Health Improvement Coalition led by the Howard County Health Department, which includes more than 100 local organizations invested in health, and the Association of Community Services, which represents local nonprofit health and social service organizations
- Well-respected national health organizations, such as the American Heart Association and the American Diabetes Association
- Influential state health organizations, such as the Maryland Dental Action Coalition; the Maryland Chapter of the American Academy of Pediatrics; MedChi, the Maryland State Medical Society; Sugar Free Kids; and the YMCA

Within the health care community, providers with an acute sense of how the community environment impacts health and prevents illness (e.g., pediatricians and hygienists) were key voices on behalf of children's health and needed little convincing to join the coalition. Other providers, more focused on sick care, needed additional data on both the health and economic consequences of a poor diet before joining the coalition.

All of these organizations joined because they care about children, social justice, and equity, and they were instrumental in showing broad and deep support for community changes that would improve health for children. They boldly took a stand even in the midst of sometimes intense opposition. The coalition successfully engaged and activated residents not only through media engagement (see following), but also in mobilizing thousands of people to sign petitions, write letters/emails to lawmakers, show up at school board meetings and local and state legislative hearings, plan visits with lawmakers, and take time for phone banking to elected officials, all of which created an overall buzz that the community wanted to make healthy choices the easy choices in Howard County. (The Horizon Foundation and its other 501(c)(3) partners abide by federal Internal Revenue Service rules that allow insubstantial lobbying activity.) This grassroots engagement of coalition members gave them a deeper level of commitment to the cause and, once they saw big wins, gave them the satisfaction of having a meaningful impact in their community (Box 40.1).

## Anticipating Opposition Responses

Going after Big Soda at the local level requires thick skin and constant scenario planning ("If we do X, how might our opponents respond, and then how should we react?"). In campaigns around the country, the industry tends to use legal threats, sympathetic surrogates, campaign contributions, highly paid lobbyists, and deep marketing pockets to respond to potential legislative actions that threaten its bottom line. In Howard County, beverage executives made verbal promises to build new playgrounds at local African American churches, made contributions to local elected officials, and verbally threatened legal action against the Foundation. In San Francisco, the beverage industry legally challenged an ordinance requiring advertisements of sugary drinks to include a warning to consumers that they contribute to obesity, diabetes, and tooth decay. Similarly, the industry filed lawsuits to stop a sugary drink tax to fund Pre-K programs in Philadelphia and also encouraged state lawmakers to file preemption legislation to invalidate the tax. In Chicago, the industry launched a massive "Can the Tax" campaign and has made targeted campaign contributions to lawmakers in Cook County, Illinois, which led to the Cook County Commissioners repealing the county's sugary drink tax.

In lieu of deep pockets, local campaigns have the ability to stay a few feet ahead of the industry by learning from its actions in other communities, strategically planning for different scenarios, and fostering deep community connections and solidarity with partners. Keeping in touch with other campaigns around the country enabled the coalition to anticipate the industry's response and to prepare community leaders beforehand. In fact, in Howard County, the community felt besieged by industry leaders who did not live or work in the community, and it heightened the sense that they were outsiders preying on *our* children. The coalition could not outspend the industry, but it could hold tighter community hands to reinforce local will for change.

## Framing and Reframing the Message

Limiting sugary drink consumption via public policy mechanisms unveils deep philosophical differences between the role of government versus individual decision-making. As localities try to use local laws and regulations to improve health, the industry bombards lawmakers with threats of unjustified interference with people's lives or groundless limits on commercial freedom.

### Box 40.1 | Health Equity and Sugary Drink Policy

Low-income youth and youth of color, particularly African Americans and Latinos, disproportionately carry the burden of unhealthy weight and the impact of chronic diseases such as type 2 diabetes, heart disease, and stroke. In addition, data show that African Americans and Latinos consume higher amounts of sugary drinks on a daily basis. Campaigns that look at public policy solutions to our national epidemics related to obesity and chronic disease must look at both policy solutions and coalition-building with an equity lens.

The Horizon Foundation and a large social justice coalition partner, People Acting Together in Howard County (PATH), intentionally looked at policies that would remove barriers related to health outcomes for low-income communities and communities of color. The coalition assessed each of the sugary drink policy options with the question of whether enacting policies would both help *all* children and/or residents and *particularly* children of color and low-income children.

For example, legislation to create healthy vending machines on government property and in youth-oriented programs particularly impacted lower income and minority youth who make up a significant portion of participants in county after-school programs and summer camps.

The Howard County School Wellness Policy implemented Institute of Medicine nutrition standards for more than 50,000 children during the school day. Nearly 60% of these students are youth of color, and 23% are eligible for free and reduced-price meals.

The Howard County Unsweetened campaign also assessed the diversity of its coalition members and made a concerted effort to reach out to communities of color to discuss mutual health-related goals. Extensive engagement with the Howard County Chapter of the NAACP, the African American Community Roundtable, the Association of Community Services (which represented nonprofits serving lower income communities), Head Start, and the Latino Parent Association helped the campaign to better understand pressing health issues and gained buy-in and support from these organizations. These partners proved critical to moving the needle on legislative efforts, reinforcing the importance of reducing health disparities, and serving as respected champions for our very diverse community.

The fallacy of exercising individual choice can certainly be challenged in an environment in which sugary drinks and advertising for sugary drinks are omnipresent. For example, the beverage industry spent $866 million in marketing its unhealthy beverages in 2013, and children and teens were a key target.[19] Black children and teens saw twice as many sugary drink ads as whites.[19]

The campaign undertook extensive market research to better understand how to counter the barrage of industry marketing and to frame our messages to resonate with residents, particularly parents. Based on extensive focus group research, early campaign efforts focused on factual education and parent support, including the following:

- Providing data related to the amount of excessive sugary drink consumption in the community
- Showing how much added sugar was contained in everyday sugary drinks
- Sharing evidence related to the severe health consequences (e.g., diabetes, heart disease, obesity) linked to sugary drink consumption
- Being supportive of parents by not judging
- Pointing parents toward healthier drink alternatives (Figure 40.1)

Early efforts were informative, factual, data-driven, and almost emotionless. As our research evolved, focus groups continued to emphasize how words such as "ban," "prohibit," "restrict," or "limit" felt like a nanny-state intervention and still

**Figure 40.1** ▼

Howard County unsweetened drinks advertising during debate on healthy vending legislation.

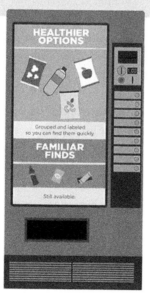

felt judgmental and self-righteous. In 2015, when the coalition focused on healthy vending legislation that would make healthier food and beverages more widely available, accessible, and noticeable on county property and in county children's programs, the coalition reframed the message to focus on the following:

- Making healthy options more widely available
- Encouraging healthy choices
- Giving children the same healthy food and drinks they get at home and in other locations
- Being at the forefront of a movement with other cities around the country that are making changes

These messages resonated with parents and voters. The messages more effectively countered the nanny-state framing, more forcefully showed parental desire to control their children's nutrition environment, and tapped into a sense of community pride by celebrating the passionate people who care about kids and making their lives better. The message framing and reframing helped lead to successful passage of the healthy vending machine bill, which earned enough votes in the county council to overturn a veto by the county executive and become law.

The coalition's messaging has continued to evolve as community members increasingly have become more aware of the facts of sugary drinks. More recently, the campaign has elevated messages that further enhance the emotional appeal of our work. Ads have featured community leaders (e.g., soccer coach, pastor, educator, and day care provider) showing how much they care about our community's children by taking steps to switch their drinks. Spanish-language ads have also focused on switching at home to water as a way of reinforcing parental love for their children. The coalition has also deepened its reach with tweens and teens (not just parents) and built off their sense of independence and authenticity. Recent campaign advertisements have shown teens uncovering and decoding the deceptive practices of and rebelling against the industry for hurting their generation. This focus on anger and calling out the hypocrisy of the beverage industry might be considered risky, but it ultimately is driven to help the coalition lift up the youth voice as other successful public health campaigns (i.e., anti-tobacco and more recently gun violence) have done as well.

By continuously assessing the campaign's messaging and resonance with families, the coalition continually ensured that messages were fresh, current, and engaging. We remained responsive to the evolving needs and understanding of our community.

## Deploying a Successful Media Strategy

Public health advocates have had to become savvy media specialists to engage with the public, not only around general awareness of these issues, but also on how to get specific policy campaigns covered and shared in the traditional news media and on social media. The coalition used the *paid, earned, shared, and owned (PESO)* media model, developed and championed by Gini Dietrich (Figure 40.2),

# Figure 40.2 ►

Paid, Earned, Shared, and Owned (PESO) media model developed by Gini Dietrich.

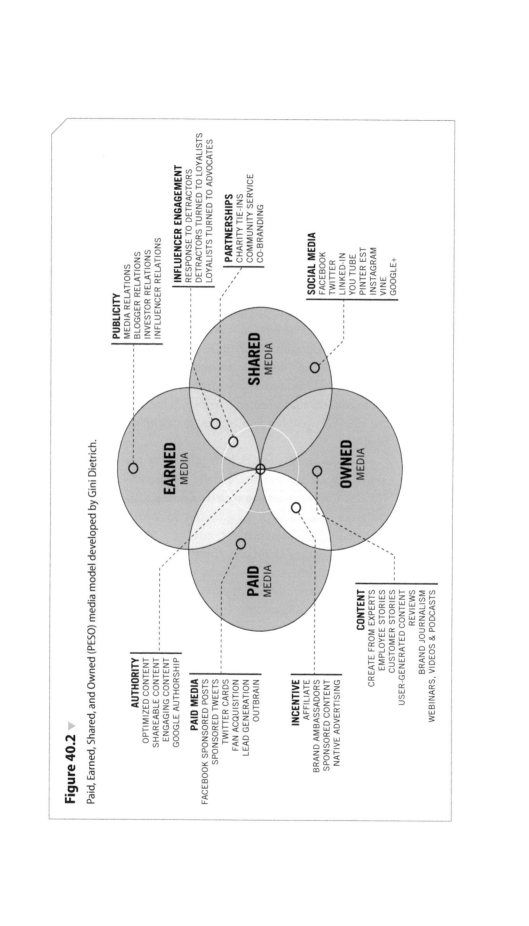

**AUTHORITY**
OPTIMIZED CONTENT
SHAREABLE CONTENT
ENGAGING CONTENT
GOOGLE AUTHORSHIP

**PAID MEDIA**
FACEBOOK SPONSORED POSTS
SPONSORED TWEETS
TWITTER CARDS
FAN ACQUISITION
LEAD GENERATION
OUTBRAIN

**INCENTIVE**
AFFILIATE
BRAND AMBASSADORS
SPONSORED CONTENT
NATIVE ADVERTISING

**CONTENT**
CREATE FROM EXPERTS
EMPLOYEE STORIES
CUSTOMER STORIES
USER-GENERATED CONTENT
REVIEWS
BRAND JOURNALISM
WEBINARS, VIDEOS & PODCASTS

**PUBLICITY**
MEDIA RELATIONS
BLOGGER RELATIONS
INVESTOR RELATIONS
INFLUENCER RELATIONS

**INFLUENCER ENGAGEMENT**
RESPONSE TO DETRACTORS
DETRACTORS TURNED TO LOYALISTS
LOYALISTS TURNED TO ADVOCATES

**PARTNERSHIPS**
CHARITY TIE-INS
COMMUNITY SERVICE
CO-BRANDING

**SOCIAL MEDIA**
FACEBOOK
TWITTER
LINKED-IN
YOU TUBE
PINTER EST
INSTAGRAM
VINE
GOOGLE+

EARNED MEDIA

SHARED MEDIA

PAID MEDIA

OWNED MEDIA

to develop a comprehensive strategy that used data analytics to drive decisions about where to invest time and funding, and was adaptable to a rapidly changing campaign environment.[20]

The coalition trained spokespeople, such as pastors, parents, pediatricians, and philanthropists, who conducted press interviews and participated in radio call-in shows and television appearances to deliver consistent messages about the campaign legislation. These spokespeople proved to be persuasive champions who explained how the changes would increase healthy options for residents and children. They were supported by trained staff who strategically placed paid media pieces and who engaged reporters to pitch provocative and timely stories as well as major media events that earned coverage in a competitive Baltimore–DC media market. The coalition also effectively used social media to continue the drumbeat on the importance of legislative efforts, share images and materials, engage residents in expressing their opinions, and undertake targeted ad buys to further elevate the message. A constant barrage of opinion editorials, letters to the editor, and commentary from bloggers ensured that legislators saw the sentiment of the public debate in key influential outlets. The *coup de grâce* from the healthy vending effort was a newspaper editorial that asked, in reference to the county executive's intent to veto the bill, "Why pull out your big gun to defend high-calorie vending machine fare?"[21]

A youth-oriented push to highlight the beverage industry's deceptive marketing tactics also successfully integrated PESO media. Ads showed Howard County teens in a variety of settings, such as outside the American Beverage Association's headquarters in Washington, DC, on the phone with industry representatives, and in a makeshift "kitchen" assembling the ingredients of Gatorade. These ads, some of which mimicked the approach of anti-tobacco youth ads, received media coverage from local and national news outlets, such as WBAL-TV and *Politico,* and have earned regional marketing awards. Other sugary drink initiatives from across the country shared the ads extensively through their own networks. And on social media, the Gatorade-making videos proved the campaign's most-watched ads to date.

## EMERGING PHILANTHROPIC ROLE IN SUPPORTING ADVOCACY AND PUBLIC POLICY

Local public health advocacy efforts often have to be cobbled together from disparate and often paltry funding sources. Funding can be particularly challenging when, as in our case, the county health department could not support efforts that did not match the executive's leadership priorities. In many cities and jurisdictions around the county, national, regional, and local philanthropies are filling the void and supporting local efforts to engage in public policy, to advocate for executive and legislative action, and to directly engage citizens in voter-driven referendums. Many of these philanthropies believe strongly in the power of advocacy and recognize that policy and systems change lead to longer lasting, more transformative social change (Box 40.2).

---

## Box 40.2 | Advocating for Health, Starter Kit

*Viviana Martinez-Bianchi*

Where do you start with advocating for a health message, policy, or strategy? Follow these steps to get started

### 1. DEVELOPING YOUR VISION AND GOAL

- What do you want to achieve?
- Have you used an Equity and Empowerment Lens for your plan? https://multco.us/diversity-equity/equity-and-empowerment-lens
- What is the impact?
- How do you see yourself being successful?
- Are you applying principles of Community Engagement?
  - https://www.atsdr.cdc.gov/communityengagement/pdf/PCE_Report_508_FINAL.pdf

### 2. ASSESSING THE POLITICAL AND SOCIAL ENVIRONMENT

- How possible is it to achieve your goal?
- Who makes the decisions re your topic of interest?
- What is the risk of your actions?
- Style of government of the country/state, or governance of the organization.
- Is there more than one avenue?
- Community Factors
- Economic Characteristics
- Demographics
- Has there been previous support to this issue?
- Focus on community

### 3. LEARN ABOUT YOUR AUDIENCE
*Policymakers*

- What (or who) influences them?
- How did they get into office?
- Which jurisdiction do they serve?
- What are their personal interests?

*Organizations*
- What are the "core values" of your audience?
- Rules re legislative

*Academia*
- What are the "core values" of your audience?

## 4. PREPARE THE MESSAGE

- Be specific
- Know your audience
- Frame the message
- Focus on benefits
- Make it real and tangible

Have a 20 seconds elevator talk, and a 2 minute follow up ready to go.

## 5. CREATE A NETWORK

1. Who will be the advocates?
Friends, trustees, funders, visitors, volunteers, employees, local partners, educators, students

2. How can we organize the advocates?
   - Logistics (database)
   - Key contacts / leaders in advocacy
   - Skills (volunteer intake form)
   3. Training How can we activate the advocates?
      Tools for activation
   - On-line (e-mail, social networks, etc.)
   - Off-line (leaflets, posters)

   4. Determine when activation is required
   What are you going to ask them to do?

## 6. BUILD / CREATE COALITION

- Who is best to deliver your message?
  - Based on knowledge of the audience and the message
  - Is it necessary to "tweak" the message depending on who makes the delivery?
- Identification potential coalition partners
- Approaching coalition partners
- Using coalition partners to build on strengths

## 7. DELIVERING THE MESSAGES

*Meetings*
- When and where meetings can happen?
- Who should deliver the message?
- How to adapt the message?
- What will happen at the meeting?
- How will you monitor effect

### Phone calls

- Prepare advocates
- Pros and cons of scripts
- Always ask for a response!

### Written communications (including email)

- Call to action
- personal history
- relevance
- Be brief

### Social Media

- professional use
- Conveying the message in a powerful way

### Blogs

- Writing for policy change

### 8. MONITOR AND EVALUATE PROGRESS

- What measures will you use to evaluate the impact of your work?
- Has your advocacy changed outcomes for your target population? If so, which ones?
- Have there been any unintended effects?
- What changes need to be made to move you closer to your goals?

*Adapted from "Embracing Cultural Humility, Competency, and Advocacy to Decrease Health Disparities" by Viviana Martinez-Bianchi, MD, FAAFP, presented at National Conference of Residents and Students. AAFP. 2015. Contact: viviana.martinezbianchi@duke.edu Tweeter: @vivimbmd.*

The Horizon Foundation, like many philanthropic organizations, used to strongly avoid advocacy. In fact, many foundations have traditionally thought their role was to fill the holes or the void left by failed government and/or private sector interventions. Today, many philanthropic organizations are rethinking how to engage with government at all levels and recognize that a stronger public sector is good for social change. Fred Ali, the president and CEO of the Weingart Foundation in California recently said that "Foundations can—[and] should be—doubling down on supporting organizations involved in advocacy and organizing, as well as using their voice, influence, and resources to directly engage with government around issues of common concerns."[22] Public and private foundations are educating themselves about how they can better inform, educate, and/or lobby within Internal Revenue Service standards and limits. As a result, local advocacy campaigns can now look to philanthropy not only as a source of funding, but also as a voice to help uplift causes, catalyze issues, convene partners, and influence debate.

## CONCLUSION

Recent evidence shows obesity rates continuing to rise, undercutting hopes that obesity rates had started to decline.[23] Diabetes rates are still climbing, and research suggests that up to half of all African American and Latino youth will have diabetes in their lifetimes unless we, as a nation, do something to stem the tide.[24] Public health professionals, researchers, and advocates are calling for a comprehensive national strategy to fight these ongoing epidemics and to double down on necessary public policy changes at the local, state, and national levels. The health of our children depends on courageous adults taking action. Around the country, local efforts to tackle Big Soda have made progress, culminating in successful campaigns to curb sugary drink consumption. Let us hope that these successful local campaigns lead to bigger national changes. Our kids depend on us.

### REFERENCES

1. Nielsen SJ, Popkin BM. Changes in beverage intake between 1977 and 2001. *Am J Pre Med.* 2004;27(3):2–5,201.

2. Malik VS, Popkin BM, Bray GA, Després JP, Willett WC, Hu FB. Sugar-sweetened beverages and risk of metabolic syndrome and type 2 diabetes: A meta-analysis. *Diabetes Care.* 2010;33(11):2477–83.

3. Mallik VS, Popkin BM, Bray GA, Després JP, Hu FB. Sugar-sweetened beverages, obesity, type 2 diabetes mellitus, and cardiovascular disease risk. *Circulation.* 2010;121(11):1356–64.

4. American Heart Association. Understanding Childhood Obesity. http://www.heart.org/idc/groups/heart-public/@wcm/@fc/documents/downloadable/ucm_304175.pdf. 2010. Accessed January 22, 2019.

5. Testimony Before the Subcommittee on Competition, Infrastructure, and Foreign Commerce Committee on Commerce, Science, and Transportation United States Senate "The Growing Epidemic of Childhood Obesity" Statement of Richard H. Carmona, MD, MPH, FACS, Surgeon General, US Public Health Service, US Public Health Services, US Department of Health and Human Services. 2004. www.surgeongeneral.gov/news/testimony/childobesity03022004.html. Accessed January 22, 2019.

6. McGuire S, Institute of Medicine. Accelerating progress in obesity prevention: Solving the weight of the nation. *Adv Nutr.* 2012;3(5):708–9.

7. Institute of Medicine Committee on Assuring the Health of the Public in the 21st Century. *The Future of the Public's Health in the 21st Century.* Washington, DC: National Academies Press; 2002.

8. Sugar-Sweetened Beverages Playbook. ChangeLabSolutions. https://changelabsolutions.org/sites/default/files/SSB_Playbook_FINAL-20131004.pdf. Accessed January 22, 2019.

9. Howard County Unsweetened. http://www.hocounsweetened.org. Accessed January 22, 2019.

10. Sugar Free Kids Maryland. http://www.sugarfreekidsmd.org. Accessed January 22, 2019.

11. Piekarz E, Schermbeck R, Young SK, Leider J, Ziemann M, Chriqui JF. *School District Wellness Policies: Evaluating Progress and Potential for Improving Children's*

Health Eight Years after the Federal Mandate. School Years 2006–07 through 2013–14. Volume 4. Chicago, IL: Bridging the Gap Program and the National Wellness Policy Study, Institute for Health Research and Policy, University of Illinois at Chicago; 2016. www.go.uic.edu/NWPSproducts.

12. Gardner CD, Whitsel LP, Thorndike AN, et al. Food-and-beverage environment and procurement policies for healthier work environments. *Nutr Rev.* 2014;72:390–410. doi:10.1111/nure.12116.

13. Robert Wood Johnson Foundation, Healthy Eating Research. Promoting Good Nutrition and Physical Activity in Child-Care Settings (Research Brief) 2007 May; http://healthyeatingresearch.org/wp-content/uploads/2013/12/HER-Child-Care-Setting-Research-Brief-2007.pdf. Accessed January 22, 2019.

14. Nielsen SJ, Popkin BM, Bray GA, Despres' JP, Willett WC, HU FB. Sugar-sweetened beverages and risk of metabolic syndrome and type 2 diabetes; a meta-analysis. *Diabetes Care.* 2010;33(11):2477-2483.

15. Nielsen SJ, Popkin BM. Changes in beverage intake between 1977 and 2001. *Am J Pre Med* 2004;27(3):2-5-201.

16. Schwartz MB, Schneider GE, Choi YY, et al. Association of a community campaign for better beverage choices with beverage purchases from supermarkets. *JAMA Intern Med.* 2017. doi:10.1001/jamainternmed.2016.9650.

17. Md. Code Ann., Family Law § 5-573 (2014).

18. Howard County, Maryland. Code of Ordinances § 12.1800 (2015).

19. Sugary Drink Food Advertising to Children and Teens Score. 2014. Rudd Center for Food Policy and Obesity. November 2014. http://www.sugarydrinkfacts.org/resources/sugarydrinkfacts_report.pdf. Accessed January 22, 2019.

20. Dietrich G. PR pros must embrace the PESO Model. [Blog] *SpinSucks: Professional Development for PR and Marketing Pros.* 2018. https://spinsucks.com/communication/pr-pros-must-embrace-the-peso-model/ Accessed January 22, 2019.

21. Baltimore Sun. Editorial. July 16, 2015.

22. Ali F. Speech at the Forum of Regional Association of Grantmakers Annual Conference. July 19, 2017. http://www.weingartfnd.org/Philanthropys-Role-in-Supporting-Advocacy-and-Engaging-in-Public-Policy. Accessed January 22, 2019.

23. Skinner AC, Ravanbakht SN, Skelton JA, et al. Prevalence of Obesity and Severe Obesity in US Children, 1999–2016. *Pediatrics.* 2018;141(3):e20173459.

24. May AL, Kuklina EV, Yoon PW. Prevalence of cardiovascular disease risk factors among US adolescents, 1999–2008. *Pediatrics.* 2012 Jun;129(6):1035–41. doi:10.1542/peds.2011-1082. Epub May 21, 2012.

# Chapter 41

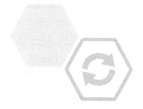

# Building Off of Evidence-Based Policies: The CDC's Health Impact in 5 Years (HI-5) Initiative and CityHealth, an Initiative of the de Beaumont Foundation and Kaiser Permanente

ELIZABETH SKILLEN AND SHELLEY HEARNE

Successful policymaking does not have to be mysterious. The science and art of good policymaking involves identifying evidence-based options, conducting feasibility assessments, and fostering strategic partnerships.[1] Understanding these elements allows public health leaders to more successfully use policy as a population-wide approach for better health*.

## CRITICAL FACTORS IN DEVELOPING AND IMPLEMENTING POLICY

Policy is developed, enacted, and implemented within a broad context and is the product of many factors and players.[2] These include the following:

- *Development of an evidence base* and making evidence available to inform action is the primary subject of this chapter. Experts note that

---

\* Note: The findings and conclusions in this chapter are those of the authors and do not necessarily represent the official position of the Centers for Disease Control and Prevention decision-makers can achieve substantially better results by using evidence to select policies, inform budget decisions, and strategically implement programs.[3] Using evidence to understand, substantiate, and analytically assess the nature of health problems and their potential solutions can make policies more acceptable to policymakers, the public, and potential opposing interests. Furthermore, the evaluation of experiences of early adopters is critical to this step.

- *Innovation* by early adopters allows for the evolution of evidence of impact and informs decision-making by other jurisdictions. The progression from problem identification, to proposed intervention, to research and demonstration, to initial adoption, and then to broader acceptance requires risk-taking by early adopters.[4] For example, sufficient evidence existed that documented the severity and cost of escalating obesity rates in New York City. Using these data, Mayor Michael Bloomberg adopted many policies to address the epidemic escalation of childhood obesity, including calorie labeling in chain restaurants, trans-fat bans, cup size limits, and nutrition mandates in schools. There was evidence that the interventions would work, supported by the health department working collaboratively across government to make the case to decision-makers to adopt these strategies.[5]

- *Alignment of political, economic, and social factors* that impact the policy process. The best evidence-based policies may be exceedingly difficult to implement in a particular jurisdiction without accounting for a set of favorable sociopolitical conditions, such as community context, economic costs, and political feasibility. Modeling and economic analysis can provide critical information for "making the case" for policy solutions by assessing the health and economic impacts from both the perspective of those implementing the interventions (i.e., budgetary costs) and the larger benefits of the interventions to society (e.g., health and safety).[6] Political feasibility, in turn, can be a product of cultural, ideological, and personal factors that are subjective and hard to quantify, with limited treatment in public debate or in the literature.[7] For example, policies designed to reduce consumption of tobacco,[8] alcohol,[9] and sugar[10] by increasing their costs can be challenging to pass despite evidence of health and economic benefits. Purtle et al. reported that Philadelphia recently was able to address this by framing the passage of a sugar-sweetened beverage tax as a means toward funding highly popular universal, high-quality early-education programs.[11] The range of interests informing policy-making and potential partners to forge policy alliances is shown in Figure 41.1.[12]

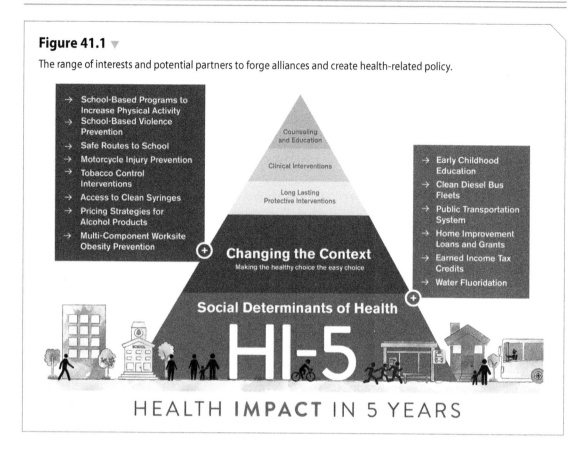

**Figure 41.1** ▼

The range of interests and potential partners to forge alliances and create health-related policy.

## ACCESSING AND USING EVIDENCE IN ADVANCING POLICY

When policymakers use evidence-informed approaches, they can better aim scarce resources toward effective programs, invest in innovative new approaches, and stop investing in approaches that do not work. There are several key points in the policy process[13] where credible data and evidence could increase the opportunity for better results:

- *Problem identification*: Know the prevalence, location, severity, and causes of a given health issue and the disproportionate burden on certain populations (e.g., children, those in poverty).
- *Policy and equity analysis*: Identify and evaluate different policy options to address the problem using quantitative and qualitative methods to determine the most effective, efficient, and feasible options; assess the identified health impact and costs of policy solutions with special attention to health equity and potential variation in social determinants.[14]
- *Evaluation of policy implementation*: Identify indicators and metrics to evaluate the implementation and impact of the policy.[15]

Evidence is critical but not always readily accessible to decision-makers at the state and local levels, particularly where analytic capacity may be limited. The daunting array of policy options and the ambiguity of many sources of evidence often complicates movement toward consensus and action. The balance of this chapter discusses two approaches to help decision-makers accelerate the policy process by distilling evidence and making it more accessible.

## Using Evidence-Based Policies to Improve Health: The CDC HI-5 and CityHealth Approaches

It is well-known that evidence-based policies have the best chance for impact, but how can the evidence be catalyzed into action? The first steps of selecting effective policies and assessing how to apply policies to particular settings can be formidable. For example, a Google Scholar search on "early childhood education policy" returned about 3,620,000 results in total and 17,100 in 2018 alone.[16] There are numerous federal, academic, and not-for-profit clearing houses of evidence-based policies, including the Community Guide, County Health Rankings & Roadmaps: What Works for Health, and The Washington State Institute for Public Policy, yet there is still a large volume of information to cull through. The following describes two different initiatives designed to help decision-makers and practitioners identify approaches that work in their communities.

### What Is HI-5?

Putting science into action to prevent disease is one of the core roles of the Centers for Disease Control and Prevention (CDC) to achieve its mission as the nation's health protection agency.[17] The CDC is well known for being expert at handling some of the world's most dangerous infectious, chemical, biological, and environmental threats.[18] CDC experts also protect the United States from chronic diseases that are responsible for 6 in 10 deaths each year and for the vast majority of the nation's health care costs.[19] The CDC brings together data, health care systems, and communities to support healthy choices and reduce risk behaviors to prevent the burden of diseases. Providing the best science on effective policy[20] is a critical component of the CDC's role, as well as informing decision-makers on what works to prevent disease. The CDC also works to enhance the policy fluency of health officials in choosing those policy and community-wide interventions that have the greatest potential for impact. How do public health practitioners and policymakers know where to begin to find the best science?

In 2016, to meet state and local health officials' requests for evidence-based policy approaches, the CDC launched the Health Impact in 5 Years (HI-5) initiative, which highlights nonclinical, community-wide interventions that can improve the places where "we live, learn, work, and play." HI-5 policies can help communities achieve healthy outcomes in 5 years or less and have demonstrated cost effectiveness over the lifetime of the population or earlier. The CDC developed the HI-5 tool through a careful and methodical process.[21] The HI-5 project team consulted two frameworks to select, translate, and package the findings for public health practitioners and decision-makers. The Three Buckets of Prevention Framework informed the development of the criteria by characterizing interventions along a continuum from clinical care to community-wide policy interventions.[22] In addition, the Public Health Impact Pyramid provided a framework for public action[23] that groups the HI-5 interventions into those that address the social determinants of health and those that "change the context to make the healthy choice the easy choice." Interventions focusing on these two lower levels of the pyramid have the potential to be more effective because they reach more members of society and do not require as much individual effort.

One goal of the HI-5 Initiative was to have a "short-list of evidence-based policy interventions" to provide a starting point for public health practitioners. The HI-5 project team initially compiled a list of interventions with the highest evidence rating from the Community Guide to Preventive Services ("Recommended")[1] and the Robert Wood Johnson Foundation-funded County Health Rankings & Roadmaps (CHRR): What Works for Health ("Scientifically Supported") database.[2] Interventions from the Community Guide were based on recommendations from the Community Preventive Services Task Force (CPSTF). The CPSTF was established by the US Department of Health and Human Services (DHHS) in 1996 to develop guidance on which community-based health promotion and disease prevention intervention approaches work and which do not work. These recommendations are based on hundreds of studies that meet rigorous standards. After the HI-5 project team selected the interventions from these databases, they then screened out duplicates and patient-focused clinical interventions, leaving 118 community-wide interventions. They then assessed this initial list of 118 against five inclusion criteria (listed here) and chose to include interventions that:

- Have evidence of a measurable impact on health within 5 years
- Have evidence reporting cost-effectiveness and/or cost savings over the lifetime of the population or earlier
- Focus on whole populations or communities
- Have not yet been implemented in at least 85% of communities and/or states nationwide
- Had evidence of implementation through federal-, state-, or local-level policies

1 The Community Guide rated an intervention as "Recommended" if, after conducting a systematic review of the available studies, it determined that they provided strong or sufficient evidence that the intervention was effective. Their systematic reviews consider several factors, including study design, number of studies, and consistency of the effect across studies.
2 County Health Rankings and Roadmaps rated an interventions as "Scientifically Supported" if it was supported by one or more systematic reviews, or at least three experimental studies, or three quasi-experimental studies with matched concurrent comparisons. Supporting studies had to include strong designs and statistically significant positive findings.

| Table 41.1 ▼ The Health Impact in 5 Years Initiative: 14 Community-Wide Interventions for Population Health Improvement—change the context: making the healthy choice the easy choice |
| --- |
| • School-based programs to increase physical activity |
| • School-based violence prevention |
| • Safe routes to school (SRTS) |
| • Multicomponent worksite obesity prevention |
| • Motorcycle injury prevention |
| • Tobacco control interventions |
| • Access to clean syringes |
| • Pricing strategies for alcohol products |
| Address the social determinants of health |
| • Early childhood education |
| • Clean diesel bus fleets |
| • Public transportation system introduction or expansion |
| • Home improvement loans and grants |
| • Earned income tax credits |
| • Water fluoridation |

Finally, the HI-5 project team then consulted with subject matter experts from across the CDC to verify findings and identify any additional community-wide interventions supported by systematic reviews that met the inclusion criteria but were not included in the original interventions identified in the Community Guide or CHRR database. One intervention was included during this phase. Table 41.1 shows the resulting 14 community-wide interventions included in HI-5 (see also Figure 41.2).

The CDC developed and shared on its website and through webinars and presentations a series of HI-5 evidence summaries outlining the health impact and cost data for each community-wide intervention, many of which address multiple health issues. The CDC has continued work with federal partners, foundations, and state and local health departments to share the evidence on policies that drive population health impact. Partnerships continue to grow, as do emerging efforts to gather practice-based evidence so that public health practitioners can better use policy as a tool for improving health and well-being.

## Figure 41.2 ▼

The 14 community-wide interventions included in HI-5.

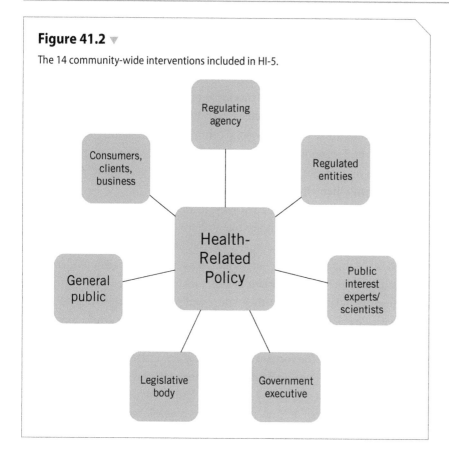

## CityHealth Strategy for Catalyzing Evidence-Based Policies to Promote Healthier, Thriving Environments

Cities are increasingly in a prime position to innovate and lead with policy initiatives that improve the lives and health of their residents while supporting culture change and incubating policies that drive state and national change. For instance, Chicago, Duluth (Minnesota), Los Angeles, and New York led the nation in regulating electronic cigarettes in public settings.[24] Increasingly, leaders are recognizing that vibrant, thriving economies require an architecture of policies that builds a healthy place to live, work, eat, and play. However, that can be a daunting task for government officials who are often overwhelmed by the daily challenges and stress of governance.

In feedback from health officials and mayors when preparing for first release of CityHealth findings in 2017, many appreciated a curated, evidence-based list of because leaders had felt "paralyzed" by the hundreds of different policy options and lack of resources to target best practices for their jurisdiction.[3] CityHealth, an initiative of the de Beaumont Foundation and Kaiser

*This study showcases our work toward creating a healthy city for all Boston residents, and also identifies other cities that are leading in each policy area, creating opportunity for collaboration and learning from one another.*
*—Monica Valdes Lupi, Executive Director, Boston Public Health Commission*

---

3 Personal communication from health officials and mayors when preparing for first release of CityHealth findings in 2017.

Permanente, is designed to give city leaders a policy blueprint to use as a lever to improve residents' lives and help their cities to thrive. CityHealth rated the nation's largest cities based on their progress in adopting an evidence-based policy package. This policy package was derived using a three-part process that considered (1) the evidence base of policies addressing the key social determinants of health, (2) cities' jurisdictional authority and precedent, and (3) analysis by a policy advisory committee representing key partners, influencers, and community representatives. The goal was to provide city leaders with a pragmatic, achievable, yet aspirational package of policies that could align with their city's priorities and needs.

Similar to CDC's HI-5 initiative, CityHealth started with all those policies that leading authorities—such as the Robert Wood Johnson Foundation's County Health Rankings & Roadmaps, the National Academy of Medicine, and the CDC's Community Guide—determined as having sufficient evidence/expert opinion to provide important health benefits.[25] Policies were sorted into key categories related to how they addressed social determinants of health along with key preventable causes of death and disability: education, transportation, housing, public safety, education, financial security, environment, and tobacco control. The focus was exclusively on upstream policies that prevent health problems, not on medical treatment and care. CityHealth also determined that at least one policy should be under the direct authority of the local public health agency (rather than a city council, zoning board, or other decision-maker). Policies were further filtered by jurisdictional authority—only policies that could potentially be actionable at the city level were used. CityHealth conducted a feasibility assessment, drawing from national subject matter experts and a policy advisory committee representing influential parties in a local policymaking process, which included a mayor, a chamber of commerce representative, a public health dean, and community leaders.

CityHealth's nine policy recommendations are as follows:

- Paid sick leave
- High-quality, universal pre-kindergarten
- Affordable housing/inclusionary zoning
- Complete streets
- Alcohol sales control
- Smoke-free air
- Tobacco 21
- Food safety/restaurant grading
- Healthy food procurement

The CityHealth package is not intended to be an exhaustive list; instead, nine policies were selected that met the specific criteria of being largely under city jurisdiction, being backed by evidence, and showing a track record of bipartisan support. The project team also looked for those policies that were ready to be adopted in the most places with the greatest potential to improve people's lives.

*A healthy city measures itself not only by life expectancy, but by access to nutritious food and park space, by traffic policies that reduce serious accidents, by child care affordability for working parents, and by the beauty of its neighborhoods. [The CityHealth] assessment of LA, as one of America's healthiest big cities, speaks to the effectiveness of our work.*

*—Eric Garcetti, Mayor, Los Angeles*

Following this assessment, CityHealth created a public accountability tool to convey the status of the nine policies in each of the nation's largest cities. Working with leading subject matter experts, CityHealth developed criteria for scoring individual policies as gold, silver, bronze, or no medal (see Cityhealth. org for descriptions of scoring methodology in the "deep data dive" section for each policy). For instance, the early education medal status reflected the quality and access benchmarks established by the nation's leading expert in that domain—the National Institute for Early Education Research, which produces an annual state-level assessment. Cities were awarded an overall city-wide medal based on how many policy medals they had earned: gold is awarded for five or more gold medal policies, silver is awarded for five or more silver or gold, and bronze is awarded for four of any combination of medals. Recognizing that cities have different needs, priorities, and realities, CityHealth does not weight policies and only requires a plurality of policies winning top marks in order to award a medal.

Recognizing that policy does not happen in a vacuum, CityHealth also includes an action phase to provide support for city partners, technical assistance, and communication to spur policy adoption by city leaders.[26] In doing so, CityHealth places a particular emphasis on supporting local health department officials to serve as health strategists who can help champion policies that best align with their city's needs and interests. In addition, CityHealth provides grants to appropriate local organizations with experience in promoting health policies; these range from nonprofit advocacy organizations to local chambers of commerce.

While passage of new policies routinely takes multiple years, city leaders have quickly embraced the CityHealth model and have made remarkable progress in adopting these nine evidence-based policies. In the year since CityHealth launched its initial assessment, 24 policy improvements were made, resulting in 10 cities moving their overall medal status.[27] (See Chapter 43 for the work in Kansas City as one example.)

CityHealth's ratings present an opportunity for city leaders to begin conversations about how to help residents' live healthier lives and make their cities the best places to live, work, and do business. Working with national experts, CityHealth does more than award medals: it helps city leaders understand—and ultimately adopt—strong policies and recognize the full range of considerations that impact policymaking. Public accountability is a powerful force—by seeing that peer cities have enacted key policies, city leaders in government, community organizations, and business can use information to help generate will for change.

## Similarities and Differences

Accelerating the use of evidence in policy development is at the core of both HI-5 and CityHealth. Yet the roles of the two organizations provide different approaches for informing local decision-making. The HI-5 Initiative is an example of the CDC's role as a federal agency putting science into action to prevent disease by synthesizing the evidence on what works. HI-5 captures the evidence on health and cost related to 14 community-wide interventions in keeping with the CDC's role to inform on the *science* of policymaking, yet the decisions about choosing specific policies are left up to state and local governments. In keeping with this role, the HI-5 criteria did not include consideration of readiness for or willingness of state or local jurisdictions to enact any of the policies. In contrast, CityHealth's stated goal was to create a "new gold standard for health and well-being in cities" and provide annual assessments of the nation's 40 largest cities on policies that can have lasting impacts in people's everyday quality of life. CityHealth, as an initiative implemented by a nongovernmental organization, had greater license to incorporate other factors, such as political context. These two initiatives use different strategies to motivate state and local officials to get started on policies. The CDC uses its role as a trusted source for information, and CityHealth provides public accountability, technical assistance, and city leader support to encourage adoption of specific policies. Both are important to accelerate evidence-based policymaking.

## CASE STUDIES OF DIFFERENT POLICY TARGETS THAT CAN IMPROVE HEALTH IN DIFFERING POLICY ENVIRONMENTS

The range of sectors addressed by upstream, evidence-based policy is increasingly outside the jurisdiction of health agencies and even outside traditional definitions of public health. This is particularly true as these policies tackle many of the underlying social factors that contribute to health. From early education to earned sick leave, the next generation of policies that will make the greatest impact on health are in a wide range of areas, such as transportation, housing, the business community, and the financial sector. While evidence may be strong that these policies will make valuable population health improvements, public health agencies do not have direct oversight. Public health leaders can find ways to engage, convene, and support cross-sector efforts to support good policy. Partnerships with health systems, community organizations, foundations, businesses, and other influential leaders are key for generating strategic policies and getting them to decision-makers to inform evidence-based policy.

### Economic Policy—Earned Income Tax Credit: An Example of Refundable Credits

*It is our job as public health professionals to use data to tell the whole story about what creates health.*
*—Jeanne F. Ayers, Assistant Commissioner, Minnesota Department of Health*

The relationship between income and health, and between poverty and poor health in particular, has been well established[28–30] with documented adverse health outcomes for infants and children.[31–33] According to the US Census Bureau, 5.8% of workers aged 18–64 years were in poverty in 2016.[34] Tax credits such as earned income tax credit (EITC), one of the HI-5 interventions,[35] provide benefits for working people with low to moderate incomes.[36] EITC is an income tax credit—often refundable—that can be levied at federal, state, and local levels to reduce the tax burden for low-income working people.[37,38] Twenty-nine states and the District of Columbia have their own EITCs.[39] For example, Minnesota increased the total value of its Minnesota Working Family Credit by 25% and expanded eligibility for workers aged 21–24 years (see Minnesota Statutes, §290.0671).[40] State-specific or local data can be critical for making the case to policymakers during the policy enactment phase, which is a key role for public health. In 2014, the Minnesota Department of Health (MDH) wrote a white paper including local data on the relationship between income and poverty and their relationship to health outcomes,[41] as well as a report to the legislature on health equity.[42] These types of data provide critical tools for partners and advocates to make the case to policymakers about policy options. This work by the MDH continues with targeted reports on important policy issues for Minnesotans.[43]

Policy enactment is just one stage of the policy process: Then what?[44] How does a law, regulation, or administrative action come to life to make a difference? Once any policy is enacted, there is an opportunity for broad coalitions of partners to make it work. Public health practitioners have a vital role in helping to translate enacted policies "into action, monitor uptake, and ensure full implementation."[45] Partners such as health care providers or tax preparers can ensure that eligible people are aware of policy changes and able to access benefits. For example, in Minnesota, the United Way provides free tax services to help Minnesota low-income residents, and critical partners, such as the Mille Lacs Band of the Ojibwe, provide critical outreach to ensure uptake of changes to tax credit law.[46] In Boston, primary health care providers provide screening for linking to vital tax preparation services in Massachusetts.[47]

Policy enactment and implementation is challenging work and getting started can be difficult. Many national organizations provide data, tools, and training for practitioners. EITC partners, such as the nonpartisan Center on Budget and Policy Priorities, provide singular research on state budget and tax issues.[48] Organizations, such as Health Impact Partners, provide critical training, technical assistance, and leadership development "to build a will to act on the social determinants of health," as well as stories from the field at HealthEquityGuide.org.

## Advancing the Next Generation of Tobacco Reforms: San Antonio's Leadership and Key Partners Strategy

Tobacco use remains the single most preventable cause of death and disease in this country, resulting in approximately 480,000 deaths, more than $156 billion in lost productivity costs,[49] and nearly $170 billion in direct medical care expenditures each year.[50] The CDC recommends a comprehensive strategy for preventing and reducing tobacco use in each state (described in CDC's *Best Practices for Comprehensive Tobacco Control Programs—2014*).[51]

Three of the strategies are included in HI-5: (1) mass-reach health communication interventions, (2) state and community interventions (e.g., increasing the price of tobacco products), and (3) comprehensive smoke-free indoor air policies that prohibit smoking in all indoor public areas including worksites, restaurants, and bars (which is consistent with CityHealth's smoke-free indoor air recommendation). States such as California have comprehensive smoke-free policies receiving a grade of "A" according to rankings by the American Lung Association. Additional local approaches can assist when feasible.

Evidence shows that people who begin using tobacco in youth and young adulthood are at greater risk of lifetime use.[52] Because the brain continues to develop into young adulthood, adolescents and young adults are more susceptible to addiction.[52] Approximately 90% of adult cigarette smokers first try smoking before the age of 18 years, and about 95% first try smoking before they are 21 years old.[53] Therefore, delaying the age at which young people first experiment with or begin using tobacco can reduce the risk that they will become addicted smokers.[54] Research shows that raising the minimum age for tobacco sales 21 years has the potential to decrease tobacco retailer and industry sales, which in turn could contribute to a reduction in tobacco use and addiction.[54]

A 2015 report by the Institute of Medicine (now the National Academy of Medicine) projected significant health benefits from raising the tobacco purchase age to 21 nationally. Key projections included the following:

- A 25% decline in cigarette smoking initiation by 15- to 17-year-olds
- A 12% drop in adult cigarette smoking prevalence once today's youth reach adulthood[55]
- A total of 16,000 cases of preterm birth and low birth weight would be averted within 5 years

The Academy also predicted that increasing the age of sale for cigarettes to age 21 years could save 4.2 million years of life for today's youth. Other research models estimate that increasing the legal smoking age from 18 to 21 years could lead to $212 billion in savings over 50 years, driven largely by reduced medical costs.[56]

In 2017, San Antonio, Texas, appointed Colleen Bridger, MPH, PhD, to be the director of the Metropolitan Health District. In this position, Dr. Bridger is responsible for implementing policies aimed at improving the health of the population in San Antonio and Bexar County and managing nearly two dozen programs, including the Women, Infants, and Children [WIC] program; vector control; air quality; sexually transmitted diseases and HIV prevention; and tuberculosis control and prevention. As part of San Antonio's commitment to be the healthiest city in Texas, Dr. Bridger used the CityHealth policy package and accountability system as a roadmap for strategically advancing the city's health policies. In 2017, San Antonio had no overall medal under CityHealth scoring. With support from the mayor, city manager, and key city council members, Dr. Bridger championed a commitment for achieving a bronze medal in 1 year, a silver medal in 2 years, and a gold medal in 3 years. Recognizing the city's high youth smoking rate, the Tobacco 21 (T21) policy was an initial objective.

Although more than 300 US cities and five states have raised the tobacco age to 21 years as of July 2018, all previous city and statewide efforts to pass T21 in Texas had been unsuccessful.[57] San Antonio changed that equation by becoming the first Texas city to pass legislation restricting tobacco purchases to those age 21 years and older. As the city's chief health strategist, Dr. Bridger developed support with key governmental leaders for the T21 policy. She also cultivated partners such as the University of Texas/MD Anderson, which committed staff time to provide expertise on best practices and educational outreach. Public health advocates also joined the effort by forming a coalition to provide support, public engagement, and public opinion research to assist with the statewide T21 efforts. This included partners such as the American Heart Association, the American Cancer Society Cancer Action Network, and the Campaign for Tobacco Free Kids, among others. CityHealth supported these efforts, providing technical assistance and funding for educational outreach.

Key community influencers provided input during the San Antonio City Council hearings, ranging from the San Antonio Chamber of Commerce to high school and middle school students who spoke out on the need to reduce tobacco use on campus as well as among their friends and peers. In February 2018—following a robust city council deliberation and months of efforts to inform the public about the benefits of T21—the San Antonio City Council adopted a T21 ordinance to increase the tobacco purchasing age from 18 to 21 years. The strong partnerships, authentic and highly credible community voices, and exceptional city leadership allowed San Antonio to step forward as the first city in Texas to adopt a T21 policy. The success in San Antonio has helped inform similar efforts in other cities, as well as efforts to pursue a statewide T21 policy.

## Final Thoughts

Shrinking resources coupled with demands for better health outcomes provide an opportunity for state and local public health decision-makers to become adept at identifying and implementing high-impact and cost-effective approaches to address the drivers of health and well-being. Evidence-based policies such as high-quality universal pre-kindergarten[58] and EITCs[59] can have a significant impact on population health, yet awareness across disciplines about their value is often underrecognized.[60] Policy development and implementation can be important tools to promote community-wide health and well-being by addressing the social determinants of health and the contextual influences that can affect the health decisions people make. Engaging in these "upstream" efforts, however, involves more than knowledge of the evidence; it also requires knowledge of what works, for whom, in what circumstances. What is even more important is an improved understanding of how policy can be used as a tool to address public health concerns. The most vital ingredient to successfully developing, establishing, and implementing policies that make a difference in improving health, vitality, and wellness will be to use the best available science in strategic partnership with a broad coalition of community stakeholders and decision-makers.

## REFERENCES

1. Centers for Disease Control and Prevention. The CDC Policy Process.: https://www.cdc.gov/policy/polaris/policy-cdc-policy-process.html. Accessed January 18, 2019.

2. Centers for Disease Control and Prevention. The CDC Policy Process.: https://www.cdc.gov/policy/polaris/policy-cdc-policy-process.html. Accessed January 18, 2019.

3. Brownson, RC, Baker, EA, Deshpande AD, Gillespie, KN. *Evidence-based Public Health* (3rd ed.). New York: Oxford University Press; 2018.

4. Centers for Disease Control and Prevention. The CDC Policy Process.: https://www.cdc.gov/policy/polaris/policy-cdc-policy-process.html. Accessed January 18, 2019.

5. Kelly PM, Davies A, Greig AJM, Lee KK. Obesity prevention in a city state: Lessons from New York City during the Bloomberg Administration. *Front Public Health*. 2016;4:60. http://doi.org/10.3389/fpubh.2016.00060.

6. Centers for Disease Control and Prevention. The CDC Policy Process.: https://www.cdc.gov/policy/polaris/policy-cdc-policy-process.html. Accessed January 18, 2019

7. McLaughlin CP, McLaughlin CD. *Health Policy Analysis: An Interdisciplinary Approach. Chapter 9: The Policy Analysis Process—Evaluation—Political Feasibility*. Sudbury, MA: Jones and Bartlett Publishers; 2008:233.

8. The Community Preventive Services Task Force. Tobacco use and secondhand smoke exposure: Mass-reach health communication interventions. https://www.thecommunityguide.org/findings/tobacco-use-and-secondhand-smoke-exposure-mass-reach-health-communication-interventions.

9. The Community Preventive Services Task Force. Alcohol—Excessive consumption: Increasing alcohol taxes. https://www.thecommunityguide.org/findings/alcohol-excessive-consumption-increasing-alcohol-taxes.

10. County Health Rankings & Road Maps. Sugar sweetened beverage taxes. http://www.countyhealthrankings.org/take-action-to-improve-health/what-works-for-health/policies/sugar-sweetened-beverage-taxes.

11. Purtle J, Langellier B, Lê-Scherban F. A case study of the Philadelphia sugar-sweetened beverage tax policymaking process: Implications for policy development and advocacy. *J Public Health Manag Pract*. 2018;24(1):4–8.

12. McLaughlin CP, McLaughlin CD. *Health Policy Analysis: An Interdisciplinary Approach. Chapter 9: The Policy Analysis Process—Evaluation—Political Feasibility*. Sudbury, MA: Jones and Bartlett Publishers; 2008:240.

13. Centers for Disease Control and Prevention. The CDC Policy Process.: https://www.cdc.gov/policy/polaris/policy-cdc-policy-process.html. Accessed January 18, 2019.

14. Centers for Disease Control and Prevention. A Practitioner's Guide for Advancing Health Equity, Community Strategies for Preventing Chronic Disease. https://www.cdc.gov/nccdphp/dch/pdf/HealthEquityGuide.pdf. Accessed January 18, 2019.

15. Centers for Disease Control and Prevention. The CDC Policy Process.: https://www.cdc.gov/policy/polaris/policy-cdc-policy-process.html. Accessed January 18, 2019.

16. Google Scholar Search. Early childhood education policy. https://scholar.google.com/scholar?hl=en&as_sdt=0%2C11&q=early+childhood+education+policy&btnG=&oq=early+child. Accessed July 2, 2018.

17. Centers for Disease Control and Prevention. Mission, Role and Pledge. https://www.cdc.gov/about/organization/mission.htm. Accessed January 18, 2019.

18. Centers for Disease Control and Prevention. 2015 CDC Saving lives. Protecting People. Keeping America, Save, Healthy, & Secure. https://www.cdc.gov/about/report/2015/docs/2015HealthSecurityREPORT18_508.pdf. Accessed January 18, 2019.

19. Centers for Disease Control and Prevention. About Chronic Diseases. https://www.cdc.gov/chronicdisease/about/index.htm. Accessed January 18, 2019.

20. Bauer UE, Briss PA, Goodman RA, Bowman BA. Prevention of chronic disease in the 21st century: Elimination of the leading preventable causes of premature death and disability in the USA. *Lancet.* 2014;384:45–52.

21. Centers for Disease Control and Prevention. About the Evidence Summaries, Health Impact in 5 Years. https://www.cdc.gov/policy/hst/hi5/aboutsummaries/index.html. Accessed January 18, 2019

22. Auerbach JA. The 3 buckets of prevention. *J Public Health Mgmt Pract.* 2016;22(3):215–8.

23. Frieden TR. A framework for public health action: The Health Impact Pyramid. *Am J Public Health.* 2010;100(4):590–5.

24. Cox E, Rachel B, Glantz S. E-cigarette policymaking by local and state governments: 2009–2014: E-cigarette policymaking: 2009–2014. *Milbank Q.* 2016;94:520–96. doi:10.1111/1468-0009.12212.

25. Centers for Disease Control and Prevention. Health Impact in 5 Years. https://www.cdc.gov/hi5/index.html. Accessed January 18, 2019. Centers for Disease Control and Prevention. The Community Guide. https://www.thecommunityguide.org. Accessed January 18, 2019. University of Wisconsin Population Health Institute and Robert Wood Johnson, County Health Rankings & Roadmaps, What Works for Health. http://www.countyhealthrankings.org/take-action-to-improve-health/what-works-for-health. Accessed January 18, 2019.

26. Brownson RC, Chriqui JF, Stamatakis KA. Policy, politics and collective action: Understanding evidence-based public health policy. *Government Politics Law.* 2009;99:1576–83. https://ajph.aphapublications.org/doi/pdf/10.2105/AJPH.2008.156224.

27. CityHealth. Press release. New CityHealth report shows city leaders are putting policies in place to help residents thrive. May 22, 2018. http://www.cityhealth.org/press-release-2018-report.

28. Marmot M, Wilkinson R. *Social Determinants of Health.* Oxford: Oxford University Press; 2005.

29. Bosworth B, Burtless G, Zhang K. *Later Retirement, Inequality in Old Age, and the Growing Gap in Longevity Between Rich and Poor.* Washington, DC: The Brookings Institution; 2016.

30. Blackburn C. *Poverty and Health: Working with Families.* Maidenhead, UK: Open University Press; 1991.

31. Strully KW, Rehkopf DH, Xuan Z. Effects of prenatal poverty on infant health: state earned income tax credits and birth weight. *Am Sociol Rev*. 2010;75(4):534–62.

32. Brooks-Gunn J, Duncan GJ, Leventhal T, Aber JL. Lessons Learned and Future Directions for Research on the Neighborhoods in Which Children Live. In: Brooks-Gunn J, Duncan GJ, Aber JL, eds. *Neighborhood Poverty: Context and Consequences for Children* (vol. 1). New York: Russell Sage Foundation; 1997:279–97.

33. Hair NL, Hanson JL, Wolfe BL. Association of child poverty, brain development, and academic achievement. *JAMA Pediatrics*. 2015;169(9):822–9.

34. Semega JL, Fontenot KR, Kollar MA. *US Census Bureau, Current Population Reports, P60-259, Income and Poverty in the United States: 2016*. Washington, DC: US Government Printing Office; 2017.

35. https://www.cdc.gov/policy/hst/hi5/taxcredits/index.html.

36. Internal Revenue Service. Earned Income Tax Credit (EITC). 2018. https://www.irs.gov/credits-deductions/individuals/earned-income-tax-credit. Accessed April 13, 2018.

37. Hathaway J. Tax credits for working families: Earned Income Tax Credit (EITC). 2016. http://www.ncsl.org/Portals/1/Documents/Labor/workingfamilies/EITC_Jan2016Update_FINAL.pdf. Accessed June 6, 2016.

38. New York State Department of Taxation and Finance. New York City credits. 2014. https://tax.ny.gov. Accessed June 6, 2016.

39. https://www.cbpp.org/blog/new-federal-tax-law-reduces-value-of-state-eitcs.

40. Minnesota. 2017 Minnesota Statutes, section 290.0671. Minnesota Working Family Credit. https://www.revisor.mn.gov/statutes/cite/290.0671. Accessed July 3, 2018.

41. Minnesota Department of Health. White Paper on Income and Health. http://www.health.state.mn.us/divs/opa/2014incomeandhealth.pdf. Accessed January 18, 2019.

42. Minnesota Department of Health. Advancing Health Equity in Minnesota, Report to the Legislature. 2014. http://www.health.state.mn.us/divs/che/reports/ahe_leg_report_020114.pdf. Accessed January 18, 2019.

43. Minnesota Department of Health. Health Equity Reports and Publications. http://www.health.state.mn.us/divs/che/reports/index.html. Accessed January 18, 2019.

44. Centers for Disease Control and Prevention. The CDC Policy Process.: https://www.cdc.gov/policy/polaris/policy-cdc-policy-process.html. Accessed January 18, 2019.

45. Centers for Disease Control and Prevention. The CDC Policy Process.: https://www.cdc.gov/policy/polaris/policy-cdc-policy-process.html. Accessed January 18, 2019.

46. Mille Lacs Band of Ojibwe. State of Minnesota Working Family Tax Credit 2017 Update. https://www.millelacsband.com/news/state-of-minnesota-working-family-tax-credit-2017-update. Accessed January 18, 2019.

47. Hole MK, Marcil LE, Vinci RJ. Improving access to evidence-based antipoverty government programs in the United States: A novel primary care initiative. *JAMA Pediatrics*. https://jamanetwork.com/journals/jamapediatrics/fullarticle/2596272. Accessed January 18, 2019.

48. https://www.cbpp.org/topics/state-budget-and-tax

49. Xu X, Bishop EE, Kennedy SM, Simpson SA, Pechacek TF. Annual healthcare spending attributable to cigarette smoking: An update. *Am J Prev Med.* 2015;48(3):326–33.

50. Centers for Disease Control and Prevention. 2014 Surgeon General's Report: The Health Consequences of Smoking—50 Years of Progress. https://www.cdc.gov/tobacco/data_statistics/sgr/50th-anniversary/index.htm. Accessed January 18, 2019.

51. Centers for Disease Control and Prevention. Best Practices for Comprehensive Tobacco Control Programs-2014. https://www.cdc.gov/tobacco/stateandcommunity/best_practices/index.htm. Accessed January 18, 2019.

52. Institute of Medicine (IOM). *Public Health Implications of Raising the Minimum Age of Legal Access to Tobacco Products.* Washington, DC: The National Academies Press; 2015.

53. United States Department of Health and Human Services. Substance Abuse and Mental Health Services Administration. Center for Behavioral Health Statistics and Quality. *National Survey on Drug Use and Health, 2014.* Ann Arbor, MI: Inter-university Consortium for Political and Social Research [distributor]; March 22, 2016. https://doi.org/10.3886/ICPSR36361.v1.

54. Winickoff JP, Hartman L, Chen ML, Gottlieb M, Nabi-Burza E, DiFranza JR. Retail impact of raising tobacco sales age to 21 years *Am J Public Health.* 2014;104(11):e18–21. doi:10.2105/AJPH.2014.302174. Epub September 11, 2014.

55. Institute of Medicine of the National Academies. Public Health Implications of Raising the Minimum Age of Legal Access to Tobacco Products. 2015. http://www.nationalacademies.org/hmd/~/media/Files/Report%20Files/2015/TobaccoMinAge/tobacco_minimum_age_report_brief.pdf. Accessed January 18, 2019.

56. Ahmad S. Closing the youth access gap: The projected health benefits and cost savings of a national policy to raise the legal smoking age to 21 in the United States. *Health Policy.* 2005;75(1):74–84.

57. Campaign for Tobacco-Free Kids. States and localities that have raised the minimum legal sale age for tobacco products to 21. https://www.tobaccofreekids.org/assets/content/what_we_do/state_local_issues/sales_21/states_localities_MLSA_21.pdf. Accessed June 17, 2018.

58. http://cityhealthdata.org/policy/cityhealth-pre-k-1518113514-37.

59. Centers for Disease Control and Prevention. Earned Income Tax Credits. https://www.cdc.gov/policy/hst/hi5/taxcredits/index.html. Accessed January 18, 2019.

60. Oliver K, Lorenc T, Innvær S. New directions in evidence-based policy research: A critical analysis of the literature. *Health Res Policy Syst.* 2014;12:34.

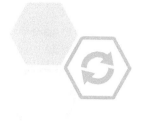

# Chapter 42

# The Impact of State and Territorial Public Health Policy: Interventions to Prevent Opioid Misuse and Addiction

MICHAEL R. FRASER, PHILICIA TUCKER, AND JAY C. BUTLER

## PREVENTION, POLICY, AND STATE PUBLIC HEALTH

State public health leaders have broad responsibility for the health of their jurisdictions, working around the clock to protect and promote the public's health and prevent illness and disease. This involves implementation of a broad spectrum of prevention programs and services and the development of comprehensive policies to improve health statewide. Communicable and chronic disease prevention and control, surveillance and monitoring of health threats, assessing health risks and environmental hazards, and enforcing public health laws and regulations are just some of the policy areas in which state public health agencies are engaged (Box 42.1). Taking a "health in all policies" approach, state health agencies collaborate with many different sectors to address health challenges, including housing, education, transportation, and, most frequently, health care systems and health care providers. For example, Figure 42.1 illustrates the many partners that state public health agencies engage with in developing policy to prevent substance misuse and addiction and to expand access to treatment and recovery services in their jurisdictions.

Public health policy interventions are a critical tool in a state health leader's toolbox. The importance of public health policy interventions is highlighted by former Director of the Centers for Disease Control and Prevention (CDC), Thomas R. Frieden, in his "Health Impact Pyramid"[1] which emphasizes the wide reach of prevention and public health policy interventions and social-economic change in influencing population health compared to individual-based

## Box 42.1 | New Hampshire's All-Payer Claims Database

*Theresa Chapple*

*Problem*: New Hampshire policymakers were finding it hard to make informed health policy decisions around health care spending, utilization, and access to care, and they found a lack of price transparency for health services. They also expressed that the absence of price transparency negatively impacted the consumer's ability to make informed decisions regarding health care cost and quality, as well as where to receive services. The lack of a central authority responsible for aggregating data from the numerous payers was seen as the underlying problem, making it difficult for the state to regularly, accurately, and transparently track total health care spending.

*Solution*: In order to address the issues caused by a lack of data on health care utilization, claims, and cost, the state decided to create an All-Payer Claims Database (APCD) to house claims data derived from medical claims, pharmacy claims, eligibility files, provider files, and dental claims from public and private payers.

*Medicaid and public health collaboration*: The New Hampshire Insurance Department (NHID) and Medicaid collaborated to provide language to be included in the legislation. They were also jointly responsible for carrying out the directives of the statute. NHID had the authority and was in the position to enforce the regulations by holding the insurance carriers responsible. NHID could impose penalties such as fines or revocation of a carrier's license for those that did not submit claims. Medicaid had the personnel and capabilities to collect and manage the data from all the insurers.

In 2007, 4 years after the APCD had been written into law, NH Medicaid received a 5-year CDC innovation grant to determine the best way to incorporate traditional public health data sets, such as vital records, hospital discharge data, and behavioral risk factor surveillance system surveys, into the APCD platform. As a result of this grant, a leadership team was created that consisted of the director of the division of public health services, the state epidemiologist, the director of the bureau of policy and performance management, and the data management lead from NH Medicaid. They met regularly to discuss how best to incorporate and make use of APCD data for public health purposes. These meetings resulted in a web-based query tool that produces both standard indicator reports and has the ability to make custom reports relating to chronic conditions and the care for those chronic conditions.

*Statutory changes*: NHID and NH Medicaid proposed language for the statute that created an APCD in 2003. The statute did not include steps on how to create the database, but it did call for NH Insurance Department and NH Medicaid to create a memorandum of understanding to jointly develop the APCD. The legislation merely required that data be collected and the information be made available to insurers, employers, providers, purchasers of health care, and state agencies.

To read more about this project, visit http://www.astho.org/Health-Systems-Transformation/Medicaid-and-Public-Health-Partnerships/Case-Studies/New-Hampshire-All-Payer-Claims-Database/.

counseling and education and patient-based clinical interventions. Frieden's framework, and its emphasis on policy change to improve health, informs our analysis of state policy work and its current and potential impact in the specific case of America's current opioid crisis.

## STATE RESPONSES TO THE OPIOID MISUSE AND ADDICTION CRISIS

The opioid misuse and addiction epidemic has left no segment of the American population untouched. The National Institutes of Health (NIH) estimates that 115 Americans die daily of an opioid-related overdose, with CDC data indicating 46 deaths a day due to prescription opioid overdose.[2,3] While a comprehensive etiology and epidemiology of the opioid epidemic is well beyond the scope of this chapter, it is important to note that multiple factors have led to the explosive scale and spread of addiction to prescription and illicit opioids. These factors include treating pain as the "fifth vital sign,"[4] unrealistic patient expectations about reducing pain using nonopioid alternatives, health care providers' varied prescribing practices, pharmaceutical and drug distribution industry marketing behavior, and the wide availability of relatively inexpensive heroin and fentanyl. Most critically, however, widening economic and social inequality in America has led many to conclude that the opioid epidemic is "not just a crisis of health, it is a crisis of hope." That is, the current crisis is largely the result of individuals and neighborhoods facing lack of opportunity, uneven economic prosperity, and weak familial and social ties that decrease both individual and community resilience as a protective factor in preventing addiction.[5,6]

Informed by an evidence-based approach to disease prevention and health promotion, public health leaders widely agree that America will not arrest or treat its way out of the current epidemic. Instead, as with other disease outbreaks, the more promising approach is to prevent opioid use disorder in the first place using sound public health policy interventions focused on individual and community health improvement. States have long been the incubators of innovation in American policy development, including public health policy. Important successes in infection control, sanitation, tobacco control, and motor vehicle safety are all the result of state policy actions that brought clinical

**Figure 42.1** ▼

The many partners that state public health agencies engage with in developing policy to prevent substance misuse and addiction.

## Cross-Sectoral Collaboration is Key

| Public Health Agencies | Attorneys General Offices | Justice and Corrections | Medical Boards |
| --- | --- | --- | --- |
| Healthcare Providers | Hospitals and Clinics | Community Coalitions 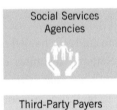 | Businesses and Labor |
| Media | Emergency Medical Services | Social Services Agencies | Faith Communities |
| Pharmaceutical Industry | Educators | Third-Party Payers | Others |

and community health together with other partners to impact and improve the health of the public. State leadership to address opioid misuse is no exception.

State public health agencies and their partners in federal, state, and local governmental public health and health care are involved in an extensive array of policy interventions to respond to the many facets of the crisis, including monitoring and surveillance, treatment and recovery services, managing access to opioids, and public awareness and education activities.[7] Specifically, these include policies to increase the availability of the overdose reversal drug naloxone and accompanying "Good Samaritan" laws that provide waiver of civil and, in some states, criminal liability; policies requiring prescribers and dispensers to use prescription drug monitoring programs (PDMP); policies supportive of increasing access to addiction treatment and recovery support services; policies expanding drug courts and law enforcement diversion to treatment prior to incarceration on first offence; policies that integrate recovery and treatment with incarcerated populations; policies that support public awareness and education campaigns; policies to expand sober housing options; policies to expand access to medication-assisted treatment (MAT) providers and programs; stricter policies to regulate pain clinics; and policies to promote harm reduction strategies, including syringe exchange.

Although extremely important, few state or territorial efforts have focused on public health policies that support building community resiliency or addressing the social and economic conditions that influence individuals' drug use, although work in this area holds great promise in terms of primary prevention of opioid use disorder, addiction, and many other public health issues (e.g., suicide and chronic disease prevention). Public health practitioners are keenly aware that social and economic factors, as well as individual behaviors, play a role in influencing how people cope with emotional, physical, and social trauma that is the result of what Cohen terms "adverse community events" (i.e., violence, lack of economic opportunity, limited resources, racism, and income inequality).[8,9] As this chapter suggests, future work on these issues and effective policy development to address them are sorely needed to truly address the root causes of opioid misuse and addiction nationwide. States and territories, as laboratories of policy development and disease prevention work, are doing just that.

A public health policy approach to addressing the opioid crisis is based on disease surveillance, which has always been a vital component to understanding the impact of a public health problem among a population. Surveillance data inform policymaking and provide the evidence for developing, framing and focusing, and evaluating policy interventions. Surveillance also provides evidence of impact and success, forming the basis for taking successful policies to scale from one jurisdiction to others. As such, surveillance and monitoring of opioid-related morbidity and mortality has been used to help understand the opioid crisis mostly through state efforts to monitor opioid prescriptions, monitor overdose deaths, and, through working with law enforcement agencies and other partners, to identify and intervene in high intensity drug trafficking areas (HITDA) and related overdose "hot spots." Using these data, state and territorial health officials have a key role in informing governors, peers at cabinet and subcabinet levels, and state and territorial policymakers regarding evidence-based policymaking to address disease trends; they have also worked to create effective public health policy solutions to address a variety of specific priorities related to the epidemic.

Eight states (Arkansas, Arizona, Florida, Massachusetts, Maryland, Pennsylvania, South Carolina, and Virginia)[10] have declared the opioid crisis a state of emergency or have executed a similar disaster declaration to catalyze statewide action and provide government with the optimal flexibility to address opioid-related issues, including preventing overdose deaths and expanding access to addiction treatment and recovery programs. In support of the state and territorial responses to the opioid crisis, and the Association of State and Territorial Health Official's (ASTHO) President's Challenge[11] created a Substance Misuse and Addiction Framework (Figure 42.2) using the three levels of prevention (primary, secondary, tertiary), and the program and policy options are available to public health leaders to implement within each level.[11] Tactics at these three levels of intervention are supported by five strategic priorities at

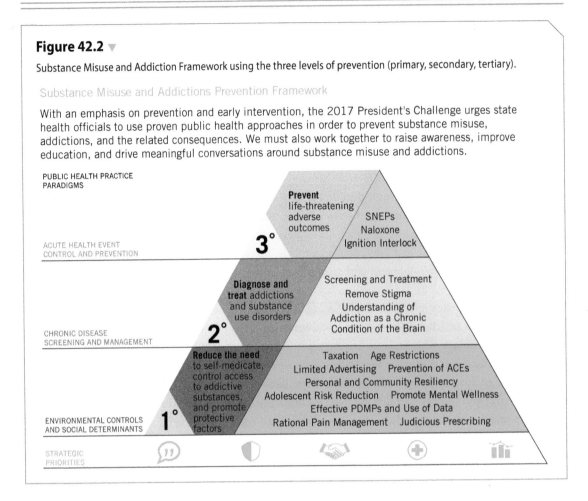

**Figure 42.2** ▾

Substance Misuse and Addiction Framework using the three levels of prevention (primary, secondary, tertiary).

Substance Misuse and Addictions Prevention Framework

With an emphasis on prevention and early intervention, the 2017 President's Challenge urges state health officials to use proven public health approaches in order to prevent substance misuse, addictions, and the related consequences. We must also work together to raise awareness, improve education, and drive meaningful conversations around substance misuse and addictions.

PUBLIC HEALTH PRACTICE PARADIGMS

**Prevent** life-threatening adverse outcomes

SNEPs
Naloxone
Ignition Interlock

ACUTE HEALTH EVENT CONTROL AND PREVENTION

**3°**

**Diagnose and treat** addictions and substance use disorders

Screening and Treatment
Remove Stigma
Understanding of Addiction as a Chronic Condition of the Brain

CHRONIC DISEASE SCREENING AND MANAGEMENT

**2°**

**Reduce the need** to self-medicate, control access to addictive substances, and promote protective factors

Taxation    Age Restrictions
Limited Advertising    Prevention of ACEs
Personal and Community Resiliency
Adolescent Risk Reduction    Promote Mental Wellness
Effective PDMPs and Use of Data
Rational Pain Management    Judicious Prescribing

ENVIRONMENTAL CONTROLS AND SOCIAL DETERMINANTS

**1°**

STRATEGIC PRIORITIES

the base of the pyramid that cross-cut the levels of prevention: (1) reduction of stigma and changing social norms related to addiction, (2) increasing protective factors and reducing risk factors, (3) strengthening multi- and cross-sector collaboration, (4) improving the prevention infrastructure, and (5) optimizing the use of cross-sector data for decision-making.

Although the ASTHO Framework applies to broad substance misuse and addiction prevention, it was designed to be directly applicable to the specific case of opioid misuse and addiction prevention. State public health policy interventions at each level of prevention are part of the ASTHO Framework, several of which are described in the following text in more detail to illustrate the importance of using state public health policy as a key prevention strategy to end the crisis. These policies leverage the power of both the clinical and community perspectives to support population health improvement efforts at the local and state levels. These policies also involve state public health and clinical leaders working together to coordinate advocacy in state legislatures to authorize and appropriate resources to support them.

# "DOWNSTREAM" OR TERTIARY PREVENTION POLICY: EXPANDING ACCESS TO OVERDOSE REVERSAL MEDICATIONS AND SYRINGE AND NEEDLE EXCHANGE PROGRAMS

Tertiary prevention involves interventions to prevent the immediate life-threatening effects of existing disease and to increase quality of life. Typically, tertiary prevention involves efforts to prevent acute morbidity associated with advanced medical conditions long after they have become manifest. With both illicit and prescription opioid misuse, sudden death due to overdose is often an initial presentation, and, as such, tertiary prevention (i.e., overdose reversal) is a life-saving prevention approach. The US Surgeon General's recent public health advisory urging more Americans to keep overdose reversal medications on hand is an example of the importance of this prevention strategy, but also of the extent to which opioid overdose has become a national public health crisis.[12] Two examples of state public health policies that promote tertiary prevention strategies are (1) expanding the use of opioid reversal medications and (2) the implementation of syringe and needle exchange programs (SNEPs) at the local and state levels.

Naloxone is a medication that attaches with high affinity to opioid receptors in the central nervous system, displacing opioids from the receptor and restoring the respiratory depression that causes death in opioid overdose.[13] When administered to a person experiencing an overdose, naloxone may be successful in reviving the individual. As attention to opioid overdose prevention has increased, more "user-friendly" forms of naloxone administration were developed to be administered by individuals without clinical training (e.g., law enforcement officers and friends or family members).[14] Many states and territories have taken the initiative to combat the opioid epidemic through legislative actions pertaining to naloxone, such as allowing statewide dispensing through health officer "standing orders" or direct dispensing authority for pharmacists, using the advantages of user-friendly nasal or self-injection forms. Some states have discussed requiring naloxone be dispensed whenever a patient is prescribed an opioid medication; however, co-dispensing has yet to experience widespread uptake as a policy intervention.

In 2016, after declaring the opioid crisis a public health emergency, the Commonwealth of Virginia legislated greater access to and use of naloxone by the public. Virginia HB1672 gave prescribers the authority to allow an individual to administer naloxone to another individual without the prescriber's knowledge of the individual being treated, and HB1458 expanded protection against civil liability to anyone who prescribes, distributes, and delivers naloxone in Virginia. These laws provide individuals who administer naloxone to a person experiencing an overdose the legal protections needed in case an individual is injured during the overdose response. HB1672 also includes a provision to allow pharmacies to provide naloxone to anyone in the Commonwealth of Virginia on request, without a prescription.[15] Similar policies have been widely adopted by all states and territories (Figure 42.3), which is also part of the Trump administration's Initiative to Stop Opioid Abuse, launched in March 2018.

SNEPs have been found to be effective harm reduction strategies related to preventing infectious disease among intravenous (IV) drug users,[16] but policy work in this area of tertiary prevention and harm reduction is associated with significant controversy. As the Scott County, Indiana, and similar local stories illustrate, the rise of illicit opioid use is often accompanied by a rise in HIV and hepatitis C infection as a result of family members and friends sharing each other's needles, but efforts to set up SNEPs are often thwarted by some who believe that they promote injection drug use.[16] Given the controversy, less than half of all states and only one territory[17,18] allow some form of SNEP, although other countries around the world have relied on such programs for years to successfully reduce co-infections among injection drug–using populations (see Figure 42.3).

SNEPs illustrate the role that local jurisdictions and tribal organizations often play in pushing broader state and territorial health policies. Locally, several US cities have been operating both legal (regulated) and "underground" SNEPs for years, including Phoenix, Arizona; Atlanta, Georgia; Minneapolis, Minnesota; Charleston, West Virginia; Salt Lake City, Utah; and Durham, North Carolina, thus setting the stage for state-wide debate on their expansion.[19] The city of Vancouver, British Columbia, has demonstrated the life-saving role of a variety of SNEPs, which includes monitoring of individuals while using drugs. These "safe injection sites" are staffed with trained individuals (lay people or health professionals) who monitor individuals post-injection and stand by to assist in case of overdose. Despite opposition by some in municipal and provincial governments and the Canadian federal government that such sites encourage illicit drug use, evaluations of these sites demonstrate that they effectively prevent overdose and also serve as potential gateways for referrals to treatment, housing, and other social supports.[20] Several US cities, most notably New York; Philadelphia, Pennsylvania; and Seattle, Washington, have considered developing local and state public health policies to allow for safe injection sites, but they face political opposition because of the misperceptions of their efficacy, interjection of particular political agendas and ideologies, and stigma.[21]

# Figure 42.3 ▽

The policy interventions separated by primary, secondary, and tertiary prevention that have been adopted by states and territories.[39,46]

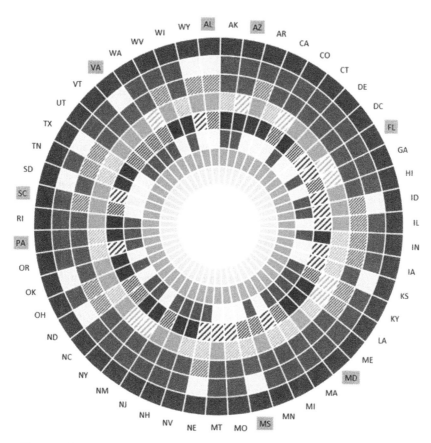

## Tertiary Prevention

- Naloxone Access[38]
- Existence of Syringe Exchange Program[39]

## Secondary Prevention

- Medicaid Coverage of Methadone, Buprenorphine, and Naltrexone Treatment[40]
- Medicaid Coverage of at least one form of MAT[40]
- Parity Law[34]
- Minimum Mandate Benefit[34]
- Mandate Offering[34]

## Primary Prevention

- PDMP, mandated for all prescribers[35]
- PDMP, not mandated for all prescribers[35]
- PDMP, voluntary for all prescribers[35]
- Mandated Initial Prescribing Guidelines[36]
- Access to Home Visiting[37]
- Drug Free Communities[44]
- Emergency Declarations[15]

# EXPANDING ACCESS TO ADDICTION TREATMENT SERVICES AND ASSURING PARITY BETWEEN MENTAL AND PHYSICAL HEALTH CARE SERVICES AS SECONDARY PREVENTION POLICY EFFORTS

Secondary prevention involves detecting and treating illness or disease before it progresses to a more advanced and severe phase, which often requires high acuity care. Taking medication to reduce hypertension or using insulin to maintain a healthy blood sugar level are classic examples of secondary prevention in the area of chronic disease prevention. As opposed to primary prevention, which aims to prevent the need for such medical or other interventions, secondary prevention aims to mitigate or resolve a health condition and prevent it from getting worse. The most common secondary prevention policies in the area of opioid misuse and addiction are policies to promote use of MAT and developing state and territorial efforts to expand access to them. Methadone has been widely used to treat heroin addiction for decades. Other MAT medications include buprenorphine and naltrexone, or a combination of buprenorphine and naloxone, which is used in the drug Suboxone to treat opioid dependence. These medicines are used in conjunction with behavioral therapy and/or counseling to address addiction, providing one of the most effective, evidence-based methods for treating addiction and promoting recovery.[20]

State and territorial policies to expand the use of MAT have been a key component in efforts to support recovery and slow the opioid epidemic. A barrier to implementing MAT in states has been federal policy that limited the number of patients a physician could manage on buprenorphine and a special waiver process to register and train providers in its use by the Drug Enforcement Agency (DEA). A lack of rural physicians who are DEA "waivered" to prescribe buprenorphine has confounded state efforts as well.[22] To address this issue, states have requested federal policy changes on the waiver process but also adopted state-based "hub and spoke" treatment models that allow specialist providers to manage patients using telemedicine modalities and that link academic medical centers and urban specialists with rural providers managing the day-to-day care of their patients.[23]

For example, in 2011, Vermont's access to treatment for opioid use disorder was at an all-time low, with few physicians providing MAT and patients being wait-listed for treatment for as long as 2 years before receiving care. The Vermont Blueprint for Health, Department of Vermont Health Access' Medicaid Health Services and Managed Care Division, and Vermont Department of Health's Division of Alcohol and Drug Abuse Programs worked with waivered primary care physicians, local drug treatment providers, and other substance abuse–related organizations to develop their hub and spoke model.[24] In this model, the "spoke" represents the link to primary care providers who work directly with patients and who consult with the "hub" that consists of a centralized and specialized MAT care team that provides guidance and assistance to physicians.[25] The model greatly expanded the number of patients that physicians were able to treat and provided needed specialty medical services in rural areas in the state. As a result, between 2013 and 2015, MAT providers have increased across Vermont by 170%.[24] Other states have developed policy to support similar hub and spoke treatment systems to address opioid use disorder statewide. Policy work in this area requires enabling the use of telemedicine to address licensure requirements, addressing reimbursement issues associated with the provision of care by the hub and the spoke, and supporting the implementation of suitable technology and standards at hub and spoke sites.

A barrier to treatment for many individuals with substance use disorder or opioid dependence is the lack of parity between physical and mental health services that creates uneven health insurance coverage for medically necessary behavioral health services. Policy interventions to promote access to treatment include enforced state parity laws requiring insurance companies to provide equal coverage for physical and mental health benefits, including number of visits, deductibles, and copayments. Unfortunately, not all states have strict parity legislation, thus stymying efforts to expand covered evidence-based treatment and recovery services for those with health insurance. Several states have established minimum mandated mental health benefits or "mandated offering" regulations (see Figure 42.3). "Mandated offering" laws have some form of mental health coverage but do not always require insurance companies to offer equal benefits for physical and mental health treatment. The Pennsylvania General Assembly passed Act 106 of 1989 to increase availability for covered alcohol and other substance use disorder treatment. Act 106 requires benefits for opioid use disorder treatment to be equivalent to what insurers cover for physical illness.[26] Parity laws are well-intentioned; however, they often fail to define exact comparability to physical illnesses, and covered benefits may not be clearly understood by patients, health care providers, and/or health insurance companies. Pennsylvania Act 106 was created to mandate that insurers cover needed recovery resources and other treatment that an individual may need. These may include withdrawal management, inpatient and outpatient rehabilitation, outpatient counseling services and recovery supports, and family treatment.[27] Despite the law, there is still confusion about exactly what parity means, and it must be defined health plan-by-health plan in the state. Another significant issue is the extent to which states and territories monitor and enforce these laws with the health insurers that operate in their jurisdictions.

In addition to pursuing policy change through law or regulation, state officials may use their administrative authority to implement policies that affect communities, agencies, or patient populations under their direction. As an example, in 2016, Rhode Island implemented statewide policy to support treatment programs for its incarcerated population to screen inmates for opioid use disorder and offer MAT to those being held or released from correctional facilities. The policy also supported 12 community-based centers connected to a MAT program that would provide support for inmates transitioning out of incarceration and refer them to recovery resources in the community. The policy encourages that patients enroll or re-enroll in health insurance just prior to release so that treatment and recovery services can be covered without interruption. Early evaluation of the policy's implementation demonstrates that the Rhode Island program has been successful in reducing overdose deaths within a year by 12%, and resulted in a 64% decrease in post-incarceration fatalities from overdose since its implementation. Partners across state government, including health, behavioral health, and corrections, implemented the policy, which has resulted in significant prevention of post-release overdose among previously incarcerated individuals.[26]

The Vermont, Rhode Island, and Pennsylvania examples are indicative of the type of policy interventions that other states and territories have introduced and implemented. Policies that support MAT expansions and parity laws are important in assuring that needed treatment services are provided to individuals with opioid use disorder. In addition to these secondary prevention measures, policies that enable prevention of opioid use disorder in the first place are vital to ending the current crisis and addressing the root causes of addiction. These are discussed in the following sections.

## THE UPSTREAM APPROACH: PRIMARY PREVENTION POLICY TO PREVENT OPIOID USE DISORDER THROUGH MONITORING AND SURVEILLANCE ACTIVITIES AND EFFORTS TO ADDRESS INDIVIDUAL, FAMILY, AND COMMUNITY RESILIENCY AS PROTECTIVE FACTORS

Primary prevention is the core work of state and territorial public health agencies and involves preventing disease though broad, population-based, community health programs and policies. Primary prevention of opioid use disorder and addiction includes preventing individuals who are taking opioid medications from becoming addicted through careful monitoring and evaluation, but also addressing the many other (nonmedical) reasons that individuals may use drugs in the first place. Policies supporting mandatory use of PDMPs, supporting compliance with provider prescribing guidelines, and enhancing clinical quality improvement have been the focus of many state efforts to prevent opioid use disorder and addiction.

PDMPs have now been implemented in every state and in several territories, allowing authorized agents to monitor prescriber and dispenser compliance with guidelines. PMDPs also allow prescribers to examine whether a patient has been prescribed opioids by other providers, what other drugs they may have been prescribed that could negatively interact with opioids, and whether that patient may be "pill-seeking" or in legitimate need of medication. Policy interventions in the area of PDMPs include both in-state use (e.g., mandated vs. voluntary, and rules and regulations related to access to data and data sharing) and cross-state use (interstate data sharing and linkages across states). State policies supportive of PDMP best practices are expertly described in a 2016 Pew Charitable Trusts report and include recommended policy interventions at the state level that mandate PDMP use, allow providers to delegate a staff member to access the PDMP, streamline prescriber enrollment in the system, and promote and educate users on state PDMP systems.[28]

In several states, policies supporting the use of PDMP have led to a reduction in statewide opioid prescribing behavior.[29] A concern, however, is that those who are addicted to prescription opioids may be inappropriately discharged from care because of pill-seeking behavior, may not be appropriately referred to addiction treatment, and subsequently may turn to illicit drugs such as heroin and fentanyl. An additional concern is that PDMPs focus on the prescriber side of the opioid epidemic (supply) without a commensurate focus on why the patient became addicted in the first place (demand).

In addition to policies on PDMP implementation, states have created policies to adopt state, national, and/or specialty-specific opioid prescription guidelines for physicians, dentists, veterinarians, and other providers. National guidelines developed by the CDC have been widely promulgated in states and territories to guide provider prescribing of opioids for chronic pain.[30] In general, prescription guidelines set a calendar limit on the number of calendar days and/or the morphine milligram equivalents (MME) of an opioid that may be prescribed, limit or prohibit automatic refills, and require periodic in-person screening and assessment for addiction. States have implemented policies supportive of both voluntary and mandatory prescribing guidelines with varying success, largely based on provider adherence to the guidelines and penalties for nonadherence.

New Jersey's work in this area has evolved to encompass some of the strictest laws regarding opioid prescribing. This should be no surprise, given former Governor Christie's interest in and leadership on addressing opioid misuse both in New Jersey and also around the country. In 2011, New Jersey Administrative Code §13:35-7.6 prevented physicians from prescribing Schedule II controlled substances that surpass 120 dosage units or a 30-day supply. The law also covered the need for reviewing a patient's medical history and the need for follow-up every 3 months. During the 2015 legislative session, legislation was approved (New Jersey Revised Statute §45:1-46.1) that mandated physicians to utilize the prescription monitoring program before prescribing opioids to a patient. In May 2017, the state legislature changed the initial opioid prescription limit for both acute or chronic pain to a 5-day supply (New Jersey Statute [Annotated] §24:21-15.2 and §45:9-22.19). Not only is the first prescription limited, but prescribers must also document the patient's medical history regarding previous opioid and nonopioid pain treatment, create a therapy plan focused on the etiology of the patient's pain, and utilize the state's PDMP.[31]

In addition to overdose surveillance and PDMP data, many states have worked to develop policies that allow for linkages across various data sets for a more comprehensive picture of the epidemic in their jurisdictions and to inform their primary prevention strategy and tactics. Between 2000 and 2016, the rate of opioid-related overdose mortality in Massachusetts quintupled.[32] To better understand the complexity of the opioid crisis and prevent it, the state created a platform for data sharing with the passage of Chapter 55 of the Acts of 2015. The bill's language demonstrates the intent of the law, which is to cross-cut categorical or population-specific data systems to provide a broad picture to inform the state's understanding of the epidemic:

> Notwithstanding any general or special law to the contrary, to facilitate the examination, the department shall request, and the relevant offices and agencies shall provide, information necessary to complete the examination from the division of medical assistance, the executive office of public safety and security, the center for health information and analysis, the office of patient protection and the chief justice of the trial court, which may include, but shall not be limited to: data from the prescription drug monitoring program; the all-payer claims database; the criminal offender record information database; and the court activity record information. To the extent feasible, the department shall request data from the Massachusetts Sheriffs Association, Inc., relating to treatment within houses of correction.[33]

With the passage of the law, Massachusetts officials can now access 10 governmental data sets and work with public, private, and nonprofit stakeholder groups to analyze data. Opioid-related data that have been used for comprehensive analysis include data on opioid prescriptions, on other scheduled drug prescriptions (opioids and benzodiazepines), prescription history, previous opioid treatment for substance use disorder and/or pain, records of denial of treatment, and information regarding whether those who were incarcerated ever received treatment. From these sources, analyses were conducted to provide a better understanding of who was at risk, and the numbers of people accurately categorized as fatal opioid overdose (FOD) and nonfatal opioid overdose (NFOD) were determined.[32]

Massachusetts Chapter 55 demonstrates that it is possible to develop policies that support and encourage private and public organizations to collaborate in addressing tough public health issues, even with frequently cited privacy and data-sharing challenges. The Act authorizes various agencies to share information without restriction while also protecting patient and individual confidentially and privacy. Chapter 55 is a major milestone for state and territorial public health efforts that are often blocked by regulation (or perceptions of regulation) over what kinds of state employees can see what kinds data and with whom those data may be shared. Other states are conducting comprehensive reviews of data sets across government; for example, West Virginia has conducted an in-depth analysis of overdose deaths to better understand the factors that may have contributed to an individual's death to inform state policy development in this area.[34] Decedents in West Virginia were much more likely to have Medicaid (71%) in the 12 months prior to their death compared to the adult population in West Virginia overall (23%); 68% of decedents with Medicaid had at least one hospital emergency department visit in the year prior to death, more than half of all decedents were ever incarcerated, decedents were more likely than the overall adult population to have a high school education or less, and decedents were more likely to be unmarried.[34]

Understanding what can be done to prevent opioid use in the first place is key to ending the epidemic. Why individuals initiate drug use is a complex and complicated subject involving individual psychology and behavior as well as the influences of genetics, family history, family functioning, social supports, and community and social factors, including educational and economic opportunity, salience of alternatives to drug use, and overall community supports and resilience. The nation's current focus on acute overdose prevention (naloxone distribution) and treatment and recovery services, however, should not deter from increased efforts to understand what works when it comes to policies that support and expand primary prevention of opioid use disorder.

Despite the success of many efforts, a compelling need exists for more research on evidence-based policy approaches to the primary prevention of addiction. If primary prevention of addiction is ultimately the best way to end the opioid epidemic in America, a commensurate investment in policies supportive of primary prevention at the federal, state, and local levels is warranted. A promising primary prevention initiative includes support for evidence-based Maternal, Infant, and Early Childhood Home Visiting (MIECHV) programs. States have embraced this approach and pursued policies to support evidence-based home visiting models that promote healthy parenting and reduce the prevalence of adverse childhood events (ACEs).[35] Federal policy to expand access to evidence-based home visitation was authorized in the Patient Protection and Affordable Care Act (ACA) through the MICHEV program, and $372 million in funding for the Health Resources and Services Administration (HRSA) to administer and implement the program was recently reauthorized.[36] In addition to policy efforts that build parenting competency and family resilience, such as home visiting programs, interventions that support community resilience and promote economic and educational opportunity are crucial to addressing the opioid epidemic. Nascent public health approaches to strengthening community engagement and resilience, such as Rhode Island's Health Equity Zones, may serve as guides for the scale and spread of effective community-based and state-sponsored primary prevention policies to improve health at the population level.[37]

## THE WAY FORWARD: COMPREHENSIVE STATE AND TERRITORIAL POLICY APPROACHES TO ADDRESS OPIOID MISUSE AND ADDICTION

ASTHO's Framework[7] illustrates the variety of policy approaches that state and territorial health officials may take to address substance misuse and addiction in their jurisdictions. The combination of tertiary, secondary, and primary prevention programs and the policies that support them are critical. No single policy will comprehensively address the complex issues involved in the current crisis, but more work in the area of primary prevention is greatly needed. A comprehensive approach that utilizes evidence-based approaches to primary, secondary, and tertiary prevention is essential. The complexity of the opioid crisis requires strong clinical and community partnerships to scale and spread successful policy interventions. State and territorial public health officials are committed and well-positioned to lead such efforts in their jurisdictions.

## REFERENCES

1. Frieden T. A framework for public health action: The health impact pyramid. *Am J Public Health*. 2010;100(4):590–5. doi:10.2105/AJPH.2009.185652.

2. National Institutes of Health. Opioid overdose crisis. Updated March 2018. https://www.drugabuse.gov/drugs-abuse/opioids/opioid-overdose-crisis. Accessed March 26, 2018.

3. Centers for Disease Control and Prevention. Prescription opioid overdose data. Updated August 1, 2017. https://www.cdc.gov/drugoverdose/data/overdose.html. Accessed March 26, 2018.

4. Baker DW. The joint commission's pain standards: Origins and evolution. May 5, 2017. https://www.jointcommission.org/assets/1/6/Pain_Std_History_Web_Version_05122017.pdf. Accessed March 26, 2018.

5. Caron B. *Remarks at the White House Opioid Summit, March 1, 2018*. The White House: Washington, DC.

6. Dasgupta N, Beletsky L, Ciccarone D. Opioid crisis: No easy fix to its social and economic determinants. *Am J Public Health*. 2018;108(2):182–6. http://ajph.aphapublications.org/doi/full/10.2105/AJPH.2017.304187. Accessed 1/17/2019.

7. The Association of State and Territorial Health Officials. ASTHO opioid framework assists health officials in combating the epidemic. September 20, 2017. http://www.astho.org/Press-Room/ASTHO-Opioid-Framework-Assists-Health-Officials-in-Combating-the-Epidemic/9-20-17/. Accessed March 26, 2018.

8. Pinderhughes H, Davis R, William M. Adverse community experiences and resilience: A framework for addressing and preventing community trauma. Prevention Institute. 2015. https://www.preventioninstitute.org/sites/default/files/publications/Adverse%20Community%20Experiences%20and%20Resilience.pdf. Accessed April 23, 2018.

9. Prevention Institute. What? Why? How? Answers to frequently asked questions about the adverse community experiences and resilience framework. 2017. https://www.preventioninstitute.org/sites/default/files/publications/What%20Why%20How%20-%20ACER%20FAQ_0.pdf. Accessed April 23, 2018.

10. The Association of State and Territorial Health Officials. Emergency declarations in eight states to address the opioid crisis. January 11, 2018. http://www.astho.org/StatePublicHealth/Emergency-Declarations-in-Eight-States-to-Address-the-Opioid-Epidemic/01-11-18/. Accessed March 26, 2018.

11. Butler JC. President's challenge: Public health approaches to preventing substance misuse and addiction. *J Public Health Mgmt Pract*.2017;23(5):531–6. doi:10.1097/PHH.0000000000000631.

12. US Surgeon General. Surgeon general's advisory on naloxone and opioid overdose. https://www.surgeongeneral.gov/priorities/opioid-overdose-prevention/naloxone-advisory.html. Accessed April 7, 2018.

13. National Institute on Drug Abuse. Naloxone for opioid-overdose: Life-saving science. March 2017. https://d14rmgtrwzf5a.cloudfront.net/sites/default/files/opioid_naloxone.pdf. Accessed March 22, 2018.

14. Wermeling DP. Review of naloxone safety for opioid overdose: Practical considerations for new technology and expanded public access. *Ther Adv Drug Safe*. 2015;6(1):20–1. http://doi.org/10.1177/2042098614564776.

15. Virginia Department of Behavioral Health and Developmental Services. REVIVE! white paper: An overview of Virginia's opioid overdose and naloxone education program. Updated January 2017. http://dbhds.virginia.gov/library/substance%20abuse%20services/04%20%20revive%20white%20paper%20v41.pdf. Accessed March 22, 2018.

16. Servies AD, Reynolds M, Silverman RD. Indiana syringe exchange program. Center for Health Policy, Richard M. Fairbanks School of Public Health. 2015;1–4. https://fsph.iupui.edu/doc/research-centers/Indiana%20Syringe%20Exchange%20Program%202015.pdf.Accessed 1/17/2019.

17. North American Syringe Exchange Network. Directory of syringe exchange programs. https://nasen.org/directory/. Accessed March 22, 2018.

18. Centers for Disease Control and Prevention. Laws related to syringe exchange. Updated September 28, 2017. https://www.cdc.gov/hepatitis/policy/syringeexchange.htm. Accessed March 22, 2018.

19. National Alliance for Model State Drug Laws. At a glance: States with needle exchange programs. February 5, 2016. www.namsdl.org/library/F6467201-A309-5B89-4FBB0A9DB2B928FE/. Accessed March 22, 2018.

20. Substance Abuse and Mental Health Services Administration. Medication and counselling treatment. Updated September 28, 2015. https://www.samhsa.gov/medication-assisted-treatment/treatment#medications-used-in-mat. Accessed March 26, 2018.

21. Vestal C. Injection sites provide safe spots to shoot up. PEW Charitable Trusts website. January 12, 2018. http://www.pewtrusts.org/en/research-and-analysis/blogs/stateline/2018/01/12/injection-sites-provide-safe-spots-to-shoot-up. Accessed March 28, 2018.

22. Roman PM, Abraham AJ, Knudsen HK. Using medication-assisted treatment for substance use disorders: Evidence of barriers and facilitators of implementation. *Addictive Behaviors*. 2011;(36)6:584–9. https://doi.org/10.1016/j.addbeh.2011.01.032.

23. Elrod JE, Fortenberry Jr JL. The hub-and-spoke organization design: An avenue for servicing patients well. *BMC Health Serv Res*. 2017;17(1):25–33. doi:10.1186/s12913-017-2341.

24. The Association of State and Territorial Health Officials. Vermont: Medication assisted treatment program for opioid addiction. http://www.astho.org/Health-Systems-Transformation/Medicaid-and-Public-Health-Partnerships/Case-Studies/Vermont-MAT-Program-for-Opioid-Addiction/. Accessed March 22, 2018.

25. Brooklyn JR, Sigmon SC. Vermont hub-and-spoke model of care for opioid use disorder: Development, implementation, and impact. *J Addict Med*. 2017;11(4):286–92. http://doi.org/10.1097/ADM.0000000000000310.

26. Green TC, Clarke J, Brinkley-Rubinstein L, Marshall BDL, Alexander-Scott N, Boss R, Rich JD. Postincarceration fatal overdoses after implementing medications

for addiction treatment in a statewide correctional system. *JAMA Psychiatry*.2018. doi:10.1001/jamapsychiatry.2017.4614.

27. National Alliance for Model State Drug Laws. Model addiction costs reduction act (ACRA). http://www.namsdl.org/library/Section_A__Model_Addiction_Costs_Reduction_Act__ACRA_/. Accessed March 21, 2018.

28. PEW Charitable Trusts. Prescription drug monitoring programs. December 2016. http://www.pewtrusts.org/~/media/assets/2016/12/prescription_drug_monitoring_programs.pdf. Accessed March 26, 2018.

29. Centers for Disease Control and Prevention. State successes. Updated October 5, 2017. https://www.cdc.gov/drugoverdose/policy/successes.html. Accessed March 26, 2018.

30. Centers for Disease Control and Prevention. CDC guideline for prescribing opioids for chronic pain. Updated August 29, 2017. https://www.cdc.gov/drugoverdose/prescribing/guideline.html. Accessed March 26, 2018.

31. Davis C. Appendix b: State-by-state summary of opioid prescribing regulations and guidelines. www.azdhs.gov/documents/prevention/womens-childrens-health/injury-prevention/opioid-prevention/appendix-b-state-by-state-summary.pdf. Accessed March 22, 2018.

32. Massachusetts Department of Public Health. An assessment of fatal and nonfatal opioid overdoses in Massachusetts (2011–2015). August 2017. https://www.mass.gov/files/documents/2017/08/31/legislative-report-chapter-55-aug-2017.pdf. Accessed March 22, 2018.

33. Commonwealth of Massachusetts. An act establishing a sick leave bank for Robert Paterwic, an employee of the department of industrial accidents. March 10, 2015. https://malegislature.gov/Laws/SessionLaws/Acts/2015/Chapter5. Accessed March 26, 2018.

34. US DHHR. 2016 West Virginia Overdose Fatality Analysis: Healthcare Systems Utilization, Risk Factors, and Opportunities for Intervention. https://dhhr.wv.gov/bph/Documents/ODCP%20Reports%202017/2016%20Overdose%20Fatality%20Analysis%20final%20rv.pdf. Accessed April 7, 2018.

35. Felitti VJ, Anda RF, Nordenberg D, et al. Relationship of childhood abuse and household dysfunction to many of the leading cause of death in adults. *AJPM*. 1998;14(4):245–58. https://doi.org/10.1016/S0749-3797(98)00017-8

36. Health Resources and Services Administration: Maternal and Child Health. Home visiting. Updated June 2017. https://mchb.hrsa.gov/maternal-child-health-initiatives/home-visiting-overview. Accessed March 26, 2018.

37. Patriarca M, Ausura CJ. Introducing Rhode Island's health equity zones. *Rhode Island Med J*. 2016:47–8. http://www.rimed.org/rimedicaljournal/2016/11/2016-11-47-health-patriarca.pdf. Accessed March 26, 2018.

38. Prescription Drug Abuse Policy System. Naloxone overdose prevention laws. Updated July 1, 2017. http://pdaps.org/datasets/laws-regulating-administration-of-naloxone-1501695139. Accessed March 22, 2018.

39. Kaiser Family Foundation. Syringe exchange programs. 2017. https://www.kff.org/hivaids/state-indicator/syringe-exchange-programs/?currentTimeframe=0&sortModel=%7B%22colId%22:%22Location%22,%22sort%22:%22asc%22%7D. Accessed April 9, 2018.

40. The Kaiser Family Foundation. Medicaid's role in addressing the opioid epidemic. February 2018. http://files.kff.org/attachment/INFOGRAPHIC-MEDICAIDS-ROLE-IN-ADDRESSING-THE-OPIOID-EPIDEMIC. Accessed March 22, 2018.

41. National Conference of States Legislatures. Mental health benefits: State laws mandating or regulating. December 30, 2015. www.ncsl.org/research/health/mental-health-benefits-state-mandates.aspx. Accessed March 22, 2018.

42. The Pew Charitable Trusts. When are prescribers required to use prescription drug monitoring programs? Updated January 30, 2018. www.pewtrusts.org/en/multimedia/data-visualizations/2018/when-are-prescribers-required-to-use-prescription-drug-monitoring-programs. Accessed March 22, 2018.

43. National Conference of State Legislatures. Prescribing policies: States confront opioid overdose epidemic. August 2017. Updated April 2018. http://www.ncsl.org/research/health/prescribing-policies-states-confront-opioid-overdose-epidemic.aspx. Accessed April 23, 2018.

44. Health Resources and Services Administration. Home visiting program: State fact sheets. Updated August 2017. https://mchb.hrsa.gov/maternal-child-health-initiatives/home-visiting/home-visiting-program-state-fact-sheets. Accessed April 9, 2018.

45. The Office of National Drug Control Policy. High intensity drug trafficking areas (HIDTA) program. https://obamawhitehouse.archives.gov/ondcp/high-intensity-drug-trafficking-areas-program. Accessed April 23, 2018.

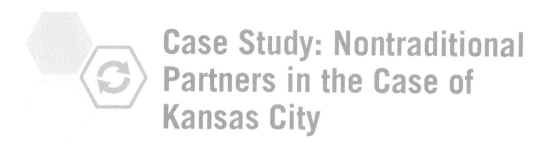

# Chapter 43

# Case Study: Nontraditional Partners in the Case of Kansas City

SCOTT HALL AND REX ARCHER

## PARTNER: THE KANSAS CITY CHAMBER OF COMMERCE

For more than 130 years, the Greater Kansas City Chamber of Commerce (KC Chamber) has been working to make its region a great place to grow a business. To do this, the KC Chamber thinks broadly, taking on more than just traditional business issues and also addressing issues that affect quality of life (e.g., education, the arts, and community health). What makes our role more complicated, though, is that we are not educators, artists, or public health experts. Instead, the great ability of the KC chamber is that of convener and partner, assembler of a diverse collective representing a variety of stakeholders and subject matter experts across a community.

This is exactly what the KC Chamber has done in its partnership with the Kansas City, Missouri, Health Department (KCMOHD).

## PARTNER: THE KCMOHD

By the time the KC Chamber was formed in 1887, the KCMOHD was already serving the residents of a growing metropolis. Over these many years, the city's health force has grown from one physician to a large team with diverse expertise, focusing on things not even imaginable as matters of public health at the KCMOHD's inception.

Today, the term "social determinants of health" is a common refrain within and by the department, espousing to all who will listen that things once not thought of as being within the sphere of public health are very much critical to its outcomes. The department's work in these areas has been recognized with the 2015 Robert Wood Johnson Foundation (RWJF) Culture of Health Prize, where its unique strength at rallying community partners, including the business community, related to a shared vision of health was applauded.

The KCMOHD continues to emphasize action on the processes and structures that generate health inequity, rather than just remediating its consequences. Reaching out to partners like the KC Chamber is one way this is happening.

## OUR HISTORY OF PARTNERSHIP

For 15 years, the KC Chamber has recognized that a healthy workforce impacts the competitiveness and productivity of its members and increases their savings on employee health care costs. As they have grown in understanding of worksite wellness, they have come to realize that because their employees are influenced by factors outside of work, the work of the KC Chamber must also focus on the outside social factors in their employees' communities that influence health. One of us (RA) was familiar with the benefits and limitations of worksite wellness programs, having worked as the leader of an internationally recognized program for Ford Motor Company in the 1980s, before returning to a governmental career in public health.

Recognizing that each organization could benefit from the other to influence healthy behaviors for Kansas City residents, in 2003, the KC Chamber and the KCMOHD began working on reducing exposure to tobacco products. KC Chamber members were able to enforce nonsmoking campuses at their worksites and created a supportive environment for employees to quit. The KCMOHD assisted in their other goals, including education on second-hand smoke and preventing residents from initiating a smoking habit.

Although many KC Chamber members had their employees' work lives covered, the KCMOHD successfully moved to prohibit the use of tobacco products first in all non-hospitality businesses. The success of those policies encouraged the KC Chamber and the KCMOHD to continue to work on tobacco legislation as well as other social factors to improve health outcomes for Kansas City residents.

More recently, the KC Chamber supported the City of Kansas City in its application for the esteemed RWJF Culture of Health Prize, which was coordinated by the KCMOHD. Essential to this award was the partnership between the KCMOHD and many community collaborators, including the KC Chamber. And the KC Chamber's association with the prize continues, as Joe Reardon, the KC Chamber's current President and CEO, sits as a member of the Culture of Health Prize Advisory Board.

## HEALTHY KC

Kansas City—really all of Greater Kansas City—is not as healthy as it should be. In Kansas City, we see huge differences in life expectancy by zip code. There can be a 14-year difference in life expectancy between residents in two zip codes. The zip codes with similar life expectancies tend to be clustered together. These differences result from socioeconomic factors, such as education, income, and structural racism. In addition, 65% of Kansas Citians are considered overweight or obese, and 20% of adults in Kansas City rated their health as "poor" or "fair."

Recognizing our community's health challenges and sharing a desire to lead by example, then-KC Chamber President and CEO Jim Heeter and Kansas City Mayor Sly James issued a public fitness challenge to each other in 2012. They competed to see who could most improve their individual health over several months. When they finished, they issued the same challenge to business, civic, and elected leaders in Greater Kansas City.

A group of about 40 high-profile business and civic leaders in our region participated in what became known as the "Not So Big KC Challenge." After several months, this effort was further broadened into a more community-wide initiative to seek health improvement for our region. This broader initiative became the KC Chamber's signature health program: "Healthy KC."

Healthy KC is a KC Chamber–supported regional health and wellness strategy whose aim is to make Greater Kansas City a destination for health and wellness. The work on this project began quietly in the summer of 2013. At the time, the KC Chamber and its project partner Blue Cross and Blue Shield of Kansas City recognized that they didn't have all of the answers to achieve this objective. Instead, they needed to seek input from experts throughout the community. One of their first meetings was with the team at the KCMOHD.

This early conversation, and many others that followed, inspired the leaders of the Healthy KC project to settle on five areas in which to focus their work: (1) healthy eating, (2) active living, (3) behavioral health, (4) workplace wellness, and (5) tobacco use cessation and prevention.

For nearly a year, the KC Chamber convened experts within each of these areas of focus to determine how the Healthy KC coalition might move our community toward regional health. Representatives from across a variety of sectors, including business, justice, not-for-profit, health insurers, health care providers, and especially health departments, were engaged in this work. At the table at each of those meetings was the KCMOHD.

During its meetings with workplace and public health experts, the Healthy KC team kept hearing that two kinds of interventions could quickly impact health outcomes in the workplace and, ultimately, the community: policy and environment. We were told that when policy was changed, behavior changed. Similarly, when the environment was changed, behavior changed.

The Healthy KC initiative was also informed by the idea that individual accountability is important, but also by the growing evidence that corporate culture (social accountability) matters in community health. It was a matter of some civic responsibility, then, that businesses lead on the issue of public health.

Finally, the KC Chamber's members recognized that most employees spend more time outside of work and are heavily influenced by their community's culture. Even if employees were surrounded by healthy environments at the workplace, the environment surrounding them outside of work was having a profound impact on their health.

Because of these influences, as well as because of its long-standing history of advocacy, the KC Chamber was encouraged to take some steps to change public policy. Within the tobacco cessation area of focus, that initial priority was "to raise the minimum age of purchase and sale of tobacco products, including alternative nicotine delivery systems, from 18 to 21." This project was soon thereafter branded "Tobacco21|KC."

## TOBACCO21|KC

Tobacco21|KC was launched publicly in October 2015, only a few days before a delegation that included both authors of this chapter would travel to Princeton, New Jersey, to accept the RWJF Culture of Health Prize on behalf of Kansas City.

Originally, the quiet goal of Tobacco21|KC was to have five cities raise their minimum legal smoking age within 3 years. We considered that progress to be ambitious. After all, no city in the Greater Kansas City area had ever passed a Tobacco21 ordinance. Both local and state laws across Missouri and Kansas had (and still have) tobacco control laws that many in the public health community would interpret as weak. And, finally, progress on local laws to remove tobacco products from bars and restaurants was solid but had been controversial and slow to gain momentum in our region a decade earlier.

Despite our modest goal, we were convinced that if we started our regional efforts in our most high-profile cities, others would take notice and might follow in our footsteps. And so the Healthy KC team and the KCMOHD began separate conversations with business leaders, elected officials, and legal experts about the possibility of passing a Tobacco21 ordinance in Kansas City.

The KCMOHD began conversations with other key city departments, such as the Law Department, to test the legality of the ordinance, and the Regulated Industries Division under the Neighborhoods and Housing Department, to consider the mechanics of implementation. Meanwhile, the KCMOHD team was also having conversations with members of the Kansas City, Missouri, City Council to make them aware that other cities across the country were beginning to consider this policy and to identify initial council sponsors for the ordinance.

At the same time, the KC Chamber and the Healthy KC team were coordinating with business leaders and other elected officials within and outside of Kansas City, Missouri, about the possibility of passing Tobacco21 laws. They made private presentations to business, civic, and elected leaders emphasizing the cost to business that tobacco imposes and how those costs could be mitigated through Tobacco21; they also asked for organizations to endorse the Tobacco21|KC effort.

While these separate meetings were happening, the KC Chamber's Healthy KC team and representatives from the KCMOHD were meeting weekly to compare notes, share feedback, further explore implementation strategies, and reinforce the strength of this multipronged approach. These meetings even happened at the RWJF Culture of Health Prize award ceremonies in Princeton.

The impact of this collaborative work is obvious from the outcome. On November 19, 2015, the Kansas City, Missouri, City Council passed an ordinance increasing the age of purchase and sale of tobacco products from 18 to 21. At that hearing, the Healthy KC team presented a list of more than 146 Kanas City area organizations that endorsed the Tobacco21|KC effort. This included hospital systems, health insurers, and health specialists, as well as organizations that just want to see Greater Kansas City as a destination for health and wellness.

At that hearing, the KCMOHD was able to quickly and simply state that they supported the ordinance and that they were available to answer any questions the city council might have about impact, implementation, and enforcement.

The notion that Kansas City, Missouri, would be the leader across the region was affirmed. Three hours after Kansas City, Missouri, City Council passed its Tobacco21 ordinance, Kansas City, Kansas, passed the same. Other cities have also followed suit.

In the nearly two and a half years since those meetings, the Tobacco21|KC effort has successfully partnered with 25 additional local communities that have raised the age of purchase and sale of tobacco products and alternative nicotine delivery systems from 18 to 21. There are now almost 1.5 million people living in Tobacco21 communities in Greater Kansas City. The KC Chamber has quarterbacked the effort in each of these communities, and the KCMOHD has served as a resource for each of those smaller cities as they thought through the implementation of this change.

## CONCLUSION

The mission of the Greater Kansas City, Missouri, Chamber of Commerce is to lead the way to the best KC region. The mission of the KCMOHD is to promote, preserve, and protect the health of Kansas Citians and their visitors. Neither one of these things can happen without the other. It is obvious to us, then, that the partnership between the KC Chamber and the KCMOHD on the Tobacco21|KC project isn't the end of our work together. And, based on our history, we know it isn't the beginning. Our partnership on Tobacco21|KC is just one chapter in a long story of collaboration between two organizations bringing health to everyone in Kansas City, Missouri.

We've even already begun collaborating on our next accomplishments together. For starters, we are working to identify and accomplish those policy changes that will advance Kansas City, Missouri, in the CityHealth initiative. Projects such as healthy vending, complete streets, and broader access to early childhood education are in our sights.

Our relationship is long-standing, and there is something to be learned from our example. You can't rush collaboration, especially when the parties have different cultures and perspectives. Develop relationships over time to cultivate trust and a shared vision. The KCMOHD and the KC Chamber have done so, and our next project together will be made easier for it. Yours could be, too.

# Training and Workforce: Preparing for the Future That Is Already Here

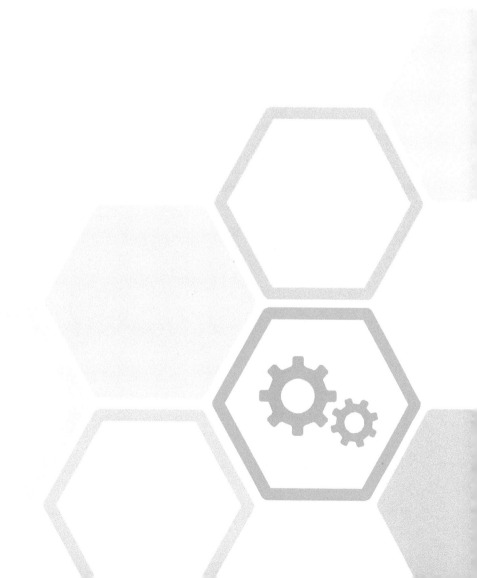

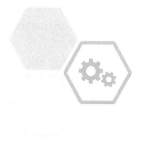

# Overview—Training and Workforce: Preparing for the Future That Is Already Here

J. LLOYD MICHENER AND CRAIG W. THOMAS

In the early days of *The Practical Playbook: Public Health and Primary Care Together* (1st edition), the roles of training and workforce were not a primary concern; the focus was on finding effective strategies and tools. But as the key elements of multisector partnerships became clear, so, too, did the need and opportunity to include students and other learners. Part of the shift was the result of the rapid growth of community partnerships, making the opportunity to include learners more than an isolated possibility. Another was the infrequent presence of learners, training programs, or professional schools in the partnerships even though many were occurring in the neighborhoods around the professional schools and programs. And a large part was the eagerness of the learners themselves when they learned of the community programs and expressed that these partnerships were central to their interests and future. The growth of multisector community partnerships, the relative absence of the schools and faculty, and the interest of learners created a challenge. Professional education and training are largely self-governed, making change a slow process of consensus-building by faculty and practitioners. But the expansion of community coalitions was not being driven by the professions, and few faculty had awareness of, much less the experience to guide or oversee, the involvement of learners.

Not all schools or programs were disengaged, however. Schools with a strong social mission have always had a deep commitment to their communities. Newer programs with strong local roots are built on local partnerships, connections, and commitments. Other, more traditional programs could become galvanized by a dynamic leader (see Chapter 46). And some specialties and disciplines have never traveled far from their beginnings as advocates for those in need, such as pediatrics and the health of children (see Chapter 45); family medicine and the health of families and communities (see Chapters 12 and 26); and nursing, with its long history of community outreach (see Chapter 48). For such groups, working with communities has been part of their history, and one that could be rediscovered and built upon.

The voice of students and residents in this process is new and has not yet reached full force. The role of learners can be seen in the student and resident sections of professional associations, and even more directly in the student essays included in this section (see Chapter 49). These essays were developed and selected through an essay contest for health professions students sponsored by the de Beaumont Foundation.

Against this backdrop of community- and student-driven training, there is the start of agreement on new and evolving competencies needed for the health care and public health workforce. Systems thinking, use of data, community engagement, team work, and knowing when to lead (and when to follow) are common, though not ubiquitous, elements and can increasingly be found in the works of the Accreditation Council for Graduate Medical Education, which accredits physician graduate training[1]; the Council on Education for Public Health[2]; and the works of the Association of American Medical Colleges[3] and Association of Schools and Programs of Public Health.[4]

Support of these changes is not being driven just by students, faculty, and associations alone. At the federal level, the Centers for Disease Control and Prevention (CDC) and the Human Resource Services Administration (HRSA) both sponsor and promote training programs to strengthen the workforce to improve population health. For governmental public health agencies, training and professional development practices are reinforced through achievement of the Public Health Accreditation Board (PHAB) national standards and measures for maintaining a competent workforce.[5] A relatively new addition is under way at the state level, and many states have become increasingly concerned about the health of their communities, especially in rural areas (see Chapter 47). The chapters that follow describe a wide array of training programs that seek to respond to those needs and build local capacity.

Yet the work of workforce development largely lies ahead. This section provides an overview and highlights of exciting practices and programs from across regions and sectors, as well as the voices of learners who see these partnerships as a key element of their future. Still to come is the systemic engagement of professional schools and programs in community partnerships, providing their expertise, learners, and services as respected and effective members of community teams for health. The engagement of schools, faculty, and students in finding, supporting, and teaching effective strategies for health will help our schools fulfill their missions, our students their calling, and our communities their visions of health.

# REFERENCES

1. Bradley D. Duke Community and Family Medicine. *Population Health Graduate Education Milestones: A Report to the Centers for Disease Control and Prevention and the Association of American Medical Colleges.* Durham, NC. 2015. https://cfm.duke.edu/files/field/attachments/Population%20Health%20Milestones%20in%20Graduate%20Medical%20Education_web_0.pdf. Accessed 1/17/2019.

2. Council on Education for Public Health. Accreditation criteria schools of public health and public health programs. 2016. https://ceph.org/assets/2016.Criteria.pdf Accessed 1/17/2019.

3. Academic Partnerships to Improve Health. AAMC-CDC cooperative agreement. 2017. https://www.aamc.org/initiatives/diversity/portfolios/cdc/.

4. Association of Schools and Programs of Public Health. Population health across all professions expert panel report. 2015. https://s3.amazonaws.com/aspph-wp-production/app/uploads/2015/02/PHaAP.pdf. Accessed 1/17/2019.

5. Public Health Accreditation Board Standards and Measures. Version 1.5. 2013. http://www.phaboard.org/wp-content/uploads/PHABSM_WEB_LR1.pdf. Accessed 1/17/2019.

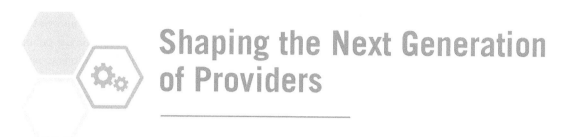

# Chapter 45

# Shaping the Next Generation of Providers

GERRI MATTSON AND KAREN REMLEY

Primary care providers are increasingly called on to expand their practice beyond the bedside and the traditional knowledge and skills of clinical medicine. Politics, economics, the physical and social environment, and structures of institutions and communities affect both access to and the outcomes of the health care services. As early as 1910, the Flexner Report emphasized that physicians should receive medical training that gives them the knowledge to prevent disease and promote health by using a wider lens than the level of the individual patient.[1] However, medical training now needs to go beyond Flexner to help providers understand the influence of social factors in affecting health disparities in the populations and communities in which our patients are born, learn, play, live, work, and age. Training that instills and cultivates the duty of social justice, an awareness and ability to reduce discrimination and bias, and the need to promote diversity and inclusion within our primary care providers is important to help us authentically and effectively work with our communities, institutions, and systems to mitigate health disparities and ultimately achieve health equity.

Today, several national groups and initiatives describe population health milestones and competencies (Population Health Graduate Education Milestones by the Accreditation Council for Graduate Medical Education [ACGME] Regional Medicine Public Health Education Centers or [RMPHEC]) for medical students and residents across a variety of primary care and specialty providers. These competencies and milestones require training programs to develop skills, knowledge, and abilities in areas such as public health, community engagement, critical thinking, and leadership development.[2] Acquiring a level of competency in each area involves multiple disciplines and cross-sector collaboration to address the "role of socioeconomic, environmental, cultural, and other population-level determinants of health on the health status and health care of individuals and populations."[1]

## PUBLIC HEALTH

Competencies in public health allow providers to apply a mix of clinical and nonclinical prevention strategies with community partners that improve the health of individuals and populations and reduce disparities. Clinical public health strategies include offering interventions such as immunizations to prevent disease and counseling and contraception to prevent teen pregnancy.[3] Nonclinical public health strategies may include reducing the impact of poverty by assisting social services with enrolling patients and their families in health insurance and public benefits and working with community partners in business and nonprofit organizations, city planning, law, and housing to change environmental structures and help make healthy choices the default.

Structural competency allows clinicians to recognize relationships among race, class, and upstream influences, such as food, zoning laws, and urban and rural infrastructure and the expression of symptoms, attitudes, illness, and disease that influence clinical interactions.[4] Training programs can include teaching about structural competency to instill in residents and students the ability to ask questions about and act on what is going on in the lives of their patients that can improve the health of both the community and the patient. Opportunities for community training and engaging community partners in clinics and hospital rounds allow for experiential learning from public health and other community partners during delivery of care and can build long-term relationships between training programs and communities. These opportunities can also attract trainees to careers in underserved areas and public health organizations.

One example of a successful partnership that supported a structural competency intervention is a New York University psychiatry residency elective that placed fourth-year residents in Brownsville, a Brooklyn community. Brownsville is a predominantly African American, low-income neighborhood with the highest density of public housing in the United States and high levels of violence. The psychiatry residents collaborated with a community development agency called Brownsville Partnership to conduct a community mental health needs assessment. The collaboration led to local churches and community centers developing trauma-informed bereavement groups and enhanced communication between mental health providers and probation officers, who prevented rearrests and hospitalizations through early treatment of their clients' symptoms.[5]

## COMMUNITY ENGAGEMENT

The Centers for Disease Control and Prevention (CDC) considers community engagement as a key effort in improving public health and defines it as "the process of working collaboratively with and through groups of people affiliated by geographic proximity, special interest, or similar situations to address issues affecting the well-being of those people,"[6] Medical students, residents in training, and health care providers can benefit from experiences with community engagement to understand and begin to use strategies to address social determinants of health and health disparities. This includes understanding that it is not enough to just screen and refer patients with identified social needs to an organization on a list. Community engagement allows providers to build relationships for respectful, collegial, interprofessional collaborations across sectors to assess for and partner in addressing a variety of concerns and challenges. Community engagement is a form of systems-based practice,[7] which is an "awareness of and responsiveness to the larger context and system of health care, as well as the ability to call effectively on other resources in the system to provide optimal health care."[7] Some academic health centers and health systems and their training programs encourage or require rotations with key community agencies for students and residents; this is a model others can emulate. One such program is the Population Health Scholar Track at Georgetown University in Washington, DC (Box 45.1).

The American Academy of Pediatrics (AAP) has a long history of encouraging and supporting its residents and providers in community engagement through its Community Access to Child Health (CATCH) program, which started in 1993. CATCH empowers pediatricians to collaborate with others,

---

**Box 45.1 | Food Matters: Medical Students Partner with a Community-Based Nonprofit to Combat Food Insecurity**

*John C. Penner, Margaret L. McCarthy, and Katherine P. Mullins*

Some students in the Population Health Scholar Track at Georgetown University in Washington, DC, are working on a program that integrates the University's web of clinics with a nonprofit called Martha's Table, as well as with pop-up food markets called Joyful Food Markets (JFM), to create a referral system, with the ultimate goal of improving the food security of populations in Washington, DC.

"As part of Georgetown's Population Health Scholar Track, we study the social determinants of health, quality improvement methods, and community partnerships in a longitudinal curriculum integrated into our medical education. Martha's Table approached us with a proposal to link local clinics to JFM, envisioning some form of referral protocol that we might design. As medical students and 'insiders' to local health care, we brainstormed methods to implement such a protocol. We envisioned our process to begin by raising local physician awareness to facilitate conversations between families and clinicians about food insecurity. We discussed ways to minimize the burden of this task on clinical resources. Eventually, we hoped physicians—through our process implementation—could encourage patients to utilize JFM as part of their overall health care goals."

adopt a population health approach, and identify promising practices that work in their communities. CATCH grants of up to $10,000 support planning or implementation of innovative community-based child health projects led by pediatricians. Pediatric residents can also receive grants of up to $2,000 to plan or implement a project. A total of more than 1,600 grants have been awarded, focused on children and adolescents who are uninsured or underinsured in rural and underserved urban areas of the United States. The projects address a variety of issues (e.g., mental health and obesity) and, most commonly, child health disparities in low-income communities. Almost 90% of CATCH projects continue beyond the initial funding. More than 25% of CATCH projects have been able to leverage additional funds to sustain their efforts; some projects have been able to receive millions of dollars in support.

Similarly, the Society of Teachers of Family Medicine has a Group on Primary Care and Public Health Integration that works toward a vision of systems of health care that increase collaborative work between primary care providers and public health professionals to improve population health, achieve health equity by eliminating health disparities, and control health care spending.[8]

## CRITICAL THINKING

Critical thinking is another important population competency. Students, residents, and primary care providers can be overwhelmed by the vast amounts of patient- and community-level data. Knowledge and skills in data collection and analysis are needed to make appropriate decisions for care and advocacy. Competency in critical thinking includes understanding the different forms of data, knowing methods for data collection and risk analysis, and understanding the limitations and costs for both quantitative and qualitative data, as well as having the ability to assess the need for and analysis of the processes and outcomes for any interventions. Collaborations between public health and primary care are helpful in understanding how to find, interpret, and use appropriate county-, state-, and community-level data to determine the epidemiology of health and to assess interventions to address the medical, social, and environmental needs of a population.

Another aspect of critical thinking is asking faculty to engage medical students and residents in critical reflection on cultural structures that lead to social and economic disadvantages and injustices, such as class bias, white privilege, and racism, and that result in health concerns in many communities. Resources for developing elements of a social justice curriculum have been used in Northeast Ohio Medical University (NEOMED), which uses humanities and bioethics. There are also examples of literature, texts, film, and clinical and community experiences that can be used in teaching.[9]

Primary care practice-based research networks (PBRNs) can help support the development of skills, knowledge, and abilities in both community engagement and in critical thinking. PBRNs exist across the country and help primary care providers engage with communities and also learn skills in clinical research, implementation and dissemination of science, and comparative effectiveness research. PBRNs investigate and answer clinical community-based practice organizational questions that are important to improve the quality of primary health care in communities; issues might include those related to discrimination and bias. PBRNs exist within national professional associations such as the AAP, the American Academy of Family Physicians (AAFP), hospital systems, academic centers, and universities and their training programs.[10]

Quality improvement science is now required as part of residency training and during the recertification of providers in multiple medical specialties (e.g., internal medicine, family practice, and pediatrics). This form of experiential learning allows providers to engage with their practices or communities to ask, assess, develop aims, and pilot small tests of change that could lead to a solution to one or more pressing health issues impacting a group of patients.

## LEADERSHIP DEVELOPMENT

Leadership development is a population health competency that includes knowledge, skills, and abilities in advocacy, communication, and working in teams. The ACGME common program requirements expect future providers to "advocate for quality patient care and optimal patient care systems," which may include addressing implicit bias or discrimination in the delivery or receipt of needed care or social services.[7] Advocacy training seems especially appropriate in pediatrics because of the story behind the founding of the national organization, the AAP, as a leading advocate for children and their families.

The Sheppard-Towner Act was passed into law in 1921 and allocated funding to establish publicly available maternal-child health centers to address topics such as hygiene and nutrition and provide services such as visits and literature. At the time, the American Medical Association (AMA) strongly opposed the legislation because of fears that it would harm the medical profession. Several years later, the law needed renewal, but the AMA continued its powerful opposition, and Congress failed to continue the funding. The Pediatric Section of the AMA House of Delegates had voted in favor of supporting renewal of the Sheppard-Towner Act, which conflicted with the AMA's position and outraged the full AMA House of Delegates. A group of pediatricians left the AMA in protest and founded the AAP in 1930. The AAP members chose the well-being of children and families as paramount. Today, the mission of the AAP is "to attain optimal physical, mental and social health and well-being of infants, children, adolescents and young adults" and to accomplish its mission to support "the professional needs of its members."[11]

Advocacy can be described as occurring at two levels. On the first level, providers "work the system" to meet a need for an individual patient. However, advocacy related to communities and social determinants of health requires more complex, coordinated strategies. Many professional associations are engaged in such advocacy,[12] but, all too often, individual primary care providers are less likely to be engaged in this level of advocacy, feeling that this is outside of what should be expected from them. However, as evidence of the need to focus beyond the clinic walls, more health care providers are choosing to "wear the hats" of community advocates, public health epidemiologists, or data explorers to help solve difficult social, economic, and other public health problems. Dr. Mona Hanna-Attisha, a pediatrician, did just that with the case of lead-contaminated water in Flint Michigan (Box 45.2).

Organizations like the AAP have initiatives with a common purpose of strengthening leadership and advocacy skills. The Community Pediatrics Training Initiative is an initiative of the AAP designed to strengthen community health and advocacy training of pediatric trainees and to develop faculty leadership and advocacy skills. The work is accomplished by providing a number of opportunities: grants that foster collaboration between residency programs and pediatric state chapters, leadership to enhance local child health efforts, scholarships to help increase opportunities for publication and presentation, and networking and mentoring opportunities. A community health and advocacy curriculum is used to help residency programs meet the Resident Review Committee advocacy training requirements. Various tools are used to improve the assessment of resident skills and to identify strengths and weaknesses in the residency program and in faculty development processes. The Community Pediatrics Training Initiative has formally provided assistance to 101 pediatric

---

**Box 45.2 | How a Pediatrician Created Awareness of the Water Crisis in Flint, Michigan**

Dr. Mona Hanna-Attisha's story of how she brought awareness and action to the Flint Water Crisis encompasses both primary care and public health principles. A pediatrician, residency program director, and public health practitioner, she learned from a childhood friend about high lead levels being found in the water of Flint, Michigan. She used electronic health records to study the blood lead levels of children before and after the change in drinking water source, demonstrating the direct correlation of the change to untreated corrosive water with an increase in blood lead levels. Rather than wait and publish her research, she used community engagement strategies coupled with science-based advocacy to force action by government at all levels. Her guided response to the crisis has included both broad evidence-based public health interventions (i.e., universal preschool, economic development) and individual child and parent clinical programs (i.e., Medicaid expansion, parenting support, nutrition education), all with the partnered involvement of children, parents, and learners at all level of training. This is an example of primary care, public health, medical education, and community engagement in action!

residency programs, awarded 183 grants, and provided support to hundreds of faculty and residents.

The ACGME program requirements also expect future providers to achieve competency in interpersonal communication that engages individual patients and families.[7] However, methods of interpersonal communication are evolving as social media allows flexibility and increased availability to patients and the public. Increasingly, interpersonal and public communication occurs through social media, and many primary care trainees and providers have become social advocates using social media.[13] With this growth has come a growing awareness of the need to appropriately frame issues so that intended messages are heard and not misinterpreted, and with the community being brought into the issue thoughtfully.[14]

With the growth of electronic communications, there are concerns about the possibilities for "violations of ethical standards, patient privacy, confidentiality, and professional codes of practice, along with the misrepresentation of information."[13] Training in appropriate interpersonal and online communication and social media has become important for medical students, residents, and currently practicing providers in both public health and medicine. It is also important to recognize situations in which computer-mediated communication tools may need to be monitored or delegated to personnel and colleagues with more experience and to create recommendations on ways to handle unprofessional or inappropriate use by patients and providers. Web-based technology, when properly used for knowledge exchange and collaboration through social media and online patient portals, allows for more access and engagement with patients, community partners, and the public.

Leadership development can have an individual focus, but good leadership has systemic influences in improving care and advancing health for patients and populations. To be effective, leadership development must be interrelated with the other population health competency areas of public health, community engagement, and critical thinking.

Primary care providers may not achieve full mastery of any competency by the end of their training, but they will continue to gain knowledge, skills, and abilities over time. Primary care providers in the community can serve as mentors for trainees, which can provide additional perspective and experience outside of the academic setting. The relationship is mutually beneficial as trainees engage in strategies rooted in public health, community engagement, critical thinking, and leadership development and address the problems of their patients *and* communities. As the saying goes, "It takes a village to raise a child," and this phrase is particularly apt in primary care as the health and well-being of the entire community depend on the collaborative work of health care providers, public health, community organizations, faith-based organizations, and the community itself. Understanding the myriad connections, competencies, and impacts of these partnerships early in training allows clinicians to engage with the community early in their careers; to deepen their engagement, understanding, and ability over time; and to be effective advocates with and on behalf of the communities they serve.

## REFERENCES

1. Maeshiro R, Johnson I, Koo D, et al. Medical education for a healthier population: reflections on the Flexner Report from a public health perspective. *Acad Med.* 2010;85(2):211–9.

2. Regional Medicine Public Health Education Centers (RMPHEC). https://www.aamc.org/download/123246/data/populationhealthcompetencies.pdf.pdf. Accessed April 28, 2018.

3. Frieden TR. The future of public health. *N Engl J Med.* 2015;373(18):1748–54.

4. Metzl JM, Hansen H. Structural competency: Theorizing a new medical engagement with stigma and inequality. *Soc Sci Med (1982).* 2014;103:126–33. http://doi.org/10.1016/j.socscimed.2013.06.032. Accessed April 28, 2018.

5. Reich AD, Hansen HB, Link BG. Fundamental interventions: How clinicians can address the fundamental causes of disease. *J Bioeth Inq.* 2016;13:185–92.

6. CDC/ATSDR Committee on Community Engagement. Principles of Community Engagement. 1997. Updated 2011. https://www.atsdr.cdc.gov/communityengagement/pdf/PCE_Report_508_FINAL.pdf.

7. ACGME Requirements. http://www.acgme.org/Portals/0/PFAssets/ProgramRequirements/CPRs_2017-07-01.pdf. Accessed April 28, 2018.

8. Society of Teachers of Family Medicine. http://www.stfm.org/Groups/GroupPagesandDiscussionForums/PrimaryCareandPublicHealthIntegration. Accessed on April 28, 2018.

9. Wear D, Zarconi J, Aultman JM, Chyatte MR, Kumagai AK. Remembering Freddie Gray: Medical education for social justice. *Acad Med.* 2017;92(3):312–7.

10. AHRQ. PBRN Fact Sheet. https://www.ahrq.gov/research/findings/factsheets/primary/pbrn/index.html. Accessed April 9, 2018.

11. AAP. Pediatric history. https://www.aap.org/en-us/about-the-aap/Pediatric-History-Center/Pages/Sheppard-Towner-Act.aspx. Accessed April 9, 2018.

12. Dobson S, Voyer S, Regehr G. Perspective: Agency and activism rethinking health advocacy in the medical profession. *Acad Med.* 2012;87(9):1161–4.

13. Grajales FJ 3rd, Sheps S, Ho K, Novak-Lauscher H, Eysenbach G. Social media: A review and tutorial of applications in medicine and health care. *J Med Internet Res.* 2014;16(2):e13. doi:10.2196/jmir.2912.

14. Frameworks Institute. http://www.frameworksinstitute.org/frame-effects.html. Accessed May 4, 2018.

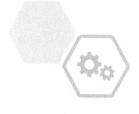

# Chapter 46

# On the Synergies That Can Generate Excellence in Public Health Education

SANDRO GALEA

Universities, broadly speaking, serve three functions. First, they generate new knowledge. Society invests in universities to generate the ideas that inform our understanding of the world and that may guide our actions toward improving the world. Second, and critically, universities are responsible for teaching students, for preparing the next generation of thinkers and doers. On this front, universities are entrusted with identifying what students need to learn and how best they can learn it, to prepare them for a life of contribution to the world that they will enter upon graduation. Third, universities are responsible for translating their knowledge. For centuries, universities were charged with preserving knowledge, a function they served principally through libraries and archives. But the digital revolution both challenged that role and created enormous new opportunities for universities to work toward ensuring that the knowledge they create does not sit idle, but is translated to the broader public conversation to contribute meaningfully to change.

In the best of times this set of functions creates synergies such that an excellent university generates knowledge, uses that knowledge to prepare the next generation, and trains that same generation to be a part of knowledge translation; this is meant to ensure that the changes that are motivated by what we know create a world that the next generation embraces and wants to live in.

In some ways, it is this confluence of responsibilities, and this opportunity for synergy, that can animate excellence in graduate public health education, which aims to best prepare the next generation of thinkers, leaders, and doers in public health.

The health of populations is a product of our social, economic, and political circumstances, and it is the role of public health to understand how we may best create the environments that generate health in populations while narrowing gaps between health "haves" and "have-nots." This suggests that public health cannot achieve its goals without an engagement in the world, without reckoning with the complex forces that create the circumstances within which we live. This urges public health to be responsive to—and engaged with—the contemporary world even as it aspires to generate knowledge that withstands the test of time.

In many respects, this creates the recipe for a dynamic subject area that can—and should—be appealing to students. Students are, understandably, interested in the contemporary world. They have a vested interest in the world they will inherit and in the conditions that will color their coming decades. That public health is concerned with the same conditions and that public health scholarship aspires to better understand the conditions to improve them—using health as our focus and lever—creates an area of inquiry that is perhaps uniquely attuned to contemporary circumstances and that, similarly, may be uniquely appealing to students.

In much the same way, public health has much to benefit from the responsibility for knowledge translation by universities. Ultimately, the creation of the social, economic, and political conditions that generate health cannot rest on publication in academic journals alone; it must also involve engagement in the tools of cultural conversation and in a full-throated engagement both in communicating these ideas to those who can make change happen and to the general public who influence them. This can and should hold enormous appeal to trainees in public health who are increasingly digital natives but are also, most importantly, concerned with entering a workforce that is responsive to their ideas, interests, and passions.

Therefore, graduate public health education stands, in my estimation, at a propitious time. The discipline rests on scholarship that is responsive to the contemporary world, and the mission of schools of public health is inextricable from an engagement in that same world. Education of the next generation of trainees sits at the heart of, and is synergistic with, both these endeavors.

The question then becomes simple: How does graduate public health education capitalize on the opportunity that this confluence of vision, mission, and circumstance presents and achieve excellence in education?

There have been several movements in recent years that point us in the right direction. The Framing the Future Task Force of the Association of Schools and Programs of Public Health (ASPPH) articulated a vision for a cross-disciplinary, dynamic, graduate public health education that resulted in changes in Council on Education in Public Health (CEPH) criteria for accreditation. These changes are steps in the right direction, offering an opportunity for graduate public health education to transcend disciplinary lines and to embed our educational efforts in the real challenges that public health trainees will grapple with in coming decades.

As a range of schools have been making changes toward achieving these goals, we have, in previous work, suggested three trends that are emerging from synergies between the goals of public health and the responsibilities of academic public health.

First, public health education is authentic and practical, is responsive to contemporary circumstances, and aspires to train students to engage with the current public conversation with the end of creating a world that can generate health. This urges an engagement of our education with cutting-edge scholarship and with the challenges that we face today as a way of informing how students will deal with the challenges they will face in future. This suggests that the opioid epidemic, the obesity epidemic, and immigration policies have to be part of graduate public health education and that students need to learn the scholarship behind these concerns as well as how action may be taken to mitigate their health consequences and how communicating this scholarship is a core part of the action.

Second, public health education is increasingly more inclusive: a big tent that encompasses and engages a range of students who represent both the populations that we serve and that is open to the ideas that such diversity brings to the table. Public health's engagement with a changing world means that we have a central, unshakeable responsibility to ensure that we put diversity and inclusion at the heart of what we do and that we aspire to grapple with the challenges and opportunities that such inclusion offers.

Third, public health education is moving beyond being a time-delimited professional master's training. Public health education must engage trainees over their lifetime (Box 46.1). Although graduate education remains the anchor experience for many, that is simply one experience among many over a lifetime, and it is the responsibility of public health educators to prepare students to be learning always, as well as to create the touchstone opportunities for students to keep refreshing their education over many decades. This recognizes that the world is changing rapidly and that it is unlikely that the problems that students will face when they are leaders in the field in 40 years much resemble those that we are facing today.

## Box 46.1 | CDC Training Programs for the Public Health Pipeline

*Patricia M. Simone, Teresa M Smith, and M. Kathleen Glynn*

The Centers for Disease Control and Prevention (CDC) advances the public health workforce through leadership development and evidence-based training programs. The CDC is committed to achieving the vision of a public health workforce prepared to meet emerging and future challenges.

Our approach to this effort requires the same rigor and comprehensive strategy as any public health challenge. Public health is evolving with advanced methodologies, new data sources, and rapidly changing technology. Training and workforce development strategies must take these changes into account and identify and address needed skills and effective models for learning.[1] For example, even as digital transformation increases the need for technological skills, demand grows for complementary skills in leadership, problem-solving, creativity, and communications.[2] How we train and develop the public health workforce must also evolve and incorporate new educational methods and advances in technology for ready access to lifelong learning.

Achieving effective solutions to the complex problems in public health requires multidisciplinary teams. An interdisciplinary learning model prepares students for collaborative, interprofessional practice. The CDC's Population Health Workforce Initiative is an example of an innovative approach to train fellows while helping health departments build capacity. In this initiative, CDC fellows from different disciplines are assigned as a team to a health department. The fellows find solutions to population health problems identified by and specific to the community by engaging and working collaboratively with experts across disciplines and community sectors (e.g., clinical care, education, public safety.). This model promotes interdisciplinary learning and supports health departments in making progress on complex population health issues.

Fellowships and other training opportunities are proven strategies that develop the workforce. The CDC offers many diverse fellowship, internship, training, and volunteer opportunities for students, graduates, and professionals to develop and enhance their public health science knowledge and skills. These opportunities provide robust on-the-job learning while filling critical gaps in the public health and health care workforce. These opportunities provide students and trainees with invaluable experience and offer paths to exciting careers in public health and health care. (For a complete list of these programs, see www.cdc.gov/fellowships.)

**Fellowships**

- *The Preventive Medicine Residency and Fellowship (PMR/F)* focuses on leadership, management, policy development, and program evaluation in public health and preventive medicine. This program is for veterinarians, nurses, physicians, and other public health professionals (www.cdc.gov/prevmed/index.html).
- *The Population Health Training in Place Program (PH-TIPP)* provides the opportunity for physicians with a master's degree in Public Health to develop population health leadership and management skills through a flexible curriculum based on the participants current work duties, and the program may qualify them for certification in the medical specialty of general preventive medicine and public health (www.cdc.gov/pophealthtraining).
- *The Epidemic Intelligence Service (EIS)* focuses on applying the science of epidemiology to solve public health problems. Candidates who are eligible for this 2-year postgraduate on-the-job training and service program include physicians, veterinarians, doctoral-level scientists, and other public health professionals (www.cdc.gov/eis/).
- *The Laboratory Leadership Service (LLS)* prepares early-career laboratory scientists to become future public health laboratory leaders. This is a 2-year competency-based public health laboratory fellowship with practical, applied investigations (www.cdc.gov/lls/).

- *The Presidential Management Fellows (PMF)* program focuses on leadership and management of public policy and programs for individuals with a masters, law, or doctoral degree. This is a 2-year fellowship program at the CDC that is coordinated with the Office of Personnel Management (OPM) (www.cdc.gov/PMF/).
- *The Public Health Informatics Fellowship Program (PHIFP)* provides training and experience applying computer and information science and technology to public health. This 2-year program is for individuals with at least a master's degree, as well as training and experience in a health-related field and information and computer science and technology (www.cdc.gov/PHIFP/).
- *The Steven M. Teutsch Prevention Effectiveness Fellowship (PEF)* provides an experiential opportunity in quantitative analyses to inform and improve public health policy and program decisions. The 2-year fellowship is for recent doctoral graduates in economics, decision sciences, policy analysis, or a related field (www.cdc.gov/PEF/index.html).
- *The Public Health Associate Program (PHAP)* provides field-based training for early-career public health professionals with little or no public health work experience who are interested in frontline public health practice (www.cdc.gov/PHAP).

## Student Programs

- *The Epidemiology Elective Program for Medical and Veterinary Students* provides a rotation opportunity in applied epidemiology, public health, and global health for medical or veterinary students. During this 6- or 8-week training, students gain hands-on experience and mentoring from CDC subject matter experts (www.cdc.gov/epielective/).

## Learning Opportunities

- *CDC Learning Connection* connects learners to a variety of public health and health care training opportunities developed by the CDC, CDC partners, and other federal agencies to help increase public health knowledge and skills and meet professional development needs. Many of the training opportunities offer continuing education credits (https://tceols.cdc.gov), and these services are free to users (www.cdc.gov/learning/).

## Reference

1. de Beaumont Foundation and the National Consortium for Workforce Development. *Building Skills for a More Strategic Public health Workforce: A Call to Action.* Published by the de Beaumont Foundation. July 18, 2017. https://www.debeaumont.org/wp-content/uploads/Building-Skills-for-a-More-Strategic-Public-Health-Workforce.pdf 1/17/2019
2. Bughin J, Hazan E, Lund S, Dahlstrom P, Wiesinger A, Subramaniam A. *Skill Shift: Automation and the future of the workforce.* McKinsey Global Institute, May, 2018. https://www.mckinsey.com/featured-insights/future-of-organizations-and-work/skill-shift-automation-and-the-future-of-the-workforce. Accessed 1/18/2019.

The good news is that these trends fit quite comfortably with the aspirations of academic institutions. This means that graduate public health training has an opportunity to rise in relevance and prominence within the academic firmament, pointing the way for other fields that are similarly interested in excellence in an education that is grounded in the present, but with an eye to the future. This should, to my mind, fill us with optimism about the promise and potential of academic public health and graduate public health education. I look forward to seeing the innovation in education that will emerge in coming decades and how the field will capitalize on these opportunities.

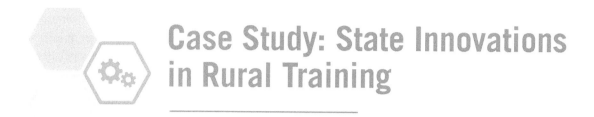

# Chapter 47

# Case Study: State Innovations in Rural Training

### KRISTI MARTINSEN AND MICHELLE GOODMAN

Rural communities are natural test beds for the development and implementation of innovative health care solutions. By virtue of their size, rural communities are often more nimble and able to make changes more quickly when something does not work. Rural health care providers also tend to have a clear understanding of the populations they are working for and are adept at coming up with innovative partnerships to come to the solutions that are needed. Nonetheless, many health care programs developed nationally are geared toward larger, urban areas that, for reasons of resources or workforce availability, cannot simply be implemented on a smaller scale for delivery in rural communities. Rural innovations, however, can be ready examples for larger urban areas.

Although there are similarities between rural communities across the United States, a community's challenges and opportunities in a small rural town in the Northeast will be very different from a rural community's experiences in the Southwest, or in a frontier area in Montana or Alaska. Additionally, economic development and health care are closely interrelated in smaller communities; the hospital is often one of the largest employers, and access to clinicians and health care services is an important consideration for employers and industries who are considering an area in which to start or grow their business.[1]

States, in particular state governments and departments of health, play an integral role in helping rural communities address these challenges through levers such as conducting statewide health needs assessments, developing targeted programs to address primary care and rural training, and undertaking scope of practice and payment system reforms. Many states have been forward thinking in their work to address rural health provider shortages and training needs. A few examples are detailed in the following text. Depending on the existing resources and challenges specific to a state or region, some solutions might prove more applicable than others.

## UNDERSTANDING THE HEALTH NEEDS OF THE COMMUNITY

Eighteen percent of the US population lives in rural communities, and residents of these rural communities tend to be older, poorer, and sicker than their urban counterparts.[2, 3] Rural communities also report a higher proportion of mental illness, serious mental illness, and substance use disorders in their population.[4] Across the United States, non-metropolitan areas have higher rates of mortality.[5] Geographic isolation, lower socioeconomic status, higher rates of underinsurance or lack of insurance, and limited job opportunities contribute to health disparities in rural communities.

In terms of provider supply, the availability of preventative services and access to health care differs across rural and urban areas of the United States. Primary care providers, in particular family physicians, provide the majority of medical care to rural and underserved areas in the United States, especially in small and remote areas.[6] However, residents of non-metropolitan areas are more likely to report less access to health care and lower quality of health care.[7] Primary care physician shortages continue to persist, particularly in rural and other underserved communities.[8] Rural behavioral health issues are complicated by a lack of access to care, and residents of rural areas often face shortages of behavioral health providers.[9] The oral health workforce also continues to face shortages in rural areas.

Beyond understanding these national trends, states can play an important role in gathering the necessary data to inform program and policy decisions and support communities to better understand and quantify their needs. The Center for Rural Health in North Dakota provided resources on strategies for conducting community health needs assessments with hospitals and public health departments, encouraging collaboration between the two facility types. The Center for Rural Health consolidated the data and shared them publicly on a website so that communities could see priorities identified across the state, could easily connect with others working on similar issues, and could see innovative ways that other communities were addressing health needs. Additionally, the website includes resources by topic to help communities develop action plans. Using their position as a facilitator, the state not only eases the burden of this process on individual communities, but the consolidated data also is useful to all state partners (Box 47.1).[10]

## USING EXISTING PROGRAMS TO TARGET PROVIDER TRAINING

The challenges to recruiting and retaining rural health care providers are many. Disproportionate numbers of medical students are choosing to practice in urban rather than rural areas because, in rural areas, salaries tend to be lower, there is cultural and professional isolation, the quality of education and housing is poorer, and spousal job opportunities are lacking.[11] The higher rates

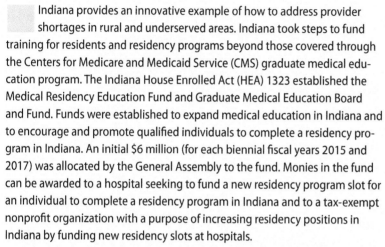

**Box 47.1 | Indiana's Response to Addressing Rural Provider Shortages**

*Eugene Johnson*

Indiana provides an innovative example of how to address provider shortages in rural and underserved areas. Indiana took steps to fund training for residents and residency programs beyond those covered through the Centers for Medicare and Medicaid Service (CMS) graduate medical education program. The Indiana House Enrolled Act (HEA) 1323 established the Medical Residency Education Fund and Graduate Medical Education Board and Fund. Funds were established to expand medical education in Indiana and to encourage and promote qualified individuals to complete a residency program in Indiana. An initial $6 million (for each biennial fiscal years 2015 and 2017) was allocated by the General Assembly to the fund. Monies in the fund can be awarded to a hospital seeking to fund a new residency program slot for an individual to complete a residency program in Indiana and to a tax-exempt nonprofit organization with a purpose of increasing residency positions in Indiana by funding new residency slots at hospitals.

In addition, the Graduate Medical Education Board created Indiana's GME Expansion Plan, which allocates funding to three separate programs to support residency in rural areas, though it is not exclusive to rural areas. Entities receive development or expansion grants for $45,000 for each new residency year, with priority given for residents in primary care or select shortage subspecialties, such as family medicine, outpatient community-based pediatrics, obstetrics/gynecology, psychiatry, emergency medicine, general surgery, or outpatient community-based internal medicine. Up to $75,000 is available to assist an entity explore the feasibility of developing a new residency program in primary care or in a selected shortage specialty (as just listed), and up to $500,000 is available to assist organizations with the investment of setting up a residency program. Priority is given to certain residency specialty programs and to those training residents in rural and underserved regions in the state, as well as for programs that include collaboration with a Federal Qualified Health Center or an Area Health Education Council organization.

of retirement of older rural primary care providers compared to their urban counterparts also adds to rural provider shortages.

Studies indicate that exposure to rural training can increase recruitment and retention; however, the bulk of training continues to take place in urban and suburban areas.[12–13] There is also evidence that physicians who receive training in community and underserved settings are more likely to practice in similar settings.[11,14] A continued focus on training of primary care, oral health, and behavioral health providers in rural communities is paramount to ensuring that there is a more equitable distribution of health care providers in rural communities across the United States. Examples of innovative programs that have taken a "grow your own" approach to addressing provider shortages in rural areas are detailed in the following text.

## Rural Health Career Opportunity Programs

A first step in creating successful health careers in a rural area is to begin exposing younger students, as early as elementary and middle school, to health careers. Arkansas is an example of how a state can help to drive and provide the needed levers for health career training in rural areas; it has more than 40 years of experience with a statewide approach. The Arkansas Area Health Education Center (AHEC), also known as the University of Arkansas for Medical Sciences (UAMS) Regional Programs, was established in 1973 through state law and is partially funded through the Health Resources and Services Administration (HRSA). Although health career opportunity programs are effective, long-term tracking of participants is a challenge. The Arkansas model, providing training along the education continuum, makes tracking participants from early entry (high school) to residency easier. One of their signature programs, Medical Applications of Science for Health (M*A*S*H), includes a 2-week intensive summer health career program for high school students to interact with a wide variety of health professionals and participate in hands-on activities. During the M*A*S*H program, students are identified and paired with regional recruiters who help to track and retain students in the long-term by investing in personal relationships, ongoing support, advising, and coaching. In fact, 30% of school of medicine students entering classes in the past 2 years were students who had been coached by M*A*S*H recruiters.[15]

## Rural Medical Education

An important next step in rural health care careers is to expose students to rural medical training experiences. As previously mentioned, students who are from rural areas or who have had a positive experience in a rural community tend to return to rural areas to practice. However, many students may not have the tools or opportunities to be able to have such rural experiences.

The UAMS Regional Programs initiative described earlier also has an innovative approach to rural medical education by recruiting, retaining, and training students in an Arkansas medical school by applying a holistic admissions process that gives preference to Arkansas students and offering preceptorships and field placements in rural settings. The Arkansas State Legislature mandates that a majority of each class admitted to UAMS be distributed equally among Arkansas's four congressional districts, and medical school admission preference is given to students from Arkansas. Recruiters are a key component to the success of this program, staying connected with students throughout their educational training and clinical rotations to ensure that they have the support needed to succeed (given that many of these students may be the first in their families to go to medical school). The state legislature, as well as foundations and health insurers, also fund loans and scholarships to incentivize medical students and residents to practice in rural areas of the state. The program has shown great results: of all former graduates, 64% remained in Arkansas, and 37% of those are practicing in small towns and rural counties.[16]

Another example of a program that has been successful in providing these opportunities to medical students is the Washington, Wyoming, Alaska, Montana, Idaho (WWAMI) Regional Medical Education model, which is a regional collaboration to address provider shortage challenges in this group of frontier states. WWAMI states cover 25% of the United States land mass but contain only 4% of the US population, and the training programs stretch over 3,000 miles. To train and prepare physicians to care for patients and communities throughout these states, WWAMI students receive foundational training from universities within their home states and clinical training at the University of Washington School of Medicine. This program is successful overall in that the majority of the students in the program stay to practice medicine in the five-state region.

To address the provider shortage challenges within rural communities, the WWAMI Regional Medical Education program operates three specific workforce programs for rural medical education. The oldest of the programs is the Rural/Underserved Opportunities Program (RUOP), a 4-week elective after the first year of medical school, in which students live in rural and urban underserved communities throughout WWAMI states and work side by side with local physicians providing health care to underserved populations. This program is designed to give the largest number of students a taste of rural medical practice and to spark interest in rural medicine. WWAMI's Rural Integrated Training Experience (WRITE) is designed to give third-year medical students a 20-week clinical education experience at a rural primary care teaching site and to provide students with an opportunity to learn how community health care systems function. Finally, the Targeted Rural Underserved Track (TRUST), the newest of the programs, provides a continuous connection between underserved communities, medical education, and health professionals in the WWAMI region and taps into the already established RUOP and WRITE. Students are picked specifically based on their likelihood of going back to rural areas. Each state in the WWAMI region picks its own students, who are matched to a community. TRUST scholars return to this same community before medical school, during the first 18 months of medical school, after the first year (for the 4-week RUOP program), and then, finally, for the WRITE program as a third-year student.

## Rural Residency Programs

The final step of ensuring an adequate supply of health care providers in rural communities, especially rural physicians, is to continue residency rotations in rural communities. Both of the programs described earlier are part of the larger group of Rural Training Tracks (RTTs)—schools nationwide with programs designed to give undergraduate- and graduate-level students practice experience at rural clinics and hospitals. Currently, nine schools of medicine are located in rural areas, and 39 medical schools have an RTT or pathway for students to train at rural sites.[17] As states think about addressing potential provider shortages, they may want to consider supporting or enhancing RTT programs (Box 47.2).

The HRSA funded a project to create an RTT Collaborative to bring RTT programs from across the country to network together, receive guidance in ways to strengthen their programs, and provide additional financial support to make it more feasible for students to participate in rural rotations. Funding for travel to interviews and stipends for housing can make a difference in a student's ability to take on a rural rotation. Although funding has ended, the RTT Collaborative continues as an online resource to share ideas of what has worked to make programs successful, share resources for schools and communities on getting new programs up and running, and act as a forum to develop an offline network of support for existing and new programs (Box 47.3).

## INTERSECTION OF PUBLIC HEALTH AND PRIMARY CARE

Given rural provider shortages, many states and communities are using innovative models that tap into existing community members to help improve the health of a population. A strong and well-trained public health workforce is integral to a state's success in addressing disparities in rural health outcomes. The following examples include models that use community lay workers to expand access to care and expand the scope of duties of emergency medical professionals and the use technology to increase public health training.

## Box 47.3 | HRSA's Teaching Health Centers Graduate Medical Education Program

The Health Resources and Services Administration's (HRSA) Teaching Health Centers Graduate Medical Education (THCGME) program began in 2010 as a new model for graduate medical education focused on primary care physician and dentist training in a team-based ambulatory care setting. The program aims to bolster the primary care workforce through support for new and expanded primary care and dental residency programs, as well as to improve the distribution of this workforce into needed areas through emphasis on underserved communities and populations. THCGME is, in most respects, an entirely different model for resident education from most other federal models of GME, which are mostly located in large, urban academic medical centers. In addition to increasing the number of primary care residents training in these community-based patient care settings, the THCGME program seeks to increase health care quality and overall access to care. In academic year 2017–2018, the THCGME program supported the training of 732 residents in 57 primary care residency programs, 12 of which are located in rural communities (https://bhw.hrsa.gov/).

## Community Health Workers

Community health worker (CHW) models engage existing community members to help extend health promotion and prevention activities from a medical setting by using trusted members of the community to achieve better population health. Although most states have activities that include community health workers, many are funded either at the state or community level through grant funding, which may not be sustainable. To address sustainability issues, some states have started to include payment for CHW services as part of their Medicaid state programs. For example, the Michigan Medicaid Managed Care contract requires a ratio of at least one full-time CHW per 20,000 covered lives, and Texas Medicaid Managed Care contract allows for CHW costs to be included as administrative costs (Box 47.4).[18]

An example of a how CHWs engage at the community level is the Health Coaches for Hypertension Control program, which addresses a population of older adults with issues of hypertension in rural Appalachia in South Carolina, where hypertension rates are higher than state and national averages. These health coaches received training via a basic hypertension education course for 8 weeks, with an optional additional 8-week session to provide education related to nutrition and physical activity. After the completion of the course, the number of patients meeting the definition for having controlled hypertension increased by 25%, which indicates significant success of the program for helping patients control their hypertension. This program started in 2010 through one of HRSA's Rural Health Outreach Grants and has continued with US Department of Agriculture funding and other funding through Clemson University Cooperative Extension.[19]

**Box 47.4 | Rural Health Information Hub**

The Health Resources and Services Administration (HRSA) funds the Rural Health Information Hub: a one-stop shop for information on funding, policies, programs, and resources specific to rural health and human services. A key feature is free Community Health Gateway toolkits designed from models that work in rural communities and available to help communities implement strategies to improve the health of their residents. In addition to a toolkit on community health workers, there are toolkits on community health, aging in place, diabetes care management, obesity, health promotion and disease prevention, mental health, HIV/AIDS, food access, transportation, and serving patients with disabilities (www.ruralhealthinfo.org/community-health).

## Expanding the Scope of Emergency Medical Professionals

Another strategy that has been effective in meeting rural health care needs is expanding the scope of emergency medical technicians (EMTs) or paramedics. Increasing the use of emergency medical professionals to treat those patients with chronic disease who are most likely to visit emergency departments can significantly reduce the costs of care. Emergency medical service (EMS) systems in rural areas experience many resource and infrastructure challenges, including lower patient volumes, greater distances, and a larger proportion of volunteer-based systems of care. Community paramedicine can be a solution to strengthen the rural EMS system and to address rural population health issues.

Many communities have adopted community paramedicine programs, mainly through grant funding. In some cases, hospital-owned ambulance services support programs through savings from reduced hospital readmissions. As a state-driven solution, in 2012, Minnesota implemented a legislative change so that community paramedics can operate under an expanded scope of practice and bill Medicaid. Community paramedics in Minnesota can do health assessments, chronic disease monitoring and education, immunizations and vaccinations, and laboratory specimen collection. Minnesota has also developed a training curriculum including 14 credits and clinic hours.[20] The Minnesota model is also seen as a method for retention, formalizing professional development that advances the provider from the designation of emergency responder to EMT and community paramedic.

## Technology in Public Health Training

Finally, a strong and well-trained primary care and public health workforce is integral to a state's success in addressing the multiple variables that influence disparities in health care outcomes in rural communities. HRSA's Regional Public Health Training Centers (PHTC) program seeks to tap into new and innovative ways of providing public health training and education to states and regions across the United States, developing resources and tailoring curricula based on local health needs assessments. The program aims to establish and enhance collaborative partnerships among state and local health departments, primary care providers, and other nontraditional partners as they work together to address critical local public health needs.

A successful PHTC model that has provided such training to rural communities across the mountain states is the Rocky Mountain PHTC, housed at the Colorado School of Public Health and using technology to deliver training to providers where they are, instead of having them travel for training. RMPHTC supports training for the public health workforce in the six-state region of Colorado, Utah, Wyoming, Montana, and North and South Dakota, and it works in collaboration with several organizations to develop, market, deliver, and evaluate a wide range of training based on current needs and public health trends. The RMPHTC has adapted the Project ECHO (Extension for Community Healthcare Outcomes) health care model for public health training, using the ECHO learning principles of creating and supporting peer-learning networks connected by live bidirectional video and employing a case-based learning approach. Topics are identified and evaluated for their fit with core ECHO model elements: peer learning and sharing, multidisciplinary panel perspectives, value of technology, and content compatibility with short didactics. ECHO courses typically include 15 learners connecting on video group sessions every 2–4 weeks for six to eight sessions (which typically last 60–90 minutes). A topic expert delivers a short, 15-minute presentation, with the remainder of the session dedicated to case presentation and discussion. Current ECHO courses focus on Local Health Agency Quality Improvement, Patient Navigation and Community Health Workers, Obesity Prevention, Tobacco Control, Foodborne Outbreak Investigations, Tuberculosis Management, and HIV Prevention (Box 47.5).[21]

---

### Box 47.5 | Project ECHO

Project ECHO (Extension for Community Healthcare Outcomes) was started by Dr. Sanjeev Arora at the University of New Mexico as a way to provide access to video training with specialists for rural primary care physicians so they could better to treat their patients with hepatitis C. This innovative model has since spread all over the country and for an increasing number of training sessions (e.g., opioids, mental health, chronic diseases). This model links up specialists (the hub) to any number of primary care providers (the spokes) for either training about a specific topic or for discussing particular cases. Not only does it help patients to receive more specialized care within their own communities, it can also help primary care providers in smaller rural communities feel less isolated (https://echo.unm.edu).

## CONCLUSION

The examples outlined in this chapter are intended to give the reader a glimpse into initiatives and programs that assess community needs, address provider shortages in rural areas, and continue to bring a population health focus to the systems of care in rural areas, given provider shortages. As state-level players are thinking about workforce challenges, these examples highlight the benefit of tapping into innovations from rural communities and the importance of considering the unique assets and challenges in developing solutions for rural health care delivery.

### REFERENCES

1. Doeksen, GA, St. Clair, CF, Eilrich, FC. Economic Impact of Rural Health Care. National Center for Rural Health Works. October 2016. http://ruralhealthworks. org/wp-content/files/Summary-Economic-Impact-Rural-Health-FINAL-100716. pdf. Accessed 1/18/2019.

2. US Department of Health and Human Services, Health Resources and Services Administration. Mortality and life expectancy in rural America: connecting the health and human service safety nets to improve health outcomes over the life course. 2015. https://www.hrsa.gov/advisorycommittees/rural/publications/ mortality.pdf. Accessed 1/18/2019.

3. Kusmin L. *Rural America at a Glance*, 2015 edition. Economic Information Bulletin No. (EIB-145). Washington, DC: US Department of Agriculture; 2015.

4. Rural Health Reform Policy Research Center. The 2014 Update of the Rural-Urban Chartbook. 2014. https://www.ruralhealthresearch.org/publications/940. Accessed 1/18/2019.

5. Moy E, Garcia MC, Bastian B, et al. Leading causes of death in nonmetropolitan and metropolitan areas—United States, 1999–2014. *MMWR Surveill Summ* 2017;66(SS-1):1–8. doi:http://dx.doi.org/10.15585/mmwr.ss6601a1. Accessed 1/18/ 2019.

6. Chen FM, Andrilla CHA, Doescher MP, Morris C. Family medicine residency training in rural locations. Final Report #126. WWAMI Rural Health Research Center, University of Washington. 2010. http://depts.washington.edu/uwrhrc/ uploads/RHRC_ FR126_Chen.pdf. Accessed August 27, 2015.

7. Agency for Healthcare Research and Quality. National Healthcare Quality and Disparities Report hartbook on rural health care. 2017: AHRQ Pub. No. 17(18)-0001-2-EF. Department of Health and Human Services. City Rockville, MD. https:// www.ahrq.gov/sites/default/files/wysiwyg/research/findings/nhqrdr/chartbooks/ qdr-ruralhealthchartbook-update.pdf. Accessed 1/18/2019.

8. US Department of Health and Human Services, Health Resources and Services Administration. National and regional projections of supply and demand for primary care practitioners: 2013–2025. November 2016. https://bhw.hrsa.gov/sites/ default/files/bhw/health-workforce-analysis/research/projections/primary-care-national-projections2013-2025.pdf. Accessed 1/18/2019.

9. Larson EH, Patterson DG, Garberson LA, Andrilla CHA. *Supply and Distribution of the Behavioral Health Workforce in Rural America. Data Brief #160*. Seattle, WA: WWAMI Rural Health Research Center, University of Washington; September 2016.

10. Center for Rural Health, University of North Dakota. https://ruralhealth.und.edu/projects/community-health-needs-assessment. Accessed February 21, 2018.

11. Mc-Ellistrem-Evenson A. Informing rural primary care workforce policy: What does the evidence tell us?: A review of rural health research center literature, 2000–2010. Rural Health Research Gateway. 2011. https://www.ruralhealthinfo.org/assets/1145-4634/informing-rural-primary-care-workforce-policy.pdf. Accessed 1/18/2019

12. Rabinowitz H, Diamond J, Markham F, Wortman J. Medical school programs to increase the rural physician supply: A systematic review and projected impact of widespread replication. *Acad Med*. 2008;83(3):235–43.

13. Patterson DG, Schmitz D, Longenecker R, Andrilla CHA. *Family Medicine Rural Training Track Residencies: 2008–2015 Graduate Outcomes*. Seattle: WWAMI Rural Health Research Center, University of Washington. February 2016.

14. Phillips RL, Petterson S, Bazemore, A. Do residents who train in safety net settings return for practice? *Acad Med*. 2013;88(12):1934–40.

15. US Department of Health and Human Services, Health Resources and Services Administration, Bureau of Health Workforce. Workforce Grand Rounds. November 2017. Strengthening the rural health workforce: Tools, resources and outcomes. https://bhw.hrsa.gov/grants/technicalassistance/grand-rounds-webinarseries. Accessed February 28, 2018.

16. University of Arkansas for Medical Sciences (UAMS) Regional Program. Regional Programs Annual Report (2016–2017). http://regionalprograms.uams.edu/files/2015/06/2017_REP_AnnualReport_FINAL_Nov27.pdf. Accessed: March 1, 2018.

17. The Rural Training Track Collaborative. Rural programs. https://rttcollaborative.net/rural-programs/. Accessed March 1, 2018.

18. National Association of State Health Policy. Community health worker models 2017. https://nashp.org/state-community-health-worker-models/. Accessed February 21, 2018.

19. Rural Health Information Hub. Health coaches for hypertension control. 2017. https://www.ruralhealthinfo.org/community-health/project-examples/753. Accessed February 22, 2013.

20. Minnesota State Department of Health. Community paramedics. http://www.health.state.mn.us/divs/orhpc/workforce/emerging/cp/index.html. Accessed February 26, 2018.

21. Scallan E, Davis S, Thomas F, et al. Supporting peer learning networks for case-based learning in public health: Experience of the Rocky Mountain Public Health Training Center with the ECHO Training Model. *Pedagogy in Health Promotion*. 2017;3(1):52S–58S.

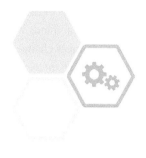

# Chapter 48

# Better Together: Engaging Nursing Leaders in Community Collaborative Efforts

ANH N. TRAN AND ANNE DEROUIN

The evidence supporting partnership between public health and health care systems has been overwhelming, and the movement to build partnerships through efforts such as *The Practical Playbook* has demonstrated effective and positive change. The first edition of this book highlighted the tremendous opportunities to improve health by connecting public health and primary care providers, using data to understand the social determinants of health and gaps in care, and bringing other services together to improve overall health of communities, as recommended by the Institute of Medicine (IOM) in 2010.[1] The energy to bring public health providers, physicians, and community leaders to the table has been substantial; this momentum is impacting communities across the nation to improve health. To sustain this trend and have an even larger impact in the future, it's become increasingly evident that a key member of the health care team has all too often been absent from the conversation and must join the table: the nurse.

## WHERE HAVE THE NURSES BEEN?

As the largest segment of the health care workforce, and for more than a decade the "most trusted" professional in the nation and member of the health care team,[2] one might wonder why nurses haven't been consistently at the decision-making table from the beginning of the integration evolution. There are many possible answers to this question, but the most likely is that they have been busy delivering day-by-day, moment-by-moment care, compassion, and education to patients, families, and communities. The truth is, however, that in most health care systems, nurses simply have not been invited to the table. They have been the invisible, but necessary, member of the health care decision-making team: carrying out many innovative solutions to the health care crisis and being the sounding board for patient or community response to many efforts. Professional nurses serve on the front lines of every health care arena as an army of health care providers who provide the critical link for most changes that are proposed, implemented, and evaluated; they are the "glue" between patients and caregivers, physicians, researchers, public health officials, and community resources. The role that nurses have historically played has been that of servant leader, sometimes the "champion" rather than the health care integration decision-maker. Because of their unique position of trust with the public and their integration into each health care delivery team, *The Practical Playbook* call to add more chairs to the decision-making table in the first edition could not have resonated more loudly for professional nurses.

## PROMPTING LEADERSHIP FOR NURSES

Nurses have a long history of community engagement to address social determinants of health. Consider the pioneer, Florence Nightingale, who famously used epidemiology skills and scientific knowledge to improve hygienic conditions in health care settings during the Crimean War. In the United States, other pioneer nurses, such as Lillian Wald (who coined the term "public health nursing") led efforts to improve living conditions in tenement houses that contributed to significant morbidity and mortality in New York City.[3] Wald believed that nurses were responsible for addressing social and economic problems, not just caring for the sick. Mary Breckenridge was a nurse midwife who traveled by horseback to provide health care to women and children living in rural Kentucky. She later founded the Frontier School of Nursing,[4] still active today in preparing nurses and advanced practice nurses to provide community-focused health care that is culturally sensitive to promote the health and well-being of families, women, and children. Clara Barton, another famous nurse and humanist, worked to organize relief efforts during wars and countless national crises. Her advocacy ultimately led to the establishment of the Red Cross—which continues to provide emergency response care, often through nursing care and coordinated community resources—that supports and reduces the risk of negative health consequences among communities facing natural and man-made disasters. These historic nurse leaders often deflected their fame, emphasizing that collaboration with other stakeholders was critical to promoting public safety and reducing social conditions that posed risks to health; they are typically depicted through images of service at the frontlines with individuals and in community, rather than as individual icons.

Although the public health focus of professional nursing practice, illustrated by these historic nursing figures, remains central to delivery of care, the trend of nurses serving solely "in the trenches" is evolving. More and more nursing professionals are being tapped to share their intimate wisdom of patient care issues as well as to act as sounding boards, innovators, and creative thinkers and to act as leaders and change agents, working collaboratively with the public and primary care health providers to improve health care systems and patient outcomes. The greatest push for nursing leadership was prompted by physician colleagues at the IOM who published *The Future of Nursing* report (2011). This report, along with recommendations from the American Association of Colleges of Nursing (AACN)[5] and other national organizations, calls for expanded opportunities for nurses at all levels to serve as leaders within the health care setting. The IOM also urges nurses to design, implement, and evaluate improvements to current health systems and to disseminate successful attempts in transforming practices.

## INFLUENCE OF NURSING ACADEMIA

Though lagging, partnership and collaboration with public and primary care providers is a natural fit for nurses: all are educated in foundations of both public health and medical concepts, thus preparing them to work with patients and health systems of all kinds, ranging from critical care to community health centers (Figure 48.1). Nurses at the front lines of patient care delivery are educated in epidemiology, surveillance of disease, social determinants of health concepts that impact patient outcomes, provision of patient education, and clinical procedures and techniques across health care settings. They are also knowledgeable of scientific concepts including pathophysiology, pharmacology, nutrition, disease processes, and evidence-based practice. Advanced-practice nurses (those with graduate degrees [MSNs]) possess advanced knowledge and skills in health care leadership, advocacy, and the management of patients and populations—abilities that have typically been built on years of clinical expertise. Nurses with doctorate degrees (PhD or Doctor of Nursing Practice [DNP])

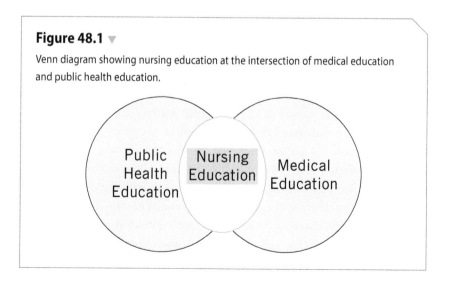

**Figure 48.1** ▼

Venn diagram showing nursing education at the intersection of medical education and public health education.

are experts in their focused topics or populations of study and have gained basic skills in technology, health care finance and management techniques, program planning, public policy, and quality improvement techniques, including evaluation strategies as well as analysis and dissemination of results. Despite knowledge bases similar to those of other health care professionals and common service-leadership goals to provide effective health care, nurses have historically been missing from many decision-making conversations about how to improve health systems through innovation to meet the care needs of communities, especially those with the greatest need.

Although the IOM report spurred meaningful action among national nursing leaders as well as dialogue with medical providers and policymakers that led to nurse leadership programming and investment of resources, the *initial* collaborations among the public health, primary care, and nursing communities was occurring quietly at many academic health systems. Nurses in academic leadership roles who were respected within their institution, such as deans of nursing programs housed among academic health centers, were among the first nursing professionals to effectively open lines of communication with their physician colleagues. Through the natural intersection of routine meetings that occur on campuses, skilled deans of nursing used this unique opportunity to promote trust and confidence between physician colleagues and academic leaders by offering thoughtful and valuable nursing insight at the decision-making tables. The results of these influential efforts led to the implementation of nurse-led community health initiatives, such as neighborhood health fairs, flu shot clinics delivered by nursing students, and school-based health clinics. All of these are considered *community-led practices* and are supported by academic partners. These efforts use the advanced-practice clinical skills of nurse faculty members (the effort is considered a part of their workload), community resources, and primary care ideology to that ensure that vulnerable populations receive care. The results of the early nurse academic leaders have been a win-win for both health care learners (academia) and community; faculty at schools of nursing enjoy applying their clinical expertise to primary care patient settings, ensuring that their certification and licensure remain active and that they are current in evidence-based practice, while community members benefit from affordable and accessible care. Most of these projects are also evaluated so that the results of the efforts are disseminated to community partners as well as to professional journals and presentations so that efforts can be replicated in other communities.

Nurse-led clinical partnerships, led by innovative nurse leaders, have proved to be effective in not only providing vital clinical services to underserved communities, but also in offering fertile opportunity for collaboration among health innovators (telemedicine), public health researchers (evaluation of integrative care, such as coaching circles, group medical visits, school-based health promotion for adolescents, and population-focused innovations for children with chronic conditions, including asthma and obesity), and community, state, and federal policymakers (reducing school absenteeism and violence as well as improving access to care across communities through funding additional community centers in underserved neighborhoods). In addition, many of the nurse-led innovations of the past decade have led to *interprofessional educational* (IPE) opportunities for a wide variety of health professional students, including those in public health, mental health, social work, medicine, and pharmacy, as well as physician assistants in training.

## INFLUENCE OF PROFESSIONAL ORGANIZATIONS

Following the IOM report and mounting evidence from academic nurse leaders demonstrating successful nurse-led models of collaborative care to address public health needs, professional nursing organizations and philanthropic health care businesses seeking partnership with nurses established leadership programs specially designed to build communication skills and confidence for nurses to lead health care innovations; this also underlined a full-fledged call to improve health outcomes through collaboration. Examples of successful nurse leadership training programs include efforts at national-level professional nursing associations, including the American Association of Colleges of Nursing (AACN) and the American Association of Nurse Practitioners (AANP), as well as at state-level associations. Promotion of nurse leadership has also occurred through funded programs, such as the Duke – Johnson & Johnson Nurse Leadership program. The program offers leadership and management training to advanced practice nurses who are committed to serving vulnerable populations, many of whom provide primary care services. The program aims to equip advanced practice nurses with the skills and competencies needed to lead health care teams to improved patient and community health outcomes, especially given the shortage and uneven distribution of primary care providers across the country.[6] All program fellows conduct a population-focused health improvement innovation in conjunction with a local partner agency. Currently hosting its sixth cohort of nurse leaders, the program boasts more than 130 individual nurse-led innovations that have impacted health outcomes in communities across the nation. The following are only a few of the many examples of health improvement initiatives born from this program.

* A project aimed to transform childhood obesity health education delivery for underserved families by merging health professionals with community partners to create an opportunity for healthy lifestyle education. The project was designed to empower families to develop sustainable health habits by providing innovative health education on obesity prevention with the use of children's literature (a book written by the nurse practitioner), as well as collaborating with community resources and local school system summer programs.

- A project aimed to improve the breadth of services offered at a nonprofit, free community health clinic by (1) increasing the breadth of patient services without having to develop new service lines and (2) providing these services in a budget-neutral manner as much as possible through the development of a replicable model using "service swaps." The project focused on leveraging community partnerships through reactivation of a dormant free clinic coalition and developing "service swaps" between clinics, which allowed stakeholders to more efficiently and comprehensively serve patients in the community.
- A project centered on the creation and implementation of the statewide chlamydia and gonorrhea screening program in one state's juvenile justice system (JJS) facilities after the state legislature approved funding. Entities involved in this project include nurses employed at a college of nursing (CON) and elsewhere within the JJS, JJS administration, CON administration, state and local health departments, and the state laboratory.
- A project focused on developing a resource center for adults with Down syndrome (DS) in association with an adult DS specialty clinic in the local area. Goals achieved included (1) developing a searchable, online resource that families and friends could peruse to find resources for an adult with DS; (2) approval by the local university medical center to host a condition-specific patient resource website; and (3) initiation of a conversation by a health system to raise awareness about the adult DS specialty clinic.
- A project that examined the billable services and actual reimbursement for perinatal services at a large, urban Federally Qualified Health Center (FQHC) to better understand the financial challenges of providing comprehensive perinatal services in this setting. The findings of this analysis helped to create a comprehensive, community-responsive model of perinatal services in an FQHC setting that is financially sustainable.

The leaderships skills promoted in both academic and leadership training programs consistently implore nurses to build collaborative partnerships with public health and primary care providers to improve the health outcomes of populations or communities

## NURSES NOW

Although professional nurses will continue to serve at the bedside of patients and families in their most vulnerable moments, they have also begun to use their advocacy and leadership skills to make positive changes and offer solutions to the challenges and choices that patients, families, and communities face in our evolving health care system. With intimate clinical knowledge and well-established trusting relationships among populations, nurses serve as a barometer for the impact that any proposed health care delivery innovation poses.

Nurses are on the forefront of community-wide health improvement initiatives through quality improvement efforts and nurse-led clinics. They have also begun to impact legislative and policy efforts at state and federal levels, serving in political office and advising lawmakers through commissions, task forces, city councils, and school boards. The Nurses on Boards Coalition (https://www.nursesonboardscoalition.org/about /), an Internet resource, is readily available for organizations seeking professional nursing collaborators, and nursing organizations, school of nursing alumni associations, and state or professional nursing organizations are excellent resources for community health innovation teams to locate a nurse for their improvement efforts. Simply asking other key stakeholders at the decision-making table about a local nursing expert will usually result in a well-trusted colleague and nursing professional who would welcome an opportunity to hear the issues, share insights, and thoughtfully collaborate with the team to promote innovations to improve health systems and population health outcomes.

Nurses invited to the decision-making table have unique opportunities to use the same leadership and communication skills that contribute to effective health care delivery in acute, chronic, outpatient, and community settings. Once at the table, nurses establish trust through careful listening and attentiveness to the social cues of the team members, attempting to understand the viewpoint of each stakeholder in a thoughtful way, and sharing unbiased information. Rather than suggesting being overlooked or left out of prior decision-making in the past, nurses joining other decision-makers can demonstrate value by agreeing to serve a designated term on the board after understanding the responsibilities and requirements for service. Nursing insight can be thoughtfully shared during board meetings using short and relevant impact stories of patient care delivery and outcomes. Other leadership habits that all nurses routinely use, such as team-based goal setting, efficient and timely completion of assigned tasks, and analyzing data carefully, lead to valuable leadership contributions and positive outcomes.

Although nurses are invaluable to the delivery of effective care to patients, they are equally willing to work with an interdisciplinary team to improve the health outcomes of communities and populations. Nurses are prepared, ready, and willing to lead and serve with others to guide population health innovations; they may be the key voice in promoting trust and ensuring consistency so that the impact of the innovation can be fully realized.

## REFERENCES

1. Institute of Medicine. *A Summary of the February 2010 Forum on the Future of Nursing: Education.* Washington, DC: The National Academies Press; 2010. https://doi.org/10.17226/12894. Accessed 1/18/19

2. Brenan M. Nurses keep healthy lead as most honest, ethical profession. 2017. https://news.gallup.com. Accessed 1/18/19

3. Fee E, Bu L. Origins of public health nursing: The Henry Street visiting nurse service. *Am J Public Health*. 2010;100(7);1206–7. doi:10.2105/AJPH.2009.186049.

4. Frontier Nursing University. About Frontier Nursing University. https://frontier.edu/about-frontier/. Accessed 1/18/19

5. American Association of Colleges of Nursing. Creating a more qualified nursing workforce. 2015. http://www.aacn.nche.edu/media-relations/fact-sheets/nursing-workforce. Accessed 1/18/19

6. US Department of Health and Human Services, Health Resources and Services Administration, National Center for Health Workforce Analysis. The future of the nursing workforce: National- and state-level projections, 2012–2025. Rockville, Maryland; 2014. https://bhw.hrsa.gov/sites/default/files/bhw/nchwa/projections/nursingprojections.pdf. Accessed 1/18/19

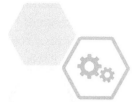

# Chapter 49

# Voices of the Next Generation

ELIZABETH CORCORAN, SARAH LAFAVE, DENNY FE GARCIA AGANA,
HALEIGH KAMPMAN, JOHN C. PENNER, MARGARET L. MCCARTHY,
KATHERINE P. MULLINS, MICHELLE VU, AND ASHTEN DUNCAN

## OVERVIEW

ELIZABETH CORCORAN

The public health workforce is a diverse team of professionals, including doctors, health educators, epidemiologists, activists, nurses, policymakers, scientists, physician assistants, and especially public health practitioners. The training backgrounds of these professionals is even more diverse, deriving from social work, public policy programs, clinical training, public health professional education, and even business schools. This diversity is a strength of the interdisciplinary field of public health, especially as we look toward a future where primary care, public health, and all health professionals work together to share the responsibility of health improvement with other sectors. However, this ideal future—where health is a shared value and a cross-sector pursuit—is not a guarantee. The workforce can only do what it is prepared to do, so there must be an intentional integration of the movement for cross-sector partnerships into the youngest members of the workforce.

Fortunately, young health students and graduates like myself are already bringing their entrepreneurial, interdisciplinary vision to their work and training. Listening to the voices of students and their perspectives on the health professions can propel us even further down the path toward population health improvement. Young people have an exciting approach to our governing systems: "Millennials do not want to destroy the system, nor do they accept it. They want to recreate it."[1] This proves true in the health field. Health students don't need to be converted to framing health in the social determinants; we are already believers. Health students don't need to be adjusted to innovations in technology and data use; we are already using and creating them. Health students don't need to be convinced that policy- and system-level changes are the answers to entrenched health disparities; we care deeply about social and systems change. Finally, health students are already looking for ways to break down silos between health professions through cross-sector partnerships. All of these characteristics are reflected by the following essays submitted by students and graduates across the country as a part of New Voices essay contest, sponsored by the de Beaumont Foundation and the Practical Playbook. This essay contest was launched to gather perspectives from students and recent graduates from the spectrum of health and health-related fields, especially as regards how they plan to work in cross-sector partnerships. Integrating the assets and voices of young workers into the rich experience of those who came before will ensure a future where cross-sector population health improvement is the new norm.

Our young writers include pharmacy students, students in medical training, public health students, epidemiologists, and combinations among these. Their essays highlight partnerships between employment services, public health departments, nonprofits, clinics, family medicine, and various social services. Each applies his or her experience in partnerships to an optimistic vision for a transformed health system where health is created outside of service delivery and supported by partnerships of all shapes and sizes. These students and recent graduates are not satisfied with the silos of their professions. Many are working to break down boundaries and form new paths to improve population health. Capitalizing on this energy is key to bending the entire health field toward partnerships for healthy populations. However, the engagement of young workers is not always a guarantee. Intentional succession planning is required in all health professions, to guide young students and workers to build on the movements already under way in population health.

### REFERENCE

1. Saratobsky KD, Feldmann D. *Cause for Change: The Why and How of Nonprofit Millennial Engagement.* New York: Jossey-Bass/Wiley; 2013.

## ENVISIONING A NEW SYSTEM

SARAH LAFAVE

I knock again on the doorframe, harder this time, and the storm door rattles. A few minutes later, an elderly man with wildly uncombed white hair cracks the door. "Not a good time, honey. We've got a problem here." He does not remember that we have met many times before, and it takes a minute to convince him that I am here to help. Cartons of Ensure tumble over a neglected basket of knitting in the dim hallway. I find Anna sitting on the far edge of the bed, her head in the palm of a paper-thin hand. I unkink the tubing connected to her oxygen concentrator and silence the alarm on her feeding pump; she and I both sigh with relief as the high-pitched beeping dissipates. I go to sit with her on the bed and realize the source of the stench in the room. Her ostomy bag has burst, its contents leaking onto the sheets and her rose-colored nightgown.

The situation I walked in on that day was not a medical problem, nor a nursing problem, nor a public health problem: it was a symptom of system failure. The home health care agency had not yet processed the referral from the skilled nursing facility by the time Anna was discharged. She was unable to open the ostomy bag with her arthritic fingers, and her husband became frustrated and confused when he attempted to the job. Her primary care physician had yet to be notified that she had even left the hospital. No one was responsible for helping Anna and her husband to maintain their home while she recovered, or for considering the implications of the couple's lack of transportation on their health. Months later, Anna's daughter would wonder aloud to me why she had urged her 96-year-old mother to pursue the complicated (and expensive) surgery: she did not know there were palliative options that could have improved her mother's quality of life.

Lori's Hands clients are older adults living with chronic illness. In their homes, I see the jarring consequences of a broken health care system that is too often disconnected from the social services system and from the communities in which our clients live. Real solutions to these challenges exist, but they will take cross-sectoral, system-level ideas.

I founded Lori's Hands as an undergraduate, naming it after my mother. My mom Lori lived with breast cancer for 8 years before dying in 2003. I saw how difficult her journey with chronic illness was despite her many financial and social resources. Our Lori's Hands students provide nonmedical in-home support to community members living in their own homes with chronic illness. The program helps students understand the challenges facing the chronically ill beyond the walls of a sterile clinical environment. One of our clients, Colleen, calls the ambulance at least once a month when she has trouble transferring from the toilet back to her motorized wheelchair. Her insurance benefits cover the expensive emergency paramedic support but do not cover routine in-home care. Another client, Gary, has diabetes and has had multiple strokes. On the evenings when the students (whom he calls his "sous chefs") are not there, he eats a sodium-laced microwaveable meal.

> The last decades of many of our clients' lives are stressful and undignified because our system is too large and too siloed to be self-aware. I believe that a system-wide shift toward coordinated, community-based care will improve health outcomes and result in cost savings, particularly in the care of vulnerable older adults. This shift will require the health care system to more effectively partner with trusted social services partners in the context of patients' "real lives" in community. Often, the health care system and the social services system see each other as external resources to list in a client's file or to refer clients to with a pamphlet and a phone number. What if we could transition to a system in which the two

entities see each other as equals, sit around the table together to partner in the care of our most vulnerable community members, and work so seamlessly that a patient hardly notices where one's services end and the other's begin? I have seen it happen, and I have seen the impact it makes on quality of life and health outcomes for patients. Over the past couple of years, a social worker at the local hospital has become a consistent referral source to Lori's Hands. When we share a client, this social worker goes the extra mile to keep the client's Lori's Hands students informed (with patient consent) when the client's health status or needs change. She also invites communication from our students: she says they are the "eyes and ears" in the community that the health care system isn't able to provide on its own. Those phone calls and emails allow us to be more effective as a community organization and, ultimately, make health care and social services more successful for our shared clients. These connections currently depend largely on the motivation of one social worker, the recognition of his or her importance by one nurse, or the time spent after hours by one physician. We need to formally make room for and fund this collaborative work in our health care system. If we can accomplish that, I believe we will save millions of health care dollars, reduce duplication of efforts, and make the United States a dignified home for older adults.

## BREAKING THE MOLD

DENNY FE GARCIA AGANA

Primary care has always acknowledged the importance of the community; however, due to divergent goals and academic achievements, primary care and public health have worked somewhat in parallel and in separate, siloed ways. This concept of silos resonated most after my master's of public health (MPH) training, when I worked as a family medicine research coordinator.

Having public health training and working in primary care research, I felt like I was being pulled in two different directions. However, the opposing forces were not intentional from either discipline; it was just how things were, in silos.

I immediately found a gap that I could potentially fill, which was to become a strong bridge between two large players whose goals were the same: to make our communities healthier. To be successful, I needed more training, and the Department of Family Medicine believed in me and offered to fully fund my epidemiology PhD.

This was step 1 in bridging the gap between public health and primary care. The Department of Family Medicine saw value in my gaining more training. And what has this led to? With this unique opportunity of belonging to two departments, one in public health and one in primary care, I have become bilingual. The ability to communicate in both languages has encouraged translational research and collaboration. For example, I helped my public health colleagues understand how a community health worker intervention can be helpful as well as the hindrances to primary care clinic workflow. I have helped family medicine physicians interested in analyzing whether their clinical interventions were significantly impacting chronic disease management and exposing them to other nonmedical interventions that public health colleagues could help with.

As a nontraditional epidemiology PhD student, I have gained uncommon skills. Being part of a clinical department, I can identify that an intervention may seem flawless when developed from data analyses and literature reviews yet will be completely inappropriate during clinical implementation. I have learned that outpatient clinics, even within the same department, have their own culture, and researchers must learn to adapt to each clinic's varying workflows. I have also learned the importance of creating working relationships with not just clinicians, but with the front-end staff and nurses, the true champions of clinic interventions.

I will admit, the decision to become a bridge between public health and primary care has felt isolating. Since I am not a traditional epidemiologist and I am not a family medicine physician, I feel eccentric. Yet, on various occasions, I have found comfort in my decision to become part of the movement to bridge the two silos. The first occurred when I had the pleasure of meeting a leader in both family medicine and public health and had some one-on-one time with him (and I do admit I volunteered myself to drive him to the airport, to pick his brain). I told him my situation of belonging to two departments and my research, and he confirmed that I was doing the right thing! Other times of confirmation have occurred when I have gone to national conferences, such as the American Public Health Association and the North American Primary Care Research Group annual meetings. Seeing other leaders aiming to bridge the two disciplines made me feel like I finally belonged and that I was not crazy to strongly believe in the natural connection between the two.

What does all of this mean? It means that what I am doing (and what all of you are doing) matters! It is making a difference. Do not feel afraid of not quite fitting into the public health mold or the primary care mold. There is a movement afoot to create a new mold: to have high-quality health care and to address the full range of factors that influence the population's health and well-being.[1]

This leads us to step 2 in bridging the gap: investing in this unique workforce. I was fortunate enough to belong in public health and primary care departments. This situation forced me and my mentors to find ways to work together, which has brought about fruitful, exciting research and quality improvement for our patient population. My call to action is directed to people with hiring and funding power: please create unique learning and training opportunities for young professionals like myself. Being trained in this uncommon way has led to my commitment to become a strong bridge and translator between primary care and public health. My hope is that more opportunities like mine will arise, and a new workforce with its own mold will emerge: the intersection of primary care and public health.

## REFERENCE

1. DeSalvo KB, Wang YC, Harris A, Auerbach J, Koo D, O'Carroll P. Public health 3.0: A call to action for public health to meet the challenges of the 21st century. *Prev Chronic Dis.* 2017;14:170017. doi: http://dx.doi.org/10.5888/pcd14.170017.

# DEVELOPING A PARTNERSHIP TO ADDRESS THE MOST CONCERNING SOCIAL DETERMINANT: EMPLOYMENT

HALEIGH KAMPMAN

It is a well-known fact that the working population is healthier than the non-working population.[1,2] After all, the overarching theme of the American lifestyle is to go to school and eventually enter into the workforce. If individuals spend more time working throughout their life than they do at home, then there needs to be a primary focus on creating partnerships with community organizations to assist individuals in providing the knowledge and resources they need to get and maintain employment.

Physicians, medical assistants, and nurses alike experience a barrier in patient care because they are not fully educated in all the resources that the outside community provides or, as I've also seen, all the resources provided to patients within their own hospital network. Bridging the gap between community resources and primary care is a vital concept to providing optimal and more personalized care for various patient populations, and that is exactly what I have been able to accomplish as a population health intern.

I began my internship with Eskenazi Health Center Cottage Corner, located in the Fountain Square neighborhood of Indianapolis. This area has long been plagued with high unemployment, low educational levels, and high rates of uninsured individuals. Knowing that many of Eskenazi's primary care clinics are located in underserved areas, the ambulatory integrated care supervisor assigned the interns to develop an intervention to identify and address the social determinant that had the greatest negative impact on the community. Using the knowledge gained from my master's classes, I was aware that educational advancement are effective means of improving community issues; however, I wanted a more hands-on approach to improving the social determinant of employment.

With no funding assistance and a lot of dedication, our clinic has been able to develop and pilot a job assistance program targeting individuals who may be struggling with securing a job or are on the path to improving their career. The partnership was developed between our clinic and WorkOne employment specialists who are contracted by Indiana's EmployIndy organization. These specialists work with individuals one-on-one to identify the barriers related to their personal situation; by pin-pointing those barriers, specialists are able to provide education and resources specific to that individual, improve employability skills, and, overall, provide long-term support so that the individual's personal goals are met.

Developing the partnership with EmployIndy was the first task; however, trying to find the right person to talk to in the organization proved to be challenging. I initially searched EmployIndy's site to gain background knowledge to ensure that this organization was the one I needed to work with to accomplish the goals of my internship. After assessing the mission and vision of EmployIndy, I determined they had the resources it would take to build a job assistance program.

It began with a website submission of a form including my name, the organization I was working with, what my role was within the organization, and what my goals were for the program I had developed. Being upfront with this information has been an encouraging experience, and, overall, it has provided our clinic with an array of community partners who would like to work with us toward the same goal: the betterment and improved health of citizens within our community. After the initial submission, I was contacted by a representative within a day. After expressing again what my goals for the program were, it was determined by the representative that they could not assist me. However, I persisted with EmployIndy, and eventually I was contacted by the district manager. I immediately invited him to a meeting to discuss the program and learn of all the support that his company could provide us. Fortunately, the goal of the program and the goal of EmployIndy aligned perfectly, and the district manager put me in touch with the WorkOne mobile team, whom I met with later that week.

Again, I reiterated the goal of the program, how I would like to address our patient population, and how both of us would benefit from this partnership. Luckily, the WorkOne mobile manager mentioned that he had met with another clinic within the Eskenazi Hospital network and determined that we had the perfect space for his team. Unfortunately, contact was lost within Eskenazi, and his mission remained incomplete until I contacted him. In our meeting, we compared resources, we discussed goals and visions for both companies, and we determined that our partnership was a perfect match. We had the space he needed, and he had the resources and additional partnerships we needed to bridge the gap between community resources and primary care.

Our partnership with WorkOne has been maintained through open lines of communication and dedication from both the community resource and the primary care roles. Although we both had concerns, we have immediately addressed these by being honest, by brainstorming ideas, and by creating a strategy to continually improve the program. Overall, having an aligned mission and set of goals is not necessarily essential to maintaining a partnership, but it is extremely beneficial for both parties. It encourages each organization to collaboratively work together to accomplish the same goal and maintain the level of dedication necessary for the benefit of the community.

After the pilot run of the program finished in March 2018, the employment specialist and I addressed how else we could improve the program for future use. In the concluding months of my internship, I presented this work to the ambulatory integrated care supervisor, who then discussed this intervention with the director. After my presentation, there was a consensus among the majority of the integrated care departmental nurses that this partnership would prove beneficial to all clinics within the Eskenazi Health System. The biggest benefit of this partnership is that both parties have come together to accomplish one and the same goal. In the coming months, this intervention will be presented to upper level management of Eskenazi Health with the hopes of implementing it systemwide.

Overall, developing this partnership has been a challenging yet extremely rewarding opportunity. When given the task initially, I was skeptical, knowing that I would have no funding to develop an intervention. My main concern was how I would persuade an organization to work with me if I couldn't provide them any incentive. But, as the partnership between Eskenazi Health Center Cottage Corner and WorkOne grew, that incentive came to be the perfectly aligned missions of our organizations, and this inspired the dedication to provide more opportunities for the less fortunate.

### REFERENCES
1. Ahonen E, Fujishiro K, Cunningham T, Flynn M. Work as an inclusive part of population health inequities research and prevention. *Am J Public Health.* 2018;108(3):306–31.
2. Baillargeon J. Characteristics of the healthy worker effect. *Occup Med.* 2001;16(2):359–66.

## FOOD MATTERS: MEDICAL STUDENTS PARTNER WITH A COMMUNITY-BASED NONPROFIT TO COMBAT FOOD INSECURITY

JOHN C. PENNER, MARGARET L. MCCARTHY, AND KATHERINE P. MULLINS

"What's your regular day of eating like?" I asked Ms. Alexander (not her real name), preparing to counsel her on the lifestyle changes that could slow the progression of her chronic diseases. If my overly starched short white coat didn't reveal my naïvety, the assumptions underneath my question did.

"It doesn't really work like that for me," she replied.

"Okay, well how about yesterday? What did you eat?"

"Not much."

"What about the day before?" I still wasn't getting it.

Her voice transitioned to the nurturing tone of a parent. "Sweetie, it's the end of the month and there's not much to go around. My kids eat before me." A single mother of three, Ms. Alexander had to choose which ends she would meet each month: gas, electricity, rent, or food. That was the only way to balance her paychecks and bills.

As red-hot shame washed over my face, I began to apologize for the fact that, despite all of the discussions in which I had offered opinions on the importance of physicians recognizing social determinants of health, I had failed to step into her reality.

I could only muster an, "I'm sorry. That was a stupid question."

"It's okay. It's not something you were thinking about."

I should have been.

Food insecurity affects 12.7% of Washington, DC's population,[1] but with unequal distribution. Wards 7 and 8 sit separated from the rest of the city, both geographically and historically, through a long tradition of racial and socioeconomic segregation. They also contain more than three-quarters of the city's "food deserts," or areas with limited access to healthy foods.[2] Families in these neighborhoods are predominantly African American and have some of the highest rates of poverty and the poorest health outcomes in our nation's capital.

Federal programs like the Supplemental Nutrition Assistance Program (SNAP) offer nutrition assistance to millions across the United States. While Ms. Alexander did not earn enough money to cover basic necessities for her family, she—like many others—earned too much to qualify for SNAP.[3] In some regions, the charitable sector has stepped in to fill these gaps. Martha's Table—a nonprofit organization in Washington, DC—launched a series of pop-up grocery markets in 2015 that bring fresh produce into elementary schools in Wards 7 and 8. At these Joyful Food Markets (JFM), students and their families practice cooking at a variety of themed stations and take home up to 23 pounds of free produce each month.[4]

Schools have managed to achieve an attendance rate of 40%, but Martha's Table is exploring ways to increase utilization. Physicians are logical partners in this since food insecurity and poor dietary patterns increase chronic disease burden. But, even for experienced, educated community leaders like the staff at Martha's Table, the health care system can be a labyrinth.

This offers a unique opportunity for medical students. As part of Georgetown's Population Health Scholar Track, we study the social determinants of health, quality improvement methods, and community partnerships in a longitudinal curriculum integrated into our medical education. Martha's Table approached us with a proposal to link local clinics to JFM, envisioning some form of referral protocol which we might design. As medical students and "insiders" to local health care, we brainstormed methods to implement such a protocol. We envisioned our process to begin by raising local physician awareness to facilitate conversations between families and clinicians about food insecurity. We discussed ways to minimize the burden of this task on clinical resources. Eventually, we hoped physicians—through our process implementation—could encourage patients to utilize JFM as part of their overall health care goals.

For many of us, you might say this was our first "consult." Through an intensive process of exploring food insecurity in DC, the structure of JFM, and geomapping of clinics and health care–seeking behavior in Wards 7 and 8, we worked with Martha's Table to develop a pilot project in a single clinic to introduce JFM to providers and facilitate a "referral" system. To examine quality, the project includes process measures for how many referrals were made to JFM by clinic providers and outcome measures tracking how many JFM users at the year's end learned of JFM or discussed JFM with their health care providers.

We are fortunate that Martha's Table created a bridge between sectors by approaching us with a specific project in mind. Martha's Table is very engaged in local nonprofit networks and outreach, but it has limited connections to the health care community. This partnership has made possible a project that our organizations would not have been capable of completing separately. As students, our responsibilities and time commitments change throughout medical school, and we do not have the benefit of regular interaction with the community outside the hospital. This project helped us make the leap from an academic understanding of social determinants of health to actual community engagement: a goal which is often a nicely theorized but poorly defined ambition of medical education. This experience has also prepared us to conceptualize and build similar partnerships in the future. In a time when the trust between providers and chronically underserved patients continues to erode in the wake of ever-changing policy, health care's economic burdens continue to increase, and subtle and not-so-subtle elements of structural racism persist in our institutions, we hope that physicians stepping out of the clinical setting and into the community can help restore the authentic interpersonal connection so critical to a meaningful patient–physician relationship. As this pilot project moves forward, we are excited to see what challenges arise. And, as the potential for lasting cross-sector partnership develops, we hope to help the Ms. Alexanders of our city to fill their own plates in addition to those of their children, even at the end of the month.

## REFERENCES

1. Feeding America. Food insecurity in District of Columbia. http://map. feedingamerica.org/county/2015/overall/districtof-columbia. Accessed February 25, 2018.

2. Smith R. Food access in DC is deeply connected to poverty and transportation. March 13, 2017. DC Policy Center. https://www.dcpolicycenter.org/publications/food-access-d-c-deeply-connected-poverty-transportation/. Accessed February 25, 2018.

3. USDA Food and Nutrition Service. Supplemental Nutrition Assistance Program. February 5, 2018. https://www.fns.usda.gov/snap/supplementalnutrition-assistance-program-snap. Accessed February 25, 2018.

4. Martha's Table. http://marthastable.org/programs/foodaccessprograms/. Accessed February 25, 2018.

# PUBLIC HEALTH PHARMACISTS: BEYOND THE COUNTER

MICHELLE VU

Pharmacists are one of the most trusted and accessible of health care providers. This pride of the profession was heavily emphasized throughout my pharmacy education. The reality is that, like the health care and public health systems, pharmacists practice in silos, partially hindered by state laws and policies that determine the scope of pharmacy. However, pharmacy has a significant role as a Public Health 3.0 stakeholder in improving social determinants of health. Strategic partnerships between health care and public health are required to achieve health in all policies and transform our health care system into one that cares and promotes health. As a Doctorate of Pharmacy/Master of Public Health student, I have witnessed the potential impact of pharmacists in public health. Within an ever-changing health care landscape, pharmacists can apply their expertise in disease state management and prevention to impact the health of the nation beyond the dispensing counter.

Expansions in health care policy have broadened the scope of pharmacy practice, with notable public health impact. For some patients, obtaining a prescription is a barrier to care. Recently, pharmacists, under collaborative practice agreements or standing orders, can dispense naloxone without a prescription and assist in curbing the opioid epidemic. Pharmacists can also promote vaccinations in the community, microbial testing for antibiotic appropriateness, and point-of-care screenings for chronic conditions. Policy is an essential infrastructure in supporting pharmacists to serve as accessible health care professionals.

Few public health professionals have elaborated on the impact of pharmacy services on the social determinants of health. From the perspective of public health, medications overall are perceived as secondary prevention. However, pharmacies can serve as a health care access point for both health promotion and disease prevention. For example, pharmacies sell nonmedication health items, and many provide community education events. Pharmacies can essentially serve as a wellness center and partner for public health educators to host screening, fitness, and healthy eating events. These events address several social determinants, including improving health literacy, community influence, and neighborhood status.

There exists a major financial challenge for pharmacy in public health: several pharmacy services are not billable and are often tied to the dispensing of medications. Currently, Medicare assigns star ratings for pharmacies based on medication adherence, and some plans pay for medication therapy management. However, this payment model reflects the process of care only, not health outcomes. Essentially, pharmacies alone cannot be reimbursed for lowering their patients' blood pressure through counseling on diet and exercise, but they can profit from improving adherence to blood pressure medications.

Realignment of incentives is necessary: a solution is for the pharmacies to join Accountable Care Organizations and share data with local hospitals, clinics, and health departments. Then, pharmacists can participate in and receive revenue from reducing hospital readmissions through medication management and referring community members to public health educational services. In collaboration with public health, pharmacies can profit from investing in infrastructure development and wellness events. Pharmacists and other stakeholders would benefit from conducting economic evaluations and "pitching" projects to administrators about the value and fiscal incentives of these collaborations to promote health.

As a rising pharmacy outcomes researcher, I can attest that pharmacy data are a valuable source of information for health care systems and public health in activities such as community health needs assessment, surveillance, and epidemiologic investigations. Data, analytics, and metrics, per Public Health 3.0, are the technological cornerstone for public and private sector collaboration. Pharmacy data represent the collection of health indicators from local environmental exposures, primary care providers, and acute care providers. A pharmacist can quickly assess the day's medication dispensing patterns and from these glean information on the severity of an influenza outbreak or a rise in asthma exacerbations and identify prescription drug abuse. Currently, few pharmacists have the time and financial incentives to report these trends to health care institutions, public health departments, and law enforcement agencies. Data-sharing agreements, consistent with privacy laws, would transform health care into a sustainable, predictive model rather than a costly, salvaging one.

The scope of pharmacy is extending more and more beyond the dispensing counter. From these examples, members of the pharmacy profession can serve as stakeholders in Public Health 3.0 and collaborate to transform our complex health care system. Pharmacist and student pharmacists can learn and apply best practices from cross-sector partnerships in achieving this aim. Pharmacists already have a well-integrated role in influenza pandemic preparedness, which has paved the way for memorandum of use agreements that allow pharmacists to distribute and administer vaccines. In the Patients, Pharmacists, Partnerships (P3) Program, through partnerships with state health plans and primary care providers, pharmacists have improved chronic disease management for public health employees.

Future pharmacy cross-sector partnerships would allow pharmacists to maximize their impact on improving health in the Public Health 3.0 model. For example, a local public health department, community pharmacy chain, primary care practice, and state Medicaid can align resources to improve asthma management for children. An environmental health team of a public health department may be funded to improve local air quality. The health department may partner with a community pharmacy chain to report patient utilization of asthma rescue inhalers. Pharmacists can follow-up with patients to assess inhaler technique and triggers for attacks. Through a shared electronic medical record, this information would be communicated to the patient's health care providers (HCPs) as well as to the health department. In the short-term, HCPs can escalate medication therapy and possibly prevent hospitalization from an asthma exacerbation. The health department could track asthma medication utilization and air quality data to generate evidence for the need to advocate for air quality improvement policies as well as a Medicaid payment model to reimburse pharmacists for improving asthma management for children. All of these cross-sector relationships would create a synergy to amplify asthma care and ultimately change the way that pharmacies and the rest of the health care industry work together.

# WITH SYNERGY, WE FLOURISH: A CASE FOR INTERDISCIPLINARY COLLABORATION TO IMPROVE HEALTH IN THE UNITED STATES

ASHTEN DUNCAN

With a rapidly increasing national population whose median age is continuing to rise, the United States faces harrowing problems in tending to the health care needs of its citizens who require substantially different services than they did during the past century.[1,2] Physicians—particularly those on the primary care front—have been embroiled for years in the issues of access to high-quality health care based on the constantly evolving needs of our nation's patients.[3,4] An unfortunate truth is that the supply of professionals coming from the "house of medicine" is unable to match the current demand for our services.[5,6] What is more is that our understanding in medicine of the bigger picture of health is limited by the nature of our still highly individualized work.

Physicians historically have not always been able to see the forest for the trees because of the way in which our training does not equip us with all of the tools necessary to fully evaluate population- or community-level health.[7-9] This is where public health comes in as a sister field to medicine: public health approaches to overarching health-related issues allow us to take our deep understanding of an individual's health and apply it more broadly.[5] On the surface, this common ground lends itself well to the development of sustainable partnerships between physicians and public health professionals, and, although some do exist, there are many partnerships that fail to last for one reason or another.[10] The barriers to sustainable partnerships are varied, but many boil down to two basic problems: a lack of resources and insufficient communication.

Partnerships between different organizations are often difficult to sustain when each side is restricted by limited resources. The inability to fulfill certain expectations associated with the partnership can lead to diminished levels of motivation toward the parties' common goals. From a health care delivery standpoint, an approach to solving this resource management issue lies in the patient-centered medical home (PCMH) model. The PCMH model is a method of co-locating multiple health care services to enhance coordination, continuity, and quality of care.[11] Apart from facilitating improved health outcomes, PCMHs also help to lower overhead costs for the different health care professionals in the practice and, ultimately, what patients must pay.[12] Through "shadowing" in different departments at the Indian Health Care Resource Center in Tulsa, Oklahoma, I have seen first-hand how this model benefits both patients and professionals. The reduction in operational costs allows for greater opportunity to collaborate with other professionals to accomplish common community health objectives. Moreover, the coordination of care has the potential to promote shared inquiry and interest in population- and community-wide interventions, both of which can be guided greatly by public health professionals working within the same model of health care delivery.

Another barrier to collaborative health care strategies lies within insufficient communication about major health-related issues and interdisciplinary intersections on those issues. In medicine, many solutions to health-related problems only contribute to about 10–15% of patients' overall health, with the social determinants of health constituting the other 85–90%.[13,14] The determinants are far-reaching, including such dimensions as environmental exposures and health-modifying behaviors.[10,15] As current and future physicians, these facts alone should signal to us the tremendous importance of engaging other professionals to promote optimal health outcomes for our patients. Effective, open communication between physicians and other professionals, such as those in public health, can be achieved in a number of ways, two of which are involvement in community-based, interdisciplinary investigation and interdisciplinary training. When different parties are brought together to answer a complex question, an exchange of different perspectives on the same issues occurs, one that can create new mutual understandings of where interests overlap and of what unique assets each side can bring to the table. A similar level of understanding can be attained when physicians choose to pursue interdisciplinary training, like a master of public health program.

The utilization of the PCMH model and improved communication through interdisciplinary investigation and training are just two ways that physicians can achieve sustainable cross-sector partnerships with other professionals in the vast realm of health-related services. For health care providers, it is tempting to keep to one's lane and to practice within one's own discipline due to strict governmental regulations and growing demands on the workforce. But it is essential for us to expand our reach to others in order to overhaul our health care system and achieve better outcomes. As a future physician, I am committed to this cause to become increasingly more involved with a team of other professionals determined to create higher standards of health.

## REFERENCES

1. Badash I, Kleinman NP, Barr S, Jang J, Rahman S, Wu BW. Redefining health: The evolution of health ideas from antiquity to the era of value-based care. *Cureus.* 2017;9(2):e1018. doi:10.7759/cureus.1018.

2. McKeown RE. The epidemiologic transition: Changing patterns of mortality and population dynamics. *Am J Lifestyle Med.* 2009;3(Suppl 1):19S–26S. doi:10.1177/1559827609335350.

3. Institute of Medicine. *A Manpower Policy for Primary Health Care.* Washington, DC: National Academy of Sciences; 1978: IOM Publication 78–02.

4. Starfield B, Shi L, Macinko J. Contribution of primary care to health systems and health. *Milbank Q.* 2005;83(3):457–502. doi:10.1111/j.1468- 0009.2005.00409.x.

5. Petterson SM, Liaw WR, Phillips RL, Rabin DL, Meyers DS, Bazemore AW. Projecting US primary care physician workforce needs: 2010–2025. *Ann Fam Med.* 2012;10(6):503–9. doi:10.1370/afm.1431.

6. Lakhan SE, Laird C. Addressing the primary care physician shortage in an evolving medical workforce. *Int Arch Med.* 2009;2:14. doi:10.1186/1755-7682-2-14.

7. Hill A, Levitt C, Chambers LW, Cohen M, Underwood J. Primary care and population health promotion. Collaboration between family physicians and public health units in Ontario. *Can Fam Physician.* 2001;47:15–25.

8. Lubetkin EI, Sofaer S, Gold MR, Berger ML, Murray JF, Teutsch SM. Aligning quality for populations and patients: Do we know which way to go? *Am J Public Health.* 2003;93(3):406–511.

9. Stevenson Rowan M, Hogg W, Huston P. Integrating public health and primary care. *Healthc Policy.* 2007;3(1):e160–e81.

10. Winters S, Magalhaes L, Anne Kinsella E, Kothari A. Cross-sector service provision in health and social care: An umbrella review. *Int J Integr Care.* 2016;16(1):10. doi:10.5334/ijic.2460.

11. AHRQ—PCMH Resource Center. Defining the PCMH. https://pcmh.ahrq.gov/page/defining-pcmh. Accessed January 15, 2018.

12. Christensen EW, Dorrance KA, Ramchandani S, et al. Impact of a patient-centered medical home on access, quality, and cost. *Mil Med.* 2013;178(2):135–41. doi:10.7205/milmed-d-12-00220.

13. Braveman P, Gottlieb L. The social determinants of health: It's time to consider the causes of the causes. *Public Health Rep.* 2014;129(Suppl 2):19–31.

14. McGinnis JM, Williams-Russo P, Knickman JR. The case for more active policy attention to health promotion. *Health Aff.* 2002;21(2):78–93. doi:10.1377/hlthaff.21.2.78.

15. Marmot M, Allen JJ. Social determinants of health equity. *Am J Public Health.* 2014;104(Suppl 4):S517–S519. doi:10.2105/AJPH.2014.302200.

# Conclusion: Taking the Next Steps Toward Population Health

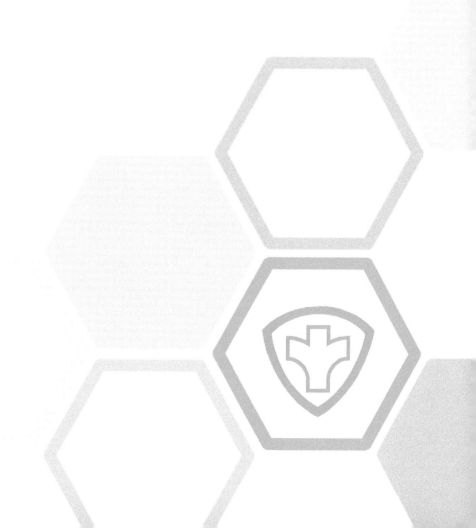

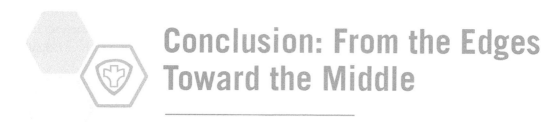

# Chapter 50

# Conclusion: From the Edges Toward the Middle

J. LLOYD MICHENER, BRIAN C. CASTRUCCI, DON W. BRADLEY, CRAIG W. THOMAS, AND EDWARD L. HUNTER

When the then Institute of Medicine launched its report on Integration of Primary Care and Public Health 6 years ago, there were few examples of community partnerships for health.[1] Now new announcements and reports about partnerships appear almost every day, data on health outcomes are available for almost all urban areas, and "playbook" has become a common term as communities seek solutions that reflect their cultures and histories. And, as described in this book, the range of partners now engaged has grown, far outstripping the earlier focus on primary care and public health.

As the movement for health has shifted toward the mainstream, the extent of the work ahead has also become clearer. We do not yet know what teams are needed to improve health, although the central role of community groups is striking in many of the successful examples. Public health is often a central convener, fulfilling the "Public Health 3.0" description,[2] while health care, both at the level of the large health care systems and at the local level with primary care, is almost always a key partner. Business, transportation, and housing groups are commonly engaged, with elected officials helping with the needed changes in policy. Pursuing equity in health, so everyone has an opportunity to live free of the burden of disease, is a particular challenge and need as it requires unraveling decades of policy and practice that have become so ingrained they are hard for those in the majority to see or comprehend.

Building teams and partnerships for health is clearly under way across the country. As we learn how they are able to improve health outcomes in diverse communities, we will need to incorporate their lessons and practices into training programs for all the health and health-related disciplines. Rather than learn what makes a difference in health, on average, we will discover and then teach what makes a difference for some and what works better for others. Rather than train only within our own fields, we will train in teams so the skills of teamwork and partnership are not just ideas, but practiced skills. And, most of all, we will relearn that health is something we can all achieve together but that no person or group can achieve alone. We hope that *The Practical Playbook 2: Accelerating Multi-Sector Partnerships for Health*, and its predecessor, *The Practical Playbook: Public Health and Primary Care Together*, have been helpful early guidebooks in the journey to health.

### REFERENCES

1. Institute of Medicine. *Primary Care and Public Health: Exploring Integration to Improve Population Health*. Washington, DC: The National Academies Press; 2012.

2. DeSalvo KB, Wang YC, Harris A, Auerbach J, Koo D, O'Carroll P. Public Health 3.0: A call to action for public health to meet the challenges of the 21st century. *Prev Chronic Dis.* 2017;14:170017. doi:http://dx.doi.org/10.5888/pcd14.170017.

## ACRONYM LIST

AACOM  American Association of Colleges of Osteopathic Medicine
AAFP  American Academy of Family Physicians
AAMC  Association of American Medical Colleges
AAP  American Academy of Pediatrics
ABFM  American Board of Family Medicine
ACA  Patient Protection and Affordable Care Act
ACGME  Accreditation Council for Graduate Medical Education
ACH  Accountable Communities of Health
ACIP  Advisory Committee on Immunization Practices
ACO  Accountable care organization
ACP  American College of Physicians
AHC  Accountable health communities
AHRQ  Agency for Healthcare Research and Quality
APHA  American Public Health Association
ASPPH  Association of Schools and Programs of Public Health
ASTHO  Association of State and Territorial Health Officials
BPC  Bipartisan Policy Center
BRFSS  Behavioral Risk Factor Surveillance System
BSCF  Blue Shield of California Foundation
CAA  Community action agencies
CAE  Center for Achieving Equity
CBO  Community-based organization
CCHH  Community-centered health home
CDC  Centers for Disease Control and Prevention
CDC  Community development corporation
CEHI  Children's Environmental Health Initiative
CHA  Community Health Assessment
CHCs  Community health centers
CHIP  Children's Health Insurance Program; Community Health Improvement Plan
CHNA  Community health needs assessment
CHWs  Community health workers
CLER  Clinical Learning Environmental Review
CMI  Center for Medicare and Medicaid Innovation
CMS  Centers for Medicare and Medicaid Services
CNA  Community needs assessment
CNF  Clinicians National Forum
CON  Certificate of need
COPC  Community-oriented primary care

CSBG  Community Services Block Grant

CSTE  Council of State and Territorial Epidemiologists

CTG  Community Transformation Grants

DASH  Data Across Sectors for Health

DHHS  US Department of Health and Human Services

DUA  Data use agreement

EHRs  Electronic health records

EHW  Environmental Health Watch

EMRs  Electronic medical records

EPA  Environmental Protection Agency

FDA  US Food and Drug Administration

FMAH  Family Medicine for America's Health

FPL  Federal poverty level

FQHC  Federally Qualified Health Center

GHHI  Green & Healthy Homes Initiative

GIS  Geographic information system

HCUP  Healthcare Cost and Utilization Project

HFF  Healthy Futures Fund

HFFI  Healthy Food Financing Initiative

HI-5  Health Impact in 5 Years

HIA  Health impact assessment

HiAP  Health in all policies

HIE  Health information exchange

HIOs  Health information exchange organizations

HIT  Health information technology

HITECH  Health Information Technology for Economic and Clinical Health Act

HL7  Health Level 7

HMO  Health maintenance organization

HNEF  Healthy Neighborhoods Equity Fund

HPSAs  Health professions shortage areas

HRSA  Health Resources and Services Administration

IHI  Institute for Healthcare Improvement

IIS  Immunization information systems

LHIC  Local Health Improvement Coalition

MAT  Medication-assisted treatment

MCH  Maternal and child health

MIECHV  Maternal, infant, and early childhood home visiting

MOU  Memorandum of understanding

MSSP  Medicare Shared Savings Program

MUAs  Medically underserved areas

NAACOS  National Association of ACOs

NGOs  Nongovernmental organizations

NHANES  National Health and Nutrition Examination Survey

NMTC  New markets tax credit

NONPF  National Organization of Nurse Practitioner Faculties

OECD  Organization for Economic Cooperation and Development

PCEP  Primary Care Extension Program

PCMH  Patient-centered medical home

PCIP  Primary Care Information Project

PCORI  Patient Centered Outcomes Research Institute

PCPs  Primary care provider

PDMP  Prescription Drug Monitoring Program

PHAB  Public Health Accreditation Board

PHI  Protected health information

PHM  Population health management

PRAPARE  Protocol for Responding to and Assessing Patient Assets, Risks, and Experiences

QALY  Quality-adjusted life year

QI  Quality improvement

RBA  Results-based accountability

RECs  Regional extension centers

RHC  Rural health clinic

SAMHSA  Substance Abuse and Mental Health Services Administration

SASH  Support and services at home

SAUP  Specialty Access for the Uninsured Program

SDHs  Social determinants of health

SHAs  State health agencies

SHIP  State health improvement process

SIM  State innovation models

SNAP  Supplemental Nutrition Assistance Program

TFAH  Trust for America's Health

TOD  Transit-oriented development

TRUST  Targeted Rural Underserved Track

USDA US  Department of Agriculture

USPSTF US  Preventive Services Task Force

WHO  World Health Organization

WIC  Special Supplemental Nutrition Program for Women, Infants, and Children

# GLOSSARY

**Accountable Care Organization (ACO)** Groups of doctors, hospitals, and other health care providers who come together voluntarily with the goal of providing coordinated high-quality care to the Medicare patients they serve. Coordinated care helps ensure that patients, especially the chronically ill, get the right care at the right time. ACOs seek to avoid unnecessary duplication of services and medical errors. When an ACO succeeds in both delivering high-quality care and spending health care dollars more wisely, it will share in the savings it achieves for the Medicare program.

**Accountable Health Communities (AHC)** Created by the CMS, the AHC works to bridge the gap between clinical and community service providers to address the health-related social needs of Medicare and Medicaid beneficiaries. It focuses on critical drivers of poor health and health care costs, seeking to reduce avoidable health care utilization and improve the health and quality of care for Medicare and Medicaid beneficiaries.

**Ambulatory Care Sensitive Conditions (ACSC)** Conditions for which good outpatient care has the potential to prevent the need for hospitalization, or conditions in which early interventions can prevent complications or more severe disease outcomes. ACSCs are calculated using age-standardized acute care hospitalization rates for conditions where appropriate ambulatory care prevents or reduces the need for admission to the hospital per 100,000 population younger than age 75 years. Hospitalization for an ACSC is considered to be a measure of access to appropriate primary health care. While not all admissions for these conditions are avoidable, it is assumed that appropriate ambulatory care could prevent the onset of this type of illness or condition, control an acute episodic illness or condition, or manage a chronic disease or condition. A disproportionately high rate is presumed to reflect problems in obtaining access to appropriate primary care.

**Behavioral determinant** A proposed or established causal factor based on individual personal choices of lifestyle or habits (either spontaneously or in response to incentives), such as diet, exercise, and substance abuse.

**Biological determinant** Often, a biological mediator variable between a determinant and an outcome, such as the role of endocrine and immunologic processes in stress. In any case, all determinants must have biological mediator variables in order to affect the organism to produce the health outcomes.

**Braiding and blending** Two approaches for funding and fiscal coordination. With a blending approach, funding from individual streams is merged by stakeholders into one award so there are no longer award-specific identities for the funding streams. In braiding, different funding streams are coordinated by stakeholders so that each individual award maintains its specific identity.

**Collaboration** The interaction of two or more persons or organizations directed toward a common goal which is mutually beneficial. From Random House Dictionary Unabridged, 2d ed., an act or instance of working or acting together for a common purpose or benefit (i.e., joint action).

**Collective impact** The commitment of a group of actors from different sectors to a common agenda for solving a complex social problem. Collective impact is a significant shift from the social sector's current paradigm of "isolated impact" because the underlying premise of collective impact is that no single organization can create large-scale, lasting social change alone. Collective impact is best employed for problems that are complex and systemic rather than technical in nature. Collective impact initiatives are currently being employed to address a wide variety of issues around the world, including education, health care, homelessness, the environment, and community development.

**Community** (1) A group of people who have common characteristics; communities can be defined by location, race, ethnicity, age, occupation, interest in particular problems or outcomes, or other common bonds.

(2) Individuals with a shared affinity, and perhaps geography, who organize around an issue, with collective discussion, decision-making, and action.

**Community Action Agency (CAA)** Private or public nonprofit organizations that were created by the federal government in 1964 to combat poverty in geographically designated areas. Status as a CAA is the result of an explicit designation by local or state government. A CAA has a tripartite board structure that is designated to promote the participation of the entire community in the reduction or elimination of poverty. They seek to involve the community, including elected public officials, private sector representatives, and especially low-income residents, in assessing local needs and attacking the causes and conditions of poverty.

**Community benefit** The federal government encourages public support for charitable activities by allowing people to deduct donations to tax-exempt organizations on their income tax returns. Tax-exempt hospitals are major beneficiaries of this policy because it encourages donations to the hospitals while shielding them from federal and state tax liability. In exchange, these hospitals must engage in community benefit activities, such as providing care to indigent patients and participating in Medicaid. The Affordable Care Act (ACA) brings a new focus on community benefit activities by requiring tax-exempt hospitals to engage in communitywide planning efforts to improve community health. The magnitude of the tax exemption, coupled with ACA reforms, underscores the public's interest not only in community benefit spending generally but also in the extent to which nonprofit hospitals allocate funds for community benefit expenditures that improve the overall health of their communities.

**Community engagement** The process of working collaboratively with and through groups of people affiliated by geographic proximity, special interest, or similar situations to address issues affecting the well-being of those people. In general, the goals of community engagement are to build trust, enlist new resources and allies, create better communication, and improve overall health outcomes as successful projects evolve into lasting collaborations.

*Community Guide* The Community Preventive Services Task Force (CPSTF; the Task Force) was established in 1996 by the US Department of Health and Human Services to identify population health interventions that are scientifically proved to save lives, increase lifespans, and improve quality of life. The Task Force produces recommendations (and identifies evidence gaps) to help inform the decision-making of federal, state, and local health departments; other government agencies; communities; healthcare providers; employers; schools; and research organizations.

*The Guide to Community Preventive Services* (*The Community Guide*) is a collection of evidence-based findings of the CPSTF. It is a resource to help you select interventions to improve health and prevent disease in your state, community, community organization, business, health care organization, or school.

*Community Guide* reviews are designed to answer three questions:

What has worked for others and how well?

What might this intervention approach cost, and what am I likely to achieve through my investment?

What are the evidence gaps?

**Community health** A perspective on public health that assumes community to be an essential determinant of health and the indispensable ingredient for effective public health practice. It takes into account the tangible and intangible characteristics of the community—its formal and informal networks and support systems, its norms and cultural nuances, and its institutions, politics, and belief systems.

The state of wellness or well-being in a defined community; affected by forces in addition to health care services, including adequate housing, quality of schools, safe streets, economic stability, and the environment.

**Community Health Assessment (CHA)**  A process that uses quantitative and qualitative methods to systematically collect and analyze data to understand health within a specific community. An ideal assessment includes information on risk factors, quality of life, mortality, morbidity, community assets, forces of change, and social determinants of health and health inequity, and information on how well the public health system provides essential services. Community health assessment data are intended to inform community decision-making, the prioritization of health problems, and the development, implementation, and evaluation of community health improvement plans.

**Community Health Center (CHC)**  Facilities that administer the delivery of health care services to people living in a community or neighborhood.

**Community Health Improvement Plan**  A long-term, systematic effort to address health problems on the basis of the results of assessment activities and the community health improvement process. This plan is used by health and other governmental education and human service agencies, in collaboration with community partners, to set priorities and coordinate and target resources. This plan is critical for developing policies and defining actions to target efforts that promote health. It should define the vision for the health of the community inclusively and should be done in a timely way. *See also* Community health improvement process. This definition of community health improvement plan also refers to a Tribal, state, or territorial community health improvement plan.

**Community Health Needs Assessment-IRS (CHNA)**  A CHNA is required under the Internal Revenue Code (IRS) by the Patient Protection and Affordable Care Act (ACA). The IRS requires hospital organizations to document compliance with CHNA requirements for each of their facilities in a written report that includes: a description of the community served, a description of the process and methods used to conduct the assessment, a description of methods used to include input from people representing the broad interests of the community served, a prioritized description of all community health needs identified in the CHNA, a description of the process and criteria used in prioritizing such needs, and a description of existing health care facilities and other resources in the community available to meet the needs identified in the CHNA (www.irs.gov/pub/irs-drop/n-10-39.pdf).

**Community Health Workers**  Community health workers should be members of the communities where they work, should be selected by the communities, should be answerable to the communities for their activities, should be supported by the health system but not necessarily a part of its organization, and will have shorter training than professional workers.

**Community-Centered Health Homes (CCHH)**  A new model for effectively bridging community prevention and health service delivery. Community health centers (CHCs) are one ideal venue for developing an integrated approach that builds on the strengths of each approach. CCHHs provide high-quality health care services while also applying diagnostic and critical thinking skills to the underlying factors that shape patterns of injury and illness. By strategically engaging in efforts to improve community environments, CCHHs can improve the health and safety of their patient population, improve health equity, and reduce the need for medical treatment. The CCHH concept takes previous models a transformative step further by not only acknowledging that factors outside the health care system affect patient health outcomes, but by also actively participating in improving them.

**Cooperation**  Association of persons for a common benefit, working toward a common effort.

**Cost-benefit analysis** A method of comparing the cost of a program with its expected benefits in dollars (or other currency). The benefit-to-cost ratio is a measure of total return expected per unit of money spent. This analysis generally excludes consideration of factors that are not measured ultimately in economic terms. Cost effectiveness compares alternative ways to achieve a specific set of results.

**Cost-effective analysis** This form of analysis seeks to determine the costs and effectiveness of an activity or to compare similar alternative activities to determine the relative degree to which they will obtain the desired objectives or outcomes. The preferred action or alternative is one that requires the least cost to produce a given level of effectiveness or that provides the greatest effectiveness for a given level of cost. In the health care field, outcomes are measured in terms of health status.

An analytic tool in which the costs and effects of at least one alternative are calculated and presented, as in a ratio of incremental cost to incremental effect. Effects are health outcomes, such as cases of disease prevented, years of life gained, or quality adjusted life years, rather than monetary measures, as in cost-benefit analysis.

**Disability-Adjusted Life Year (DALY)** A DALY lost is a measure of the burden of disease on a defined population. It is hence an indicator of population health. DALYs are advocated as an alternative to quality adjusted life years (QALYs). They are based on adjustment of life expectancy to allow for long-term disability as estimated from official statistics; the necessary data to do so may not be available in some areas. The concept postulates a continuum from disease to disability to death that is not universally accepted, particularly by the community of persons with disabilities. DALYs are calculated using a "disability weight" (a proportion less than 1) multiplied by chronological age to reflect the burden of the disability. DALYs can thus produce estimates that accord greater value to fit than to disabled persons and to the middle years of life rather than to youth or old age.

**Essential Public Health Functions/Services** The 10 services identified in Public Health in America: monitoring health status; diagnosing and investigating health problems; informing, educating, and empowering people; mobilizing community partnerships; developing policies and plans; enforcing laws and regulations; linking people to needed services; assuring a competent workforce; conducting evaluations; and conducting research. Representatives from federal agencies and national organizations developed the statement made in *Public Health in America*; this statement includes two lists, one that describes what public health seeks to accomplish and the second that describes how it will carry out its basic responsibilities. The second list, the Essential Services, provides a list of 10 public health services that define the practice of public health.

**Evaluation** The systematic investigation of a project or program by assigning value to its efforts by addressing three interrelated domains: merit (or quality), worth (or value, i.e., cost-effectiveness), and significance (or importance).

**Federal poverty level (FPL)** A measure of income that is defined each year by the US Department of Health and Human Services. It is a level of income that is used to calculate a person's eligibility for a number of programs and benefits (e.g., Medicaid or CHIP coverage).

**Federally Qualified Health Center (FQHC)** Community-based and patient-directed organizations that serve populations with limited access to health care. These include low-income populations, the uninsured, those with limited English proficiency, migrant and seasonal farm workers, individuals and families experiencing homelessness, and those living in public housing. A sliding fee scale provides accessibility to individuals who are living at or below 200% of the federal poverty level.

**Genetic determinant** A proposed or established causal factor from the genetic composition of individuals or populations that affects health outcomes.

**Geographic Information System (GIS)** An information system that incorporates digitally constructed maps and uses sophisticated modeling techniques to analyze and display information patterns. Satellite imaging and remote sensing have greatly expanded the scope of GISs (e.g., trends in specific diseases are suggested after analyzing the composition of vegetation and the amounts of precipitation in tropical regions, which relate to changes in the distribution and abundance of predators and insect vectors). Another application is digitally prepared spot maps of disease clusters using postal codes and notified cases. An important application is in geomatics.

**Health** (1) The state of complete physical, mental, and social well-being and not merely the absence of disease or infirmity (from WHO, 1994).

(2) The extent to which an individual or group is able to realize aspirations and satisfy needs, and to change or cope with the environment. Health is a resource for everyday life, not the objective of living; it is a positive concept, emphasizing social and personal resources as well as physical capabilities (from WHO, 1984).

(3) A state characterized by anatomical, physiological, and psychological integrity; an ability to perform personally valued family, work, and community roles; an ability to deal with physical, biological, and psychological stress; a feeling of well-being; and freedom from the risk of disease and untimely death.

(4) A state of equilibrium between humans and the physical, biological, and social environment, compatible with full functional activity.

**Health Care Determinant** A proposed or established causal factor in health care that affects health outcomes (e.g., access, quantity, and quality of health care services). *See also* Social Determinants of Health.

**Health care reform** Innovation and improvement of the health care system by reappraisal, amendment of services, and removal of faults and abuses in providing and distributing health services to patients. It includes a realignment of health services and health insurance to maximum demographic elements (the unemployed, indigent, uninsured, elderly, inner cities, rural areas) with reference to coverage, hospitalization, pricing and cost containment, insurers' and employers' costs, preexisting medical conditions, prescribed drugs, equipment, and services.

**Health equity [Equity]** *Equity* in health is the absence of systematic disparities in health (or in the major social determinants of health) between groups with different levels of underlying social advantage/disadvantage (i.e., wealth, power, or prestige). Equity is an ethical principle; it also is consonant with and closely related to human rights principles.

*Health equity* means that every person has an opportunity to achieve optimal health regardless of the color of their skin, level of education, gender identify, sexual orientation, the job they have, the neighborhood they live in, whether or not they have a disability.

**Health inequity** Those differences in health which are not only unnecessary and avoidable but, in addition, are considered unfair and unjust. Health inequity is related both to a legacy of overt discriminatory actions on the part of government and the larger society, as well as to present-day practices and policies of public and private institutions that continue to perpetuate a system of diminished opportunity for certain populations.

**Health Information Exchange (HIE)** A system that allows health care professionals and patients to appropriately access and securely share a patient's medical information electronically.

**Health Insurance Portability and Accountability Act (HIPAA)** Public Law 104-91, enacted in 1996, was designed to improve the efficiency and effectiveness of the health care system, protect health insurance coverage for workers and their families, and protect individual personal health information.

**Isolation** Occurring alone, and/or not working with others, as when primary care and public health entities work separately from one another.

**Meaningful use**  Using certified electronic health records technology to improve quality, safety, and efficiency; reduce healthcare disparities; engage patients and families in their health care; improve care coordination; and improve population and public health while maintaining privacy and security.

*Meaningful use* is defined by the use of certified EHR technology in a meaningful manner (e.g., electronic prescribing); ensuring that the certified EHR technology is connected in a manner that provides for the electronic exchange of health information to improve the quality of care; and that in using certified EHR technology the provider must submit to the Secretary of Health & Human Services (HHS) information on quality of care and other measures.

**Medicaid**  A US federal program, created by Public Law 89-97, Title XIX, as an 1965 amendment to the Social Security Act, administered by the states, that provides health care benefits to indigent and medically indigent persons. States have variable options on how to implement the program, using waivers and plan options to change how they administer health care to their populations. Given the number of patients using Medicaid, there have been many recent efforts to partner with, reform, and adjust the way it is administered in states. Recent trends have moved toward incorporating the social determinants of health, value-based payments, and managed care.

**Medicare**  A US federal program, created by Public Law 89-97, Title XVIII-Health Insurance for the Aged, a 1965 amendment to the Social Security Act, that provides health insurance benefits to persons over the age of 65 and others eligible for Social Security benefits. It consists of two separate but coordinated programs: hospital insurance (Medicare Part A) and supplementary medical insurance (Medicare Part B).

**Merger**  When one or more entities combine to replace formerly separate entities and operate as one unified entity.

**Morbidity**  The proportion of patients with a particular disease during a given year per given unit of population.

**Mortality rate**  The number of deaths in a population within a prescribed time, expressed as either crude death rates or death rates specific to diseases and sometimes to age, sex, and other attributes.

**Partnerships, cross-sector**  Addressing the complex challenges communities face today requires collective effort from across sectors: public, private, and nonprofit.

Relatively intensive, long-term interactions between organizations from at least two sectors (business, government, and/or civil society) aimed at addressing a social or environmental problem.

**Patient Centered Medical Home (PCMH)**  The medical home model is a potential way to improve health care in America by transforming how primary care is organized and delivered. Building on the work of a large and growing community, the Agency for Healthcare Research and Quality (AHRQ) defines a medical home not simply as a place but as a model of the organization of primary care that delivers the core functions of primary health care. The medical home encompasses five functions and attributes:

- Comprehensive care
- Patient-centered care
- Coordinated care
- Accessible services
- Quality and safety

**Patient Protection and Affordable Care Act (ACA)**  The first part of the comprehensive health care reform law enacted on March 23, 2010. The law was amended by the Health Care and Education Reconciliation Act on March 30, 2010. The name "Affordable Care Act" is usually used to refer to the final, amended version of the law. (It's sometimes known as "PPACA," "ACA," or "Obamacare.") The law provides numerous rights and protections that make health coverage fairer and easier to understand, along with subsidies (through "premium tax credits" and "cost-sharing reductions") to make it more affordable. The law also expands the Medicaid program to cover more people with low incomes.

**Policy** Whether public or private, a policy is (1) a written statement, (2) binding and enforceable, and 3) broadly applicable to a geographic area, type of institution or physical space, and/or group of people. Public health professionals play an important role in the policy process, for example, by conducting policy analysis, communicating findings, developing partnerships, and promoting and implementing evidence-based policy interventions.

**Population health** (1) A conceptual framework for thinking about why some populations are healthier than others, as well as the policy development, research agenda, and resource allocation that flow from it.

(2) The health outcomes of a group of individuals, including the distribution of such outcomes within the group.

(3) The health of a population as measured by health status indicators and as influenced by social, economic, and physical environments; personal health practices; individual capacity and coping skills; human biology; early childhood development; and health services.

The health outcomes of a group of individuals, including the distribution of such outcomes within the group.

**Population health management** There is a clear public health role for the federal and state governments to play in ensuring the health of the overall population of the nation or its several states; however, for our purposes, we assume a more limited focus; that is, that population health management means proactive application of strategies and interventions to defined cohorts of individuals across the continuum of health care delivery in an effort to maintain and/or improve the health of the individuals within the cohort at the lowest necessary cost.

**Primary care** The provision of integrated, accessible health care services by clinicians who are accountable for addressing a large majority of personal health care needs, developing a sustained partnership with patients, and practicing in the context of family and community.

**Primary prevention** Intervening before health effects occur, through measures such as vaccinations, altering risky behaviors (poor eating habits, tobacco use), and banning substances known to be associated with a disease or health condition.

**Public health** (1) Activities that a society undertakes to assure the conditions in which people can be healthy. These include organized community efforts to prevent, identify, and counter threats to the health of the public.

(2) What we do as a society collectively to assure conditions in which people can be healthy.

(3) The science and art of preventing disease, prolonging life, and promoting health through the organized efforts and informed choices of society, public and private organizations, communities, and individuals.

**Public health surveillance** Officially defined as "the ongoing, systematic collection, analysis, and interpretation of health-related data essential to the planning, implementation, and evaluation of public health practice, closely integrated with the timely dissemination of these data to those responsible for prevention and control."

**Public health system** Activities undertaken within the formal structure of government and the associated efforts of private and voluntary organizations and individuals.

**Quality improvement** The attainment or process of attaining a new level of performance or quality.

**Quality-Adjusted Life Years (QALY)** A measurement index derived from a modification of standard life-table procedures and designed to take account of the quality as well as the duration of survival. This index can be used in assessing the outcome of health care procedures or services.

**Return on investment (ROI)** A useful tool for understanding a project's costs and benefits from the perspective of an investor. ROI analysis originally was developed in a commercial, business context to assess the performance of a financial investment. Its focus is the return that a specific investor receives from his or her own financial investment. By application of a standard ROI equation, an investor who purchases goods for $1 and resells them for $3 has received a 200% return on the cost of the initial investment: (Proceeds of investment [$3] – Cost of Investment [$1]) / Cost of Investment [$1] × 100% = ROI [200%].

**Safety net providers** Providers that by mandate or mission organize and deliver a significant level of health care and other health-related services to the uninsured, Medicaid recipients, and other vulnerable patients

**Secondary prevention** The prevention of recurrences or exacerbations of a disease or complications of its therapy.

Screening to identify diseases in the earliest stages, before the onset of signs and symptoms, through measures such as mammography and regular blood pressure testing

**Shared savings** A payment strategy that offers incentives for providers to reduce health care spending for a defined patient population by offering them a percentage of net savings realized as a result of their efforts. The concept was fueled in part by Affordable Care Act provisions that create accountable care organizations and by the movement from fee-for-service to value-based payment models.

**Social determinants of health (SDHs)** Conditions in the environments in which people are born, live, learn, work, play, worship, and age that affect a wide range of health, functioning, and quality-of-life outcomes and risks.

**Teaching hospital** Hospitals engaged in educational and research programs, as well as providing medical care to the patients.

**Tertiary prevention** Measures aimed at providing appropriate supportive and rehabilitative services to minimize morbidity and maximize quality of life after a long-term disease or injury is present.

Managing disease post diagnosis to slow or stop disease progression through measures such as chemotherapy, rehabilitation, and screening for complications.

**Upstream interventions** Interventions that involve policy approaches that can affect large populations through regulation, increased access, or economic incentives. For example, increasing tobacco taxes is an effective method for controlling tobacco-related diseases. Midstream interventions occur within organizations. For example, worksite-based programs that increase employee access to facilities for physical activity show promise in improving health. Most research has been conducted on downstream interventions, which often involve individual-level behavioral approaches for prevention or disease management.

**Vulnerable populations** Groups of persons whose range of options is severely limited, who are frequently subjected to coercion in their decision-making, or who may be compromised in their ability to give informed consent.

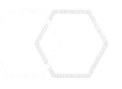

# Index

Tables, figures, and boxes are indicated by an italic *t, f,* and *b,* respectively, following the page number.

#123forEquity Campaign to Eliminate Health Care Disparities, 70–71

500 Cities Project, 189*b*

AAPHL Informatics Messaging Services (AIMS), 27

A Blueprint for a Healthy House, 25

access
to addiction treatment, 433*f*, 434–35
to health care, 10
to preventive care, 10
to providers and health insurance, 10
to therapeutic care, 10

accountability
for collaborations, lasting, 151–54
social, 7–9, 9*t*

accountable care organizations (ACO), 103–4

Accountable Community for Health (ACH), 90, 149–57
accountability, for what?, 152*f*, 154
accountability, to whom?, 151, 152*f*
accountability for collaborations, lasting, 151–54
*vs.* accountable care organization, 151
California Accountable Communities for Health Initiative, 150*b*, 150–51
collective accountability, 149, 150*b*

commitment and trust, 152, 157
community engagement, authentic, 152, 154, 157
distributed leadership, 152–53, 153*f*
early lessons, 156
feedback loops, transparent, 152, 154
inclusion, 152, 153
levels of accountability, 152*f*, 152
model fundamentals, 149
overview, 149
portfolio development, 151–54, 153*f*, 154*f*
Washington State, 356

Accountable Health Communities (AHC), 19–20

Accountable Health Community Health-Related Social Needs Screening Tool, 236

accreditation, Council on Education in Public Health, 466

acronyms, community health, 330*b*, 330

acting locally, 315–21. *See also* One Virginia Foundation

addiction treatment access, expanding, 433*f*, 434–35

adverse community events, 429

advocacy, 10, 386

communities and social determinants of health, 461–62
philanthropic, 400, 401–2*b*, 401–3 (*see also* Horizon Foundation; *specific foundations*)
provider level, 461–62
training, AAP, 461–63
transportation sector groups, 50

advocate, 106

Aetna Foundation, 287

affordability
hospitals and health systems, 68
housing developers, 335

Affordable Care Act, 103

agenda, building population health, 261–68
academic institutions, 267
for all, 267
business community, 267
community organizations, 267
Healthy Communities movement, history, 261
investors, 267
obstacles to improvement, 262
obstacles to improvement, overcoming, 262
outcome accountability, 261
partnerships, Oakland, 263

agenda, building
population health
(*cont.*)
partnerships,
Oklahoma City, 264
path forward, 264
payers, 266
policymakers, 267
providers, 266
AIM Healthy Fund
(HFF), 342
air quality, transportation
and, 48, 53*t*
Ali, Fred, 403
Alliance for Health
Equity, 271–81
collaborative focus area,
components, 280*f*
collective community
health, factors and
opportunities, 271–72
community
development,
276–77, 277*f*
community safety,
276–77, 277*f*
Data Committee, 278
history, 271
hospital
partnerships, 272–73
housing, 275
large-scale systems
change and collective
impact, 273
lessons learned,
279, 280*f*
local collaborative effort
partnerships, 273
local health department
partnerships, 272
mental health and
substance use,
275, 277*f*
Policy Committee, 278
purpose, vision, and
values, 272, 273*f*
regional and
community
partnerships, 272
strategy and impact
areas, 277*f*
structure, 272, 274*f*
violence prevention,
health care
engagement in, 277*f*
all-in approach, 266

All In: Data for
Community
Health, 163–74
All In Community, 164*f*
All In Community,
joining, 174
Altair accountable
care for people with
disabilities, 165*b*, 165
asthma rates,
childhood, 171–72*b*
Bronx Healthy
Buildings Initiative,
172–73*b*, 173
BUILD Health
Aurora, 166*b*
multisector data, cases
for, 163–64, 164*f*
multisector data
project categories,
overview, 163
multisector data
project categories,
population and
community health
and well-being,
165, 166*b*
multisector data project
categories, whole-
person systems of
care, 165*b*, 165
multisector
data-sharing
collaborations
environment, 166,
170–72*b*
multisector
data-sharing
collaborations
environment,
challenges
overview, 166
multisector
data-sharing
collaborations
environment,
honest and
mutually beneficial
relationships, 167
multisector
data-sharing
collaborations
environment,
interoperability and
social determinant
data standards, 168

multisector
data-sharing
collaborations
environment, legal
issues and legal
terms, 167
multisector
data-sharing
collaborations
environment,
meaningful data
for incorporation
into programmatic
operations, 169
multisector
data-sharing
collaborations
environment,
sustainability, 169
overview, 170*b*
shared data system,
developing, 163, 164*f*
all teach–all learn,
126–27, 132
allyship, 10
Alma Ata declaration,
WHO, 77–78
Altair accountable care
for people with
disabilities, 165*b*, 165
American Academy of
Family Physicians
(AAFP), 104, 105*b*,
236, 460–61
American Academy of
Pediatrics (AAP)
advocacy
training, 461–63
community
engagement
and CATCH
program, 459–60
Community
Pediatrics Training
Initiative, 462–63
primary care practice-
based research
networks, 460–61
American Public Health
Association, 338
Analysis Data Model
(ADaM), 180
anchor institutions,
365–73, 387. *See
also* mission, health
systems

anchor mission, 366
*Anchor Mission Playbook,
The*, 369
anchor organizations. *See
also specific types*
maximizing cultural
similarity, 134
anti-redlining, 334
applied learning,
211*f*, 307–8
Arkansas Area Health
Education Center
(AHEC), 474–75
Arora, Sanjeev, 479*b*, 479
Asian Health Services
(AHS), Oakland,
295–96*b*, 295
asset and gap analysis,
local health, energy,
and housing, 38
Association for
Community Health
Improvement, 338
Association of State
and Territorial
Health Official's
(ASTHO) President's
Challenge,
429–30, 430*f*
asthma
Lead + Asthma
Project, 25
reduction, assessing
program
effectiveness,
224–25*b*
asthma, childhood
care plan,
checking, 200*b*
housing conditions,
185–87*b*
medication prescription
filling, 214–15*b*
rates, 171–72*b*
rates, All In: Data for
Community Health,
171–72*b*
automated data exchange,
183, 184*f*. *See also*
surveillance for
community outbreak,
automation

Baltimore's B'FRIEND
initiative, 219–27
Barton, Clara, 484

Bedford Stuyvesant
Restoration
Corporation, 334
beehives, 121
behavioral health,
multisector
approach, 137–47
Behavioral Risk Factor
Surveillance System
(BRFSS), 358
belonging, sense of, 97*b*,
97, 98*f*
benchmarking, 173
Bernanke, Ben, 337
*Best Practices for
Comprehensive
Tobacco Control
Programs - 2014*
(CDC), 417–18
"Better Health Through
Housing," 275
better practices, 5
B'FRIEND
initiative, 219–27
approvals and
agreements, 222*f*, 223
data, 225
falls reduction,
via engaging
neighborhoods and
data, 219
history and origins, 219
lessons learned, 226–27
lessons learned,
consistent
approach, 227
lessons learned,
data sharing
complexity, 227
lessons learned,
hyperfocused
data and
interventions, 227
lessons learned, peer
learning, 227
lessons learned,
public health
innovations, 226
partners and
interventions,
220, 224*b*
Big Data, 106
Big Soda, fighting at local
level, 389–404
Change Lab Solution,
390, 390*t*

coalition partners,
engaging broad,
multisector, 394, 396*b*
Horizon
Foundation, 390
Horizon Foundation,
campaign
components, 391
media strategy,
398, 399*f*
message framing and
reframing, 395, 397*f*
opposition responses,
anticipating, 395
philanthropic
advocacy and public
policy role, 400,
401–2*b*, 401–3
policy lever, pulling
right, 392
policy options, sugary
drink consumption,
389, 390*t*
successful
campaigns, 392–98
Voices for Healthy
Kids, 390–91
black box framework, 129
block grants, 362
1981 Omnibus
Reconciliation Act,
354, 355*t*
budget cuts on, 354–55
history, 354–55
Medicaid or public
health funding, 351
smaller, with
administrative
flexibility, 356, 357
Blue Cross NC
Foundation, 297–98
Blue Cross of California
Foundation (BSCF)
learning loops,
308–9, 309*f*
measurement,
elements, 308*f*
one-minute message,
311*b*, 311
social determinants of
health, 303*f*, 303
Blueprint for Health,
Vermont, 359
Blue Shield of California
Foundation
(BSCF), 301–12

collaboration
for healthy
communities, 305
domestic violence
cycle, breaking, 305,
306*b*, 306
focal points, 304
"Further Forward,"
brand definition, 310,
311*b*, 311, 311*t*
future of health,
designing, 306
history and
challenges, 301–2
mission and scope, 301
new partners and
new approaches,
310*b*, 310
setting a bold goal
and learning, 306,
308*f*, 309*f*
upstream course,
charting, 306, 307*t*
upstream focus shift,
302*b*, 302,
303*f*, 303
Boelen, C., 9–10
breach procedures, 202–3
"Breaking the Mold"
(Garcia Agana), 494
Breakthrough Series
Collaborative
learning model,
IHI, 129
Breckenridge, Mary, 484
Bridger, Colleen, 418–19
Brilliant Baby
program, 263–64
Bronx Healthy
Buildings Initiative,
172–73*b*, 173
BUILD Health
Aurora, 166*b*
BUILD Health Challenge,
Cleveland, 23, 31–33
1.0, engaging
community in
healthy housing, 32
1.0, engaging
community in
healthy housing,
community impact
and outcomes, 32
2.0, Cleveland Healthy
Homes Data
Collaborative, 33

consultants, 55, 57*b*
small nonprofit
effectiveness and
intermediary
organization, 33
strategic objectives,
race-equity, 55*b*
BUILD Health Challenge,
Cleveland,
examples, 26–28
collaboration
advancement and
power and control
mitigation, 26
communication, 27
community voice, 28
inclusion, 28
BUILD Health Challenge,
Pasadena, Texas, 377
Build Healthy Places
Network,
330, 345–46
Partner Finder, 346
building population
health agenda,
261–68. *See also*
agenda, building
population health
built environment. *See
also* housing
faith community
response, 120
bundled services, 42
burnout, professional,
68, 79–80
business, public health
and, 61–65
in building population
health, 267
civic, 62
enterprise, 63
Greater Kansas
City Chamber of
Commerce, 61
Healthy KC, 61, 62
Kansas City,
history, 61
role, promoting public
health, 64
business community,
building ties with
(Pasadena, Texas),
327, 375–81
foundation for
collaboration,
building, 376

business community,
building ties with
(Pasadena, Texas)
(*cont.*)
Pasadena, Texas,
demographics, 376*t*
Pasadena, Texas,
overview, 375
strengthening ties,
funders, 377
strengthening ties,
implementation
partners, 378
strengthening
ties, strategic
partnerships, 380

California Accountable
Communities for
Health Initiative
(CACHI), 90, 149–57
accountability, to
whom?, 151, 152*f*
early lessons, 156
key elements,
150*b*, 150–51
origins, 150 (*see
also* Accountable
Community for
Health (ACH))
portfolio development,
151–54,
153*f*, 154*f*
California Endowment,
90. *See also*
Accountable
Community for
Health (ACH)
California Healthy
Places Index (HPI),
252*f*, 253*b*
Camden Coalition
of Health Care
Providers, 20
capacity, 79
care models, 77
CDC Learning
Connection, 469
Center for Care
Innovations
(CCI), 291
*Community-Centered
Health Homes:
Bridging the
Gap Between
Health Services*

*and Community
Prevention,* 291
Center for Corporate
Strategy, Boston
College, 377
Center for Medicare and
Medicaid Innovation
(CMMI), 131–32
Centers for Achieving
Equity (CAE), 30, 32
Centers for Disease
Control and
Prevention (CDC)
*Best Practices for
Comprehensive
Tobacco Control
Programs
- 2014,* 417–18
core roles, 410
Health Impact in 5
Years, 20, 386,
407–20 (*see also*
Health Impact in 5
Years (HI-5))
Health Impact Pyramid,
410–11, 425–27
Population Health
Workforce
Initiative, 468*b*
public health training
programs, 467–68*b*,
467, 468–69
Transportation and
Health Tool, 48–49
transportation design
and operational
strategies, 49
workforce training,
population
health, 454
Centers for Medicare and
Medicaid Services
(CMS). *See also
specific programs*
Accountable Health
Communities, 19–20
Center for Medicare
and Medicaid
Innovation, 131–32
Chamber of Commerce,
Pasadena, 380
chambers of
commerce, 64–65
Greater Kansas
City Chamber of
Commerce, 61, 445

chambers of health, 68–69
Change Lab Solution,
390, 390*t*
Charter Oak
communities,
342–43, 343*f*
Vita Health & Wellness
District, 342, 343*f*
Chicago, Alliance for
Health Equity, 271–
81. *See also* Alliance
for Health Equity
chief health strategist, 17
child abuse and neglect,
Loudon County,
Virginia, 317
Children's Services Act,
Virginia, 359
child restraint laws, 205
Chronic Care
Model, 131–32
chronic disease. *See
also specific issues
and types*
care and costs, 283
county and subcounty
analysis data, 211
growth, 3–4
health care
expenditures
on, 329
prevalence, 211–12
CityHealth
evidence-based policies,
for healthier, thriving
environments, 413
*vs.* Health Impact in 5
Years, 415
policymaking,
evidence-based
policies for
health, 409–10
Civic Consulting Alliance,
369, 370
Cleveland BUILD
Health Challenge.
*See* BUILD Health
Challenge, Cleveland
Clinical Data Acquisition
Standard
Harmonization
(SDASH), 180
Clinical Data Architecture
(CDA), 182*b*
Clinical Data Exchange
Standards

Consortium
(CDISC), 180
clinical partnerships,
nurse-led, 486–87
clinical population
medicine model, 105
clinical public health
strategies, 458
clinicians, in community
development, 345–47
align, 347
engage, 346
identify, 346
learn, 345
Clinician's National
Forum
(CNF), 129–30
political will,
component
integration, 130
cold spots, 82
collaboration(s), 89–91.
*See also specific topics
and types*
Blue Shield of
California
Foundation, healthy
communities, 305
BUILD Health
Challenge,
Cleveland, 26
California Endowment
and Accountable
Community for
Health Model, 90
community-centered
health homes,
292–93 (*see also*
community-centered
health homes
(CCHH))
community
engagement, 89
Community of
Solutions–Fairfax
County Public
Schools, 143*b*
co-production,
250, 251*b*
cross-sector, 265 (*see
also* cross-sector
partnerships
(collaboration))
cross-sector, value-
based health, 325
data, 125

definition, 265
Edgecombe, North
    Carolina, 90, 119–
    23 (see also faith
    community)
elected officials, 90
experiences, care
    receivers, 265
interdisciplinary, 503
local, 125
multisector, 90
Near Northside
    Community,
    Houston, 90, 109
Near Northside
    Community,
    Houston, case study,
    90, 109
policy, 386
population health, 250,
    251b
primary care, 90 (see
    also primary care,
    in population and
    community
    health)
suicide risk reduction,
    90, 137–47, 143b
    (see also suicide
    risk reduction,
    Community of
    Solutions for)
trust building, 127
work plan, 38
collaboration(s), scaling
    up, 125–35, 128b
accountability
    for, 151–54
anchor organizations,
    maximizing cultural
    similarity, 134
Clinician's National
    Forum, 129–30
Clinician's National
    Forum, political
    will for component
    integration, 130
community of
    interest, 131b
community of
    practice, 131b
community of
    solution, 131b
data, importance, 125
Health Disparities
    Collaboratives, 129

information and
    communication
    technology, 131b
local, 125
patient-centered
    medical homes, 133
    (see also patient-
    centered medical
    home (PCMH))
political will, 135
proof-of-concept
    needs, 125–26
small tests of change
    approach, 135
starting with end in
    mind, 132
teaching
    responsibility, 126
trust building, 127
collaborative
    improvement and
    innovation networks
    (CoIIN), 126–27
collective accountability,
    149, 150b
Commission on Social
    Determinants
    (WHO), 16
commitment, Accountable
    Community for
    Health model, 152
Committee of Integrating
    Primary Care and
    Public Health, 3
common data model,
    179–80b
communication,
    BUILD Health
    Challenge, 27
communities of
    solution, 102
Community Access
    to Child Health
    (CATCH)
    program, 459–60
Community Action
    for a Renewed
    Environment
    (CARE) grant, 30
Community Action
    Plan (CAP),
    Healthy Living
    Matters, 376–77
community-based
    organization (CBO)
    sector, 23–34

BUILD Health
    Challenge, Cleveland,
    23 (see also BUILD
    Health Challenge,
    Cleveland)
BUILD Health
    Challenge, Cleveland,
    examples, 26–28
Engaging Communities
    in New Approaches
    to Healthy Housing,
    23, 24f, 29
Environmental Health
    Watch, 23–25
health inequities,
    tackling root
    cause, 26–28
    (see also BUILD
    Health Challenge,
    Cleveland, examples)
leadership strength,
    multisector
    partnerships and
    initiatives, 29
community-centered
    health homes
    (CCHH), 291–98
action, 295b, 296–97
analysis, 295b, 296
Asian Health Services,
    295–96b, 295
community-level
    prevention,
    knowledge and
    skills, 294–96
Daughters of Charity
    Services of New
    Orleans, 294b
definition and
    scope, 292
early testing of
    initiatives, 297
foundational capacities,
    293, 295–96b, 295
functional
    capacities, 296
inquiry, 295b, 296
leadership, 293–94
origins and history, 291
partnerships and
    collaborations,
    292–93, 296
staffing, designated and
    diverse, 294
structure, 292, 293f
value-based system, 292

Community-Centered
    Health Homes:
    Bridging the
    Gap Between
    Health Services
    and Community
    Prevention, 291
Community
    Close-Ups, 345–46
Community
    Commons, 261
community development,
    276–77, 277f,
    326, 329–47
Build Health Places
    Network, 330
clinician and public
    health practitioner
    roles, 345–47 (see
    also clinicians,
    in community
    development)
collaboration
    importance, 329
finance institutions,
    Robert Wood
    Johnson
    Foundation, 329–30,
    331b, 331–32
funding
    streams, 332–34
funding streams,
    Community
    Reinvestment
    Act, 334
funding streams, Low-
    Income Housing Tax
    Credit, 333
funding streams,
    New Markets Tax
    Credit, 333
gentrification and
    displacement, 341
history, 329–30, 332
innovations, financing,
    investment, and
    health, 341–44 (see
    also community
    development
    financing,
    innovations)
jargon and acronyms,
    330b, 330
low- and moderate-
    income
    investments, 329–30

community development
   (cont.)
   measurement, 340
   NeighborWorks
      America, 336, 338
   organizations investing
      in, 334–36
   organizations
      investing in,
      affordable housing
      developers, 335
   organizations investing
      in, community
      development
      corporations, 334
   organizations investing
      in, community
      development
      finance institutions,
      331b, 331–32
   organizations investing
      in, community
      development
      financial
      institutions, 335
   organizations investing
      in, national umbrella
      organizations, 336
   scale and
      alignment, 340
   Stewards for Affordable
      Housing for the
      Future, 335, 336, 338
   zip code improvement,
      336–40 (see also zip
      code improvement)
community development
   corporations
   (CDCs), 334
community development
   finance institutions
   (CDFIs)
   Enterprise Community
      Partners, 338
   Local Initiative Support
      Corporation, 338
   Robert Wood Johnson
      Foundation,
      331b, 331–32
community development
   financial institutions
   (CDFIs), 335
community development
   financing,
   innovations,
   341–44

community
   development
   efforts, for multiple
   SDHs, 344
   equity funds, 342
   hospital partnerships,
      342, 343f, 344f
   loan funds, 341–42
Community Guide
   to Preventive
   Services, 411
community health. See
   also specific topics
   decision-making data
      sets, using data you
      have, 208
   Green & Healthy
      Homes Initiative, 41
   multisector data,
      165, 166b
Community Health
   Action Team
   (CHAT), 327
community health worker
   (CHW), 83–84
   faith community
      partnerships, 122
community health worker
   (CHW) models,
   477, 478b
community-led practices,
   nursing, 486
community-level
   interventions, 242
community of
   interest, 131b
community of
   practice, 131b
community of solution,
   131b, 137–38
Community of Solutions
   (CoS), 90, 137–47
   accomplishments, high-
      level, 139b, 141
   challenges, 139b
   challenges,
      Fairfax County
      Public Health
      Department, 144–46
   challenges, reticence to
      discuss suicide, 142
   challenges,
      school system
      engagement, 142–44
   challenges,
      sustainability, 146

charter, 139b
current status, 146–47
Epi-Aid, 138, 142–46
Fairfax, Virginia
   epidemic, 137–38
Fairfax County
   Public Schools
   collaboration, 143b
growth, 139
meeting locations,
   varied, 139–41
name origin, 137–38
naming, 137–38
origins and early
   history, 137–39
student
   involvement, 141
survey action foci, top
   four, 139, 140b
Community-Oriented
   Primary Care
   (COPC), 75–78, 102
Community Pediatrics
   Training
   Initiative, 462–63
Community Preventive
   Services Task Force
   (CPSTF), 411
Community Reinvestment
   Act (CRA), 334
community-wide
   health issues,
   addressing, 106
competencies, public
   health, 458
Conetoe Family Life
   Center, 121–22
Conetoe Missionary
   Baptist, Conetoe,
   North Carolina, 90,
   119–23. See also faith
   community
connectivity, equitable,
   48, 53t
Continuity of Care
   Document
   (CCD), 182b
control mitigation, BUILD
   Health Challenge, 26
co-production, population
   health, 250, 251b
Corporate Anchor
   Roundtable
   (CAR), 371
costs and expenditures
   chronic disease, 283

health care, 68
   tobacco use, to
      employers, 64
   tobacco use, to
      employers, CDC
      strategy, 417–18
Council of State
   Territorial
   Epidemiologists
   (CSTE), 27
Council on Education
   in Public
   Health (CEPH)
   accreditation, 466
Council on Hazardous
   Materials,
   24–25
County Health Rankings
   criteria, 16
County Health Rankings
   & Roadmaps, 411
critical thinking, 460
cross-sector integration,
   federal funding cuts/
   changes, 358
   South Carolina,
      352–53b, 359
   Vermont, 359
   Virginia, 359
cross-sector integration,
   state funding, 358
   South Carolina,
      352–53b, 359
   Vermont, 359
   Virginia, 359
cross-sector partnerships
   (collaboration),
   15–20
   achieving effective,
      obstacles, 17
   awareness of
      importance
      and promotion
      efforts, 15–16
   early adopters, 16
   evidence-based action
      models, 19
   future action, 20
   Green & Healthy
      Homes Initiative, 37
   leadership, public
      health sector, 16
   policy as, 385
   social determinants of
      health, 15
   ubiquity, 15

value-based health care, 325
*Crosswalk Magazine,* 345–46
Culture of Health, 5, 16
culture of health care, 83
Culture of Health Prize, 5
  Kansas City, 445, 446, 448–49

data (health and public health), 205–6. *See also specific types and topics*
  administrative, 161
  for collaborations, 125
  common data model, 179–80b
  core functions, 205
  models, 179–80b, 179–80
  overview, 161–62
  plans, 195–96b
  primary data collection, 205–6
  results, 205
  secondary data collection, 206
  sharing and integration, 18, 161
  transfer and storage, 199
  transport and exchange, 182–83b
  use after release, 199–202, 200b
data (health and public health), available, using, 208–11
  administrative and local, for program priority identification, 208
  limited, for county-level response to emerging issues, 209, 210–13f
  secondary, for county and subcounty analysis, 211, 214–15b
data (health and public health), decision-making, 205–16
  asthma medications, prescriptions filling, 214–15b

available data, using, 208–11 (*see also* data, available, using)
community health decision-making, 206
data used are data improved, 215
primary data collection, 205–6
secondary data collection, 206
sources, 206–7
using data you have, 208
data (health and public health), secondary collection, 206
  for county and subcounty analysis of, 211
  sources, 206–7
Data Across Sectors for Health (DASH), 166
data exchange, 179–80b, 185
  automated, 183, 184f (*see also* surveillance for community outbreak, automation)
  health care–public health digital, 177–85 (*see also* surveillance for community outbreak, automation)
data use agreements (DUAs), 195–96b. *See also* memorandums of understanding (MOU)
data transfer and storage, 199
data use after release, 199–202, 200b
definitions, 192, 197
goals and partnership participation capacity, 193
parties, 194
scope of services, 197, 200b
terms and agreements, 202–3
Daughters of Charity Services of

New Orleans (DCSNO), 294b
de Beaumont Foundation, 3
decision-making, data for, 205–16. *See also* data (health and public health), decision-making
decision support intermediary (DSI), 27
delivery system reform incentive payment (DSRIP), 43
department-wide change, state funding, 357
  Oregon, 358
design thinking, 250, 252f, 253b
"Developing a Partnership to Address the Most Concerning Social Determinant: Employment" (Kampman), 496
diabetes mellitus, Upstream Strategy Matrix, 82t
Dietrich, Gini, 398–400, 399f
Digital Bridge project, 183, 184f, 184–85
digital data exchange, health care–public health, 177–85. *See also* surveillance for community outbreak, automation
Dignity Health, loan funds, 342
direct primary care, 103–4
  clinics, 78
displacement, gentrification and, 341
disruptive
  innovation, 231–32
  population health improvement, 257
distributed leadership, 152–53, 153f
divergent thinking, 306b, 310b
domestic violence, breaking cycle of, 305, 306b, 306

drug overdose data, Shelby County, Tennessee, 209, 210–13f
  chronic disease, for county and subcounty analysis, 211
Duke–Johnson & Johnson Nurse Leadership program innovations, 487–88

early adopters, 16
Earned Income Tax Credit (EITC), 416
East Bay Asian Local Development Corporation (EBALDC), 334
Edgecombe, North Carolina, 90, 119–23. *See also* faith community
education
  medical, rural, 474
  nursing, 485f, 485
education, public health, 465–70. *See also* training and education
  accreditation, Council on Education in Public Health, 466
  authentic and practical, 467
  CDC training programs, 467–68b, 468–69
  engagement, 465–66
  fellowships, 468–69
  Framing the Future Task Force, Association of Schools and Programs of Public Health, 466
  inclusive, 467
  learning opportunities, 469
  lifetime training, 467
  student programs, 469
  trends, 466–70
  universities, 465, 466 (*see also* universities)

education, public health, state innovations, 471–80
community health needs, understanding, 472, 473b
community health workers, 477, 478b
emergency medical professionals, expanding scope, 478
Health Extension Rural Offices, 476b
HRSA Teaching Health Centers Graduate Medical Education program, 476, 477b
Indiana, rural provider shortages response, 473b
Project ECHO, 479b, 479
public health–primary care intersection, 476–78
rural communities, 471
rural health career pipeline programs, 474
Rural Health Information Hub, 477, 478b
rural medical education, 474
rural residency programs, 475
targeting provider training with existing programs, 472–75
technology, in training, 478
elected officials, engaging for community health improvement, 113–18
examples, 114
lobbying vs. education and advocacy, 115, 116t
motivations, 114
political engagement, 113, 117f, 118
roles, important, 113
working with, ten tips, 115, 116t

elected officials, multisector partnerships, 90, 109–11
effective, key points, 110–11
Near Northside Community, Houston, 90, 109
electronic case reporting (ECR), 181
electronic health records (EHRs), 161
HITECH and Recovery Acts, 166–67
meaningful use, 179b
social needs data, 239
whole-person systems of care, 165b, 165
electronic laboratory reporting (ELR), 181
emergency medical systems (EMS), expanding scope of, 478
emerging practice, 253–54, 254b
empaneled patient population, 103
empanelment, 103–4
employment, partnerships for, 496
engagement
health care, for violence prevention, 277f
resident, 89, 93–100 (see also resident engagement)
engagement, community, 89, 93–100, 458, 459b
Accountable Community for Health Model, 152, 154, 157
authentic, 152, 154, 157
B'FRIEND initiative, 219
clinician roles, 346
collaborations, 89
community-centered health homes, 293–94 (see also community-centered health homes (CCHH))

healthy housing, 23, 24f, 29, 32
pediatrics and CATCH program, 459–60
training population health providers, 458, 459b
engagement, public health, 465–66
education, 465–66
elected officials, for community health improvement, 113–18 (see also elected officials, engaging for community health improvement)
political, 113, 117f, 118
school system, suicide risk reduction, 142–44
transportation sector, 54
Engaging Communities in New Approaches to Healthy Housing (ECNAHH), 23, 24f, 29
Enterprise Community Partners, 338
Environmental Health Watch (EHW), 23–25
A Blueprint for a Healthy House, 25
BUILD Health Challenge, 31–33 (see also BUILD Health Challenge, Cleveland)
community role, 23–24
healthy homes pioneer, 24
Healthy House Catalog, 25
intersectionality, 25
Lead + Asthma Project, 25
leadership, multisector partnerships and initiatives, 29
mission, health in, 29–30
sustainability, 25
work, approach to, 25
environmental justice, 26

"Envisioning a New System" (LaFave), 492
Epi-Aid, Community of Solutions and suicide risk prevention, 138, 142–46
Epidemic Intelligence Service (EIS), 468
Epidemiology Elective Program for Medical and Veterinary Students, 469
epidemiology training, 494
Episcopal Health Foundation (EHF), Texas, 297–98
equity, health, 7–12, 78, 509. See also inequities
#123forEquity Campaign to Eliminate Health Care Disparities, 70–71
access to health care, 10
access to preventive and therapeutic care, 10
Alliance for Health Equity, 271–81 (see also Alliance for Health Equity)
Centers for Achieving Equity, 30, 32
community development financing, 342
connectivity, 48, 53t
definition, 7
economic survival, community, 7
health systems strategy, 365–66
high level of health, 7, 8f
hospitals and health systems, 70
IHI guide, 11
justice, 7
Multnomah County's Office of Diversity and Health Equity, 10–11
as personal value, 12
pursuing, 7

race, BUILD Health Challenge, Cleveland, 55b
social factors, 7
strategy, 365–66
teaching, 11
transportation sector partnering, 53–54 (see also transportation sector actors and advocates)
equity and empowerment lens, 10–11
Eskenazi Health Center Cottage Corner–Work One Partnership, Indianapolis, 496
EveryONE Project Provider Toolkit, 104, 105b
evidence-based action models, 19
Public Health 3.0, 17, 19
evidence-based policies, 407–8
evidence-based policies, building, 386, 407–20. See also CityHealth; Health Impact in 5 Years (HI-5)
CityHealth's evidence-based policies for health, 410
developing and implementing, 407, 409f
evidence, 409–15
final thoughts, 419
successful policymaking, 407
expenditures. See costs and expenditures
Extension for Community Healthcare Outcomes, 479b, 479
extensions, 182b

Fairfax, Virginia, suicide epidemic, 137–38. See also suicide risk reduction, Community of Solutions for

faith community, 90, 119–23
acknowledging the why, 119
flourishing, partnerships promoting, 121
gardens, beehives, and human development, 121
healing of souls, 119
members and gatherings, 119
social determinants, built environment, and healing, 120
transformative healing, 119
whole person wellness, addressing, 119
falls
older adults, public health problem, 219
reduction, initiative, 219–27
reduction, via engaging neighborhoods and data, 219
risk, Baltimore City, 219–20
Family Educational Rights Privacy Act (FErPA), 167–68
Fast Healthcare Interoperability Resource (FHIR), 179–80b, 182b
SMART on, 183b
Federally Qualified Health Center (FQHC), 129, 130
as anchor organization, 134
Clinician's National Forum, 129–30
Clinician's National Forum, political will for component integration, 130
Opportunities Industrialization Center, 122 (see also faith community)
feedback loops, transparent, 152, 154

fee-for-service payment models, 103–4
fellowships, public health, 468–69
finance and funding, 325–28. See also community development finance institutions (CDFIs); sustainability and finance
community development financing, innovations, 341–44 (see also community development financing, innovations)
health investments, acquiring and managing, 325
health investments, sustaining, 325–26
healthy homes, 43
housing finance agencies, state, 333
investors, health care, building population health, 267
loan funds, community development, 341–42
local, 315–21 (see also One Virginia Foundation)
Medicaid, state innovations, 356
obstacles, 17
Opportunity Finance Network, 336, 509
Pay for Success financing, 42, 43f, 44
state innovations, 354, 355t
state public health and prevention, 351–62 (see also state funding, public health and prevention)
flexible housing pool (FHP), 275
Flexner Report, 457
Flint, Michigan water crisis, pediatrician role, 461, 462b

FLOURISH, 51b, 54, 56f
flourishing, faith partnerships promoting, 121
Folsom, Marion, 137–38
food deserts, 17
food insecurity, combating, 498
"Food Matters: Medical Students Partner with a Community-Based Nonprofit to Combat Food Insecurity" (Penner, McCarthy, and Mullins), 498
Ford, Henry, 91
foundations, philanthropic, 4–5. See also specific types
Framing the Future Task Force, Association of Schools and Programs of Public Health, 466
Frieden, Thomas R., Health Impact Pyramid, 410–11, 425–27
Frontier School of Nursing, 484
funding. See finance and funding
"Further Forward," 310, 311b, 311, 311t
Future Centers, 263–64
future of health, designing, 306
Future of Nursing, The, 484–85

Gandhi, Pritesh, 297
gardens for health, faith community, 120–21, 122
Geiger, Jack, 132
Generate Health St. Louis, 51b, 54, 56f
gentrification, displacement and, 341
Gentrification and Neighborhood Change: Helpful Tools for Communities, 341

Georgetown University, Population Health Scholar Track, 458, 459*b*

Good Agriculture Practice, 122

Good Samaritan laws, 428

grasstops organizations, 394

Greater Kansas City Chamber of Commerce, 61, 445

Green & Healthy Homes Initiative (GHHI), 35–44
asset and gap analysis, 38
collaborative work plan, 38
community benefits, 41
cross-sector convening, 37
evidence-based model, 38
healthy homes financing, other, 43
origins and purpose, 35–36
overview, 35
payment structure, best, 41
program design, 40
purchasing, value-based, 42
purchasing, value-based, Pay for Success financing, 42, 43*f*, 44
resource integration and process flow, 36–37, 37*f*
services, bundled, 42
services, expansion, 44
services, piloting, 43
services, population served and, 35, 36*f*
training, 38

ground-softening campaign, 393

*Guide to Equitable Neighborhood Development*, 341

Hanna-Attisha, Mona, 461, 462*b*

Harris County Public Health (HCPH), 376–77

Healthy Corner Store Initiative, 378–80

Healthy Dining Matters, 378, 379–80

HealthBegins, 76*b*, 80

Healthcare Anchor Network, 368, 372

healthcarecommunities. org, 128*b*

health care groups, 4

health care investors, building population health, 267

health care parity. *See* parity, health care

health care payers, building population health, 266

Health Chicago 2.0, 275

Health Coaches for Hypertension Control, 477

Health Community50, 288–89

*Health Development Without Gentrification*, 341

Health Disparities Collaboratives (HDC), HRSA, 129
Clinician's National Forum, political will for component integration, 130

Health Eating/Active Living (HEAL), 284–85

Health Enhancement Research Organization (HERO), 64

health equity, 7–12. *See also* equity, health

Health Extension Rural Offices (HEROs), 476*b*

Health Food Financing Initiative (HFFI), 333

Health Homes Zone (HHZ), 32

Healthiest Cities and Counties Challenge (the Challenge), 287

Health Impact in 5 Years (HI-5), 20, 386, 407–12, 415–20
*vs.* CityHealth, 415
goals, 411
interventions, evidence-based, 411–12, 412*f*, 413*f*
policymaking, advancing, evidence in, 409–15
policy targets, earned income tax credit, 416
policy targets, overview, 416
policy targets, tobacco reforms, San Antonio, 417
program and scope, 410

Health Impact Pyramid, 410–11, 425–27

Health in All Policies (HiAP), 191

HealthInfoNet, 167

health information exchange (HIE). *See* All In: Data for Community Health

health information exchange (HIE), B'FRIEND fall reduction data
data and uses, 225
hyperfocus, 227
as public health innovation, 226
sharing, 223
sharing, complexity, 227
sharing, peer learning, 227
use, 220–21

health information exchange (HIE), Maine, 167

Health Information Technology for Economic and Clinical Health (HITECH) Act, 165–67

Health Insurance Portability and Accountability Act (HIPAA), 167–68

asthma medication prescription filling, 214–15*b*

asthma rates, childhood, 171–72*b*
care plan, checking, 200–1*b*
data released under, 195–96*b*
Would you like a home visit? use case, 188*b*

*Health Is a Community Affair*, 137–38

Health Level 7 International (HL7), 179–80*b*, 182*b*

Health Living Matters (HLM), 376–77

Health Resources and Services Administration (HRSA)
diabetes control program, 130–480
Health Disparities Collaboratives, 128*b*, 129
Maternal, Infant, and Early Childhood Home Visiting programs, 439
patient-centered medical homes, 481 (*see also* patient-centered medical home (PCMH))
policy strategies, 361
population health integration with primary care, 3
Regional Public Health Training Centers, 478
rural health career pipeline programs, 474
Rural Health Information Hub, 477, 478*b*
Rural Health Outreach Grants, 477
Rural Training Tracks, 475–76
Teaching Health Centers Graduate Medical Education program, 476, 477*b*

workforce training, population health, 454
health return on investment, 337, 367
health status, differences, 7–8
health systems, 67–71. *See also* hospitals and health systems; *specific types*
expenditures, 366
mission, rethinking, 365–73 (*see also* mission, health systems)
health systems, in community health improvement, 283–87
Aetna Foundation, 287
challenges, 283
chronic disease care and costs, 283
healthy communities, 283–84
Humana, 286
insurance reforms, 284
Kaiser Permanente, 284
leadership, 283–84
policy influence tools and strategies, 286*t*
Healthy Allegheny, 19
Healthy Buildings Initiative, Bronx, 172–73*b*, 173
healthy communities, 283–84
Healthy Communities movement, history, 261
Healthy Corner Store Initiative, 378–80
Healthy Dining Matters, 378, 379–80
Healthy Eating Active Living (HEAL) Buckeye, 31
Healthy Futures Fund (HFF), 342
healthy homes, financing, 43
Healthy Homes and Sustainable Communities, 25

healthy homes initiative (HHI), Nationwide Children's Hospital–Church and Community Development for All People, 343–44
Healthy House Catalog, 25
Healthy KC, 61, 62, 446
Healthy Nail Salon Collaborative, 295*b*, 295, 296–97
Healthy Neighborhoods Equity Fund (HNEF), 342
Healthy Places Index (HPI), California, 252*f*, 253*b*
healthy vending. *See* vending, healthy
Hill Community Development Corporation, 334
Homeownership Opportunities for People Everywhere (HOPE VI), 345
home visit, 187–88*b*
Hope Health, South Carolina, 352–51*b*
HOPE SF, 345
HOPE VI, 345
Horizon Foundation, 390. *See also* Big Soda, fighting at local level
advocacy, against Big Soda, 403
campaign components, 391
healthy child care certification, 393
hospitals and health systems, 67–71
affordability and value, 68
as anchor institutions, 326–27
equity of care, 70
faith community partnerships, 122
partnerships, community development financing, 342, 343*f*, 344*f*

population health, advancing, 69
"redefining the H," 67–68
roles and impacts, new, 67–68, 71
hotspotting, health care, 80–81
housing
affordable, developers, 335
affordable, on child well-being, 337
Alliance for Health Equity, 275
asset and gap analysis, 38
asthma, childhood, 185–87*b*
"Better Health Through Housing," 275
BUILD Health Challenge, Cleveland, 32
condition improvements, capitalizing on health impacts, 35–44 (*see also* Green & Healthy Homes Initiative (GHHI))
Engaging Communities in New Approaches to Healthy Housing, 23, 24*f*, 29
flexible housing pool, 275
health return on investment and research and partnership opportunities, 337, 367
healthy, community engagement, 23, 24*f*, 29, 32
insecurity, screening for, 76*b*
Low-Income Housing Tax Credit, 333
naturally occurring affordable housing, 341
Stewards for Affordable Housing for the Future, 335, 336, 338

housing finance agencies (HFAs), state, 333
Houston, TX, Near Northside Community, 90, 109
collaboration, 109
Howard County Unsweetened campaign, 396*b*
Howard County Wellness Policy, 396*b*
HRSA Health Disparities Collaboratives (HDC), 129
Clinician's National Forum, political will for component integration, 130
Humana, 286

IHI Breakthrough Series Collaborative learning model, 129
Illinois Institute of Public Health (IPHI), 272, 280–81. *See also* Alliance for Health Equity
inclusion
Accountable Community for Health model, 152, 153
BUILD Health Challenge, Cleveland, examples, 28
Indiana
Eskenazi Health Center Cottage Corner–Work One Partnership, Indianapolis, 496
rural provider shortages response, 473*b*
inequities. *See also* equity
current, degree of, 366
economic, 365
economic, poverty and, 365
health, tackling root cause, 26–28 (*see also* BUILD Health Challenge, Cleveland, examples)
tackling root causes, 26–28

Information Age, 177–78
information and
    communication
    technology
    (ICT), 131b
information pathway,
    195–96b
information point
    (entity), 196b
infrastructure owners,
    transportation
    sector, 49
innovation, 231–33
    community led, 232
    definitions, 249–50
    diffusion, 253–54
    disruptive, 231–32
    forms, 231
    funding strategies, 326
    improvement
        from, 256
    matching needs
        to, 232–33
    meaning, 231
    multisector
        partnerships for
        health, 232
    new partners and
        tools, 232
    new perspectives, 232
    old idea as, 232
    in policymaking, 408
    population health
        improvement,
        249–58 (see also
        population health
        improvement,
        innovation in)
    Public Health
        National Center for
        Innovations, 250
    in states, 427–28
    teaching public health,
        state, 471–80 (see
        also education,
        public health, state
        innovations)
    term and concept, 249
Institute for Health
    Care Improvement
    (IHI), 11
    guide to achieving
        health equity, 11
Integration of Primary
    Care and Public
    Health, 509

interdisciplinary
    collaboration, 503
International
    Classification of
    Diseases, 10th
    Revision, Clinical
    Modification (ICD-
    10-CM), 181–83
interoperability, 178
    social determinant data
        standards, 168
interprofessional
    education
    (IPE), 486–87
investors. See finance and
    funding

Joyful Food Markets
    (JFM), 459b, 461,
    499–500
justice, 7

Kaiser Permanente,
    284
    Chief Community
        Health Officer, 338
    Thriving Communities
        Fund, 339–40b
Kaiser Permanente–
    Health Leaders
    partnership, 19–20
Kansas City, 445–50
    Culture of Health Prize,
        445, 446, 448–49
    Greater Kansas
        City Chamber of
        Commerce, 445
    Healthy KC, 61, 62, 446
    Kansas City, MO Health
        Department, 445
    KC Chamber–Kansas
        City, MO Health
        Department
        partnership, 446
    Not So Big KC
        Challenge, 447
    Tobacco21 KC,
        386–87, 448
Kansas City, business and
    public health
    Greater Kansas
        City Chamber of
        Commerce, 61, 445
    history, Kansas City, 61
Kar, Sidney and Emily,
    102, 132

Kelley, Tom, 254–55
Kindig, D., 69–70

laboratory information
    management system
    (LIMS), 181–83
Laboratory Leadership
    Service (LLS), 468
La Causa, 334
Latino Health
    Access, 78–79
Lavizzo-Mourey, Risa, 337
Lawrence-Douglas
    County, Kansas, 19
Lead + Asthma
    Project, 25
leadership
    community-based
        organizations, 29
    community-
        centered health
        homes, 293–94
    cross-sector
        partnerships, 16
    distributed,
        152–53, 153f
    Duke–Johnson &
        Johnson Nurse
        Leadership program
        innovations, 487–88
    Environmental Health
        Watch, 29
    health systems, in
        community health
        improvement, 283–84
    Kaiser Permanente–
        Health Leaders
        partnership, 19–20
    Laboratory Leadership
        Service, 468
    multisector
        partnerships and
        initiatives, 29
    Neighborhood
        Leadership for
        Environmental
        Health, 30–31
    nurses, 484
    nursing leaders,
        community
        collaborative efforts,
        483–89 (see also
        nursing leaders
        in community
        collaborative
        efforts)

training population
    health providers,
    461, 462b
leading practice,
    253–54, 254b
Learning Connection,
    CDC, 469
learning loops,
    308–9, 309f
legal responsibility, or
    parties, 203
liability, 203
lifespan, poverty on, 365
loan funds. See also
    finance and funding
    community
        development
        financing, 341–42
lobbying, vs. education
    and advocacy,
    115, 116t
local funding, 315–21. See
    also One Virginia
    Foundation
Local Initiative Support
    Corporation
    (LISC), 338
locally, acting and
    funding, 315–21. See
    also One Virginia
    Foundation
Logical Observation
    Identifiers Names
    and Codes
    (LOINC), 181–83
Lori's Hands, 493–94
Loudon County,
    child abuse and
    neglect, 317
Louisiana, chronic
    disease and
    health promotion
    funding, 360
Louisiana Public Health
    Institute (LPHI),
    295–96b, 295, 297
Low-Income Housing Tax
    Credit (LIHTC), 333

Marmot, Michael, 16
Martha's Table, 459b, 498
Maternal, Infant, and
    Early Childhood
    Home Visiting
    (MIECHV)
    programs, 439

meaningful use (MU),
electronic health
records, 180
MeasureUP metrics, 346
media strategy
against Big Soda,
deploying successful,
398, 399f
Paid, Earned, Shared,
and Owned model,
398–400, 399f
Medicaid
coverage, 355–56
state–federal
partnership, 356
state funding
flexibilities, 356
Medicaid State Plan
Amendments, 356
Medical Applications of
Science for Health
(M*A*S*H), 474
medication-assisted
treatment
(MAT), 353–54b,
428, 434–35
memorandums of
understanding
(MOUs), 27, 191–204
asthma care plan,
checking, 200b
background, 194–97
benefits, 192
data plans and data use
agreements, 195–96b
definition, 191
drafting successful, 193
drawbacks, 193
parties, 194
Public Health
3.0, 191–92
purpose, 194–96, 197
scope of services,
197, 200b
terms and
agreements, 202
mental health
Alliance for Health
Equity, 275, 277f
initiative sustainability,
rural case study, 326
Milliman, 40
Mindfulness for Sports
Performance
Enhancement,
142–44

Minnesota
community
paramedics, 478
Unity Accountable
Community for
Health, 353–54b, 362
Minnesota Working
Family
Credit, 416–17
mission, health
systems, 365–73
anchor institutions, 366
anchor mission, 366
case example, 372
health care mission, 365
health equity
strategy, 365–66
national collaboration,
Healthcare Anchor
Network, 372
poverty and economic
inequities, 365
Rush University
Medical Center,
Chicago, 368
RWJBarnabas Health,
368, 370
mobility, equitable, 48
monitoring, opioid
crisis, 429
as primary
prevention, 436
Moving to Opportunity
study, 337
multidomain social and
economic needs
screening tools,
236, 237t
multisector data
cases for, 163–64, 164f
project categories,
overview, 163
project categories,
population and
community health
and well-being,
165, 166b
project categories,
whole-person
systems of care,
165b, 165
multisector data-sharing
collaborations
environment,
166–69, 170–72b.
See also All

In: Data for
Community Health
challenges, 166
honest and mutually
beneficial
relationships, 167
interoperability and
social determinant
data standards, 168
legal issues and legal
terms, 167
meaningful data for
programmatic
operations, 169
sustainability, 169
multisector initiatives, 29
multisector
partnerships, 29
access to care, 10
advocacy and advocacy
planning, 10
allyship, 10
equity and
empowerment
lens, 10–11
social obligation scale,
9–10, 9t
for upstream work, 9
Multnomah County's
Office of Diversity
and Health
Equity, 10–11

naloxone, 428,
431–32, 433f
Nashville Health, 19
National Alliance
of Community
Development
Associations
(NACEDA),
336, 346
National Coalition
for Asian Pacific
American
Community
Development
(National
CAPACD), 346
Nationally Notifiable
Condition List, 181
Nationwide Children's
Hospital–Church
and Community
Development for All
People, 343–44

naturally occurring
affordable housing
(NOAH), 341
Near Northside
Community,
Houston, TX,
90, 109
community
collaboration, 109
needle exchange, 431,
432, 433f
Neighborhood Leadership
for Environmental
Health
(NLEH), 30–31
NeighborWorks America,
336, 338, 346
New Hampshire, all-payer
claims database, 425,
426–27b
New Markets Tax Credit
(NMTC), 333, 344f
New Voices essay contest,
491–504
"Breaking the Mold"
(Garcia Agana),
494
"Developing a
Partnership to
Address the Most
Concerning Social
Determinant:
Employment"
(Kampman), 496
"Envisioning a
New System"
(LaFave), 492
"Food Matters: Medical
Students Partner
with a Community-
Based Nonprofit
to Combat Food
Insecurity" (Penner,
McCarthy, and
Mullins), 498
"Public Health
Pharmacists: Beyond
the Counter"
(Vu), 501
"With Synergy, We
Flourish: A Case for
Interdisciplinary
Collaboration to
Improve Health in
the United States"
(Duncan), 503

New York State Energy Research and Development Authority (NYSERDA), 42

New York University psychiatry residency, Brownsville program, 458

next generation, 491–504. *See also* student voices

Nightingale, Florence, 484

noise, transportation, 49, 53t

North Coast Health Improvement and Integration Network (NCHIIN), 169

Northern Virginia, 315. *See also* One Virginia Foundation
low-income resident challenges, 316
setting, 315
Stop Child Abuse Now, 317

Northern Virginia Health Foundation (NVHF), 315–16

Not So Big KC Challenge, 447

Nurse-Family Partnership Pay-for-Success Program, South Carolina, 352–53b, 359

Nurses on Boards Coalition, 488–89

nursing, 4–5

nursing leaders in community collaborative efforts, 483–89
academia, influence, 485f, 485
current status, 488
Duke–Johnson & Johnson Nurse Leadership program innovations, 487–88
key roles *vs.* decision making power, 483
leadership roles, 484
nursing education–medical

education–public health education, 485f

professional organizations, 487

Oakland, California
Asian Health Services, 295–96b, 295
East Bay Asian Local Development Corporation, 334
Oakland Promise, 263
population health partnerships, 263

Oakland Promise, 263

Object Management Group, 180b, 180

Office of the National Coordinator for Health Information Technology (ONC), 165–66

Ohio Housing Finance Agency, health return on investment study, 338

Oklahoma City, population health partnerships, 263

Omnibus Reconciliation Act (OBRA) block grants, 354, 355t

one-minute message, 311b, 311

One Virginia Foundation, 315–21
lessons learned, 318
Loudon County, addressing child abuse and neglect, 317
Northern Virginia, low-income resident challenges, 316
Northern Virginia, setting, 315
Northern Virginia Health Foundation, 315–16
systems change, upstream interventions, 316

opioid misuse and addiction
drug overdose data, Shelby County,

Tennessee, 209, 210–13f
as public health emergency, 209
as state of emergency, 429–30

opioid misuse and addiction, state and territorial public health policy, 386, 425–40
comprehensive approaches, 439
downstream or tertiary prevention, overdose reversal meds and syringe & needle exchange, 431, 433f
Health Impact Pyramid, 425–27
prevention, policy, and state public health, 425, 426–27b, 428f
primary prevention, monitoring and surveillance, 436–39
primary prevention, resiliency, 439
secondary prevention, mental & physical health care parity, 433f, 435–36
secondary prevention, treatment access, 433f, 434–35
state responses, 427, 430f

Opportunity Finance Network (OFN), 336, 509

Oregon Health Authority, Public Health Division, 358

Otho S. A. Sprague Memorial Institute, 272–73

outcomes. *See also specific topics and programs*
accountability, 261
*vs.* outputs, 340–41

outputs, 340–41

Paid, Earned, Shared, and Owned (PESO) model, 398–400, 399f

pain, as fifth vital sign, 427

Pain in the Nation, 261

Palo Alto, suicide risk reduction, 142, 145–46

panel management, 104

parity, health care
#123forEquity Campaign to Eliminate Health Care Disparities, 70–71
Health Disparities Collaboratives Clinician's National Forum, 130
HRSA Health Disparities Collaboratives, 129
mental & physical health, for addictions, 433f, 435–36
Roadmap to Reduce Racial and Ethnic Disparities in Health Care, 11–12

partnerships, 509–10. *See also* collaboration
Big Soda, against, 394, 396b
community-centered health homes, 292–93, 296
cross-sector (*see* cross-sector partnerships (collaboration))
local, 125
multisector (*see* multisector partnerships)
Oakland, 263
Oklahoma City, 264
training and workforce, 453

partnerships for health movement, 3–5
barriers, 5
barriers, cultural, 5
better practices, 5
change, need for, 4
growth, rapid, 3–4
health care groups, 4
history, 3
nursing, 4–5

philanthropic
foundations, 4–5
value and execution, 4
Pasadena, Texas
community assets, 376
demographics, 376t
economic challenges
and health
impact, 375
overview, 375
Pasadena Economic
Development
Corporation
(EDC), 380
Pasadena Vibrant
Community, 377–78
Pathways to Population
Health, 69–70
patient-centered medical
home (PCMH), 75,
78, 80, 103, 133
as anchor
organization, 134
interdisciplinary
collaborations, 503–4
Patient-Centered Primary
Care Collaborative
(PCPCC), 134
Patients, Pharmacists,
Partnerships (PE)
Program, 502
payers, health care,
building population
health, 266
Pay for Success financing
with, 42, 43f, 44
payment
delivery system
reform incentive
payment, 43
fee-for-service
models, 103–4
Green & Healthy
Homes Initiative, 41
reform, 242
structure, determining
best, 41
value-based payment
models, 83, 103–4,
242 (see also
accountable care
organizations (ACO))
PDSA cycle data, 131–32
People Acting Together
in Howard County
(PATH), 396b

People's Community
Clinic, Texas, 297
performance measures, 68
pharmacists, public
health, 501
philanthropy. See also
specific organizations
4 Ps, 392
advocacy, 400,
401–2b, 401–3
foundations, 4–5
pipeline programs, rural
health career, 474
place-based strategies,
165–66
plan-do-study-act
(PDSA), 129
policy and policymaking,
385–87. See also
cross-sector
partnerships
(collaboration);
specific types
anchor institutions,
365–73, 387 (see
also mission, health
systems)
art and science,
385, 407
business, 61–65, 387
(see also business,
public health and)
collaboration, 386
community healthy
goals, 385
contexts, 385–86
cross-sector
collaboration, 385
developing and
implementing,
critical factors,
407, 409f
elected officials,
working with,
113–18, 387 (see
also elected officials,
engaging for
community health
improvement)
emerging tool, 387
evidence, 409–15
evidence, evidence-
based policies for
health, 410
evidence base,
407–8

food and nutrition,
local level, 386,
389–404 (see also
Big Soda, fighting at
local level)
health, building
population
health, 267
health approach, 385
Health Impact in 5
Years, 386, 407–20
(see also Health
Impact in 5 Years
(HI-5))
innovation in, 408
Kansas City,
Tobacco21 initiative,
386–87, 448
public, importance, 386
state and territorial,
opioid epidemic and,
386, 425–40 (see also
state and territorial
public health policy,
opioid misuse and
addiction)
state public health, 425,
426–27b, 428f
successful, 407
transportation
sector, 49–50
political engagement, 113
ground rules, 117f, 118
political will
for component
integration,
Clinician's National
Forum, 130
harnessed appropriately
for scale-up, 135
population health, 101–3.
See also specific topics
definition, 102, 166–67
hospitals and health
systems, 69
milestones and
competencies, 457
multisector data,
165, 166b
transportation sector
partnering for,
53–54
transportation sector
partnering for,
closest transportation
sector actor, 54

transportation sector
partnering for,
established coalition
allies, 53
transportation sector
partnering for,
flexible blueprint for
change, 51b, 54, 56f
population health
improvement,
innovation in, 249–58
co-production and
collaboration,
250, 251b
cultivating or
suppressing, 254–55
design thinking, 250,
252f, 253b
disruptive
innovation, 257
improvement and, 256
innovation, emerging,
leading, and
prevailing, 251, 254b
innovation,
transformation
via, 251
innovation concept, 249
social determinants
of health, root
causes, 249
transformation
from, 258
population health
providers,
training, 457–64
community
engagement,
458, 459b
critical thinking, 460
leadership
development,
461, 462b
milestones and
competencies, 457
public health
competencies, 458
Population Health Scholar
Track, Georgetown
University, 458, 459b
Population Health
Training in
Place Program
(PH-TIP), 468
population
management, 69–70

portfolio development,
California
Accountable
Communities for
Health Initiative,
151–54, 153*f*
poverty
extremely low
income, 333
incidence, U.S., 365
on lifespan, 365
Northern Virginia,
316, 319–20
War on Poverty, 332
power
mitigation, BUILD
Health Challenge, 26
sense of, 97*b*, 98*f*, 98
sources of, 83
*Practical Playbook, The.*
*See also specific topics*
in action, 15–20 (*see*
*also* cross-sector
partnerships)
Internet-based
initiative, 3
prescription drug
monitoring
programs (PDMP),
428, 436–39
Presence Health, 41
Presence Hospital project,
Chicago, 44
President Management
Fellows (PMF), 469
prevailing practice,
253–54, 254*b*
opioid misuse and
addiction (*see*
opioid misuse and
addiction, state and
territorial public
health policy)
prevention
access, 10
community-
centered health
homes, 294–96
Community Guide
to Preventive
Services, 411
community-level,
294–96
Community Preventive
Services Task
Force, 411

monitoring, opioid
crisis, 436
primary care health
providers, 457
social needs checklist,
243*b*, 243–44
state funding,
351–62 (*see also*
state funding,
public health and
prevention)
state public health, 425,
426–27*b*, 428*f*
suicide, Epi-Aid,
138, 142–46
Three Pockets
of Prevention
Framework, 410–11
tobacco use, 417–18
tobacco use, Kansas
City, 386–87, 448
tobacco use, San
Antonio, 416–19
violence, 277*f*
Preventive Medicine
Residency and
Fellowship (MR/
F), 468
primary care,
direct, 103–4
primary care, in
population and
community health,
90, 101–7
clinical population
medicine model, 105
empaneled patients, 103
EveryONE Project
Provider Toolkit,
104, 105*b*
integrating with
community
health, pragmatic
approaches, 103–5
population and
community health
framework, 101
primary care, social
determinants of
health and, 75–84
capacity, 79
care models, 77
cold spots, 82
culture, 83
direct primary care
clinics, 78

hot spots,
community, 80–81
housing insecurity
screening, 76*b*
recent developments,
75–77, 76*b*
scope, 80–81
social determinants of
health, 76
Upstream Capability
Assessment, 80, 81*t*
Upstream Strategy
Matrix, 80–81, 82*t*
Primary Care: American's
Health in a New
Era, 103
Primary Care and Public
Health: Exploring
Integration to
Improve Population
Health, 103
primary care health
providers, disease
prevention and health
promotion by, 457
primary care practice-
based research
networks
(PBRNs), 460–61
primary data
collection, 205–6
profiles, 182*b*
Project ECHO,
479*b*, 479
*promotoras*, 78–79
proof-of-concept
needs, 125–26
protected health
information
(PHI), 41
Protocol for Responding
to and Assessing
Patient Assets, Risks,
and Experiences
(PRAPARE),
236, 239
providers, health care. *See*
*also specific types*
access to, 10
building population
health, 266
providers, transportation
sector, 49
Public Health 3.0,
17, 19, 191,
385, 509

memorandums of
understanding
in, 191–92
Public Health
Accreditation Board
(PHAB), 454
Public Health Associate
Program
(PHAP), 469
public health education.
*See* education, public
health
Public Health Impact
Pyramid,
410–11, 425–27
Public Health Informatics
Fellowship Program
(PHIFP), 469
Public Health National
Center for
Innovations
(PHNCI), 250
"Public Health
Pharmacists: Beyond
the Counter"
(Vu), 501
public health
practitioners,
in community
development, 345–47
align, 347
engage, 346
identify, 346
learn, 345
Public Health Security
and Bioterrorism
Preparedness
Response Act, 166
purchasing,
value-based, 42
Pay for Success
financing with, 42,
43*f*, 44
purpose, information
point, 196*b*
Purpose Built
Communities, 345

quality improvement (QI)
innovation, 256
residency training, 461

REAL (race, ethnicity,
language preference)
population
health, 70–71

redlining, 334
Regional Public Health
    Training Centers
    (PHTC), HRSA, 478
relationships. *See also*
    collaboration(s)
    building
    purposeful, 26–27
    honest and mutually
    beneficial,
    multisector data
    sharing, 167
reportable condition
    knowledge
    management system
    (RCKMS), 27
Representational
    State Transfer
    (REST), 182*b*
Residences at Career
    Gateway, 343–44
residency programs,
    rural, 475
resident engagement,
    89, 93–100
    belonging, sense of,
    97*b*, 97, 98*f*
    outcomes, 99*f*
    power, sense of, 97*b*,
    98*f*, 98
    Resident Engagement
    Practices Typology,
    94–97, 95*f*, 97*b*
    survey, community, 97*b*
    trust, sense of, 97*b*,
    97, 98*f*
Resident Engagement
    Practices Typology,
    94–97, 95*f*, 97*b*
resiliency, individual,
    family, and
    community, opioid
    crisis, 439
resources
    allocation
    differences, 7–8
    Green & Healthy Homes
    Initiative, integration
    and process flow,
    36–37, 37*f*
    Green & Healthy
    Homes Initiative,
    local, asset and gap
    analysis, 38
    return on investment,
    health, 337, 367

Rhode Island
    addiction treatment, for
    incarcerated, 435–36
    chronic disease and
    health promotion
    funding, 360
Roadmap to Reduce
    Racial and Ethnic
    Disparities in Health
    Care, 11–12
Robert Wood Johnson
    Foundation
    Alliance for
    Health, 272–73
    community
    development
    finance institutions,
    331*b*, 331–32
    County Health
    Rankings criteria, 16
    County Health
    Rankings &
    Roadmaps, 411
    Culture of Health, 5, 16
    Culture of Health
    Prize, 5
    Culture of Health Prize,
    Kansas City, 445,
    446, 448–49
    Digital Bridge project,
    183, 184*f*, 184–85
    Roadmap to Reduce
    Racial and Ethnic
    Disparities in Health
    Care, 11–12
    Voices for Healthy
    Kids, 390–91
Rocky Mountain
    Public Health
    Training Center
    (RMPHTC), 479
rural communities,
    327, 471
    differences, 471
    health needs,
    understanding,
    472, 473*b*
    rural health
    career pipeline
    programs, 474
    state roles, 471
Rural Health Information
    Hub, HRSA,
    477, 478*b*
Rural Health Outreach
    Grants, HRSA, 477

rural medical
    education, 474
Rural Training Tracks
    (RTTs), 475–76
Rush University Medical
    Center, Chicago, 368
RWJBarnabas Health
    (RWJBH), 368, 370

safety
    community, Alliance
    for Health Equity,
    276–77, 277*f*
    transportation, 48, 53*t*
Safe Walk Home, 89–110
San Antonio, Tobacco 21
    initiative, 416–19
scope, 80–81
scope of services, MOUs,
    197, 200*b*
screening
    for housing
    insecurity, 76*b*
    for social and economic
    needs, multidomain,
    236, 237*t*
screening, social needs
    implementing patient
    level programs,
    238–39 (*see also*
    social screening
    programs,
    implementing
    patient level)
    workflow (staff,
    modality, and
    timing), 239
Second Century
    Corp., 380
security, information
    point, 196*b*
Shaping Our Appalachian
    Region (SOAR), 327
Shelby County, Tennessee,
    209, 210–13*f*
    administrative data
    and local data, for
    program priority
    identification, 208
Sheppard-Towner
    Act, 461
small tests of change
    approach, 135
SMART, 183*b*
social accountability, 7–9
    definition, 8–9

medical education
    excellence, 9–10
    Social Obligation
    Scale, 9*t*
social and economic
    health risk
    intervention, 240–42
    community-level
    interventions, 242
    payment reform, 242
    socially informed care,
    240, 241*t*
    socially targeted care,
    241, 241*t*
social determinants of
    health (SDH), 76. *See
    also specific topics*
    Blue Cross of California
    Foundation,
    303*f*, 303
    data standards, for
    multisector data
    sharing, 168
    faith community, 120
    health care
    organizational
    competencies, 81*t*
    meaning, 78
    root causes, 249
    screening tools,
    multidomain, 236
    social factors, 7
    socially informed care,
    104, 240, 241*t*
    socially responsible,
    9–10, 9*t*
    socially responsive,
    9–10, 9*t*
    socially targeted care,
    241, 241*t*
    social needs, identifying
    and addressing
    patients', 235–44
    future, 243*b*, 243–44
    intervening, social and
    economic health
    risks, 240–42 (*see
    also* social and
    economic health risk
    intervention)
    prevention system,
    checklist for taking
    action, 243*b*,
    243–44
    socially informed care,
    240, 241*t*

ocial needs, identifying and addressing patients (*cont.*)
socially targeted care, 241, 241*t*
social risk assessment, 236, 237*t*
social screening programs, implementing patient level, 238–39 (*see also* social screening programs, implementing patient level)
social obligation scale, 9–10, 9*t*
social screening programs, implementing patient level, 238–39
  data tracking, 239
  screening workflow (staff, modality, and timing), 239
  target population, 239
social vulnerabilities, primary care assessment, 104
So Others Might Eat (SOME), 344–45
South Carolina, Nurse-Family Partnership Pay-for-Success Program, 352–53*b*, 359
South Philadelphia Community Health and Literacy Center, 329, 344*f*
Standardized Nomenclature of Medicine Clinical Terms (SNOMED CT), 181–83
standards-developing organizations (SDOs), 182*b*
starting with end in mind, 132
state and territorial public health policy, opioid misuse and addiction, 386, 425–40
  comprehensive approaches, 439

downstream or tertiary prevention, overdose reversal meds and syringe & needle exchange, 431, 433*f*
Health Impact Pyramid, 425–27
prevention, policy, and state public health, 425, 426–27*b*, 428*f*
primary prevention, monitoring and surveillance, 436–39
primary prevention, resiliency, 439
secondary prevention, mental & physical health care parity, 433*f*, 435–36
secondary prevention, treatment access, 433*f*, 434–35
state responses, 427, 430*f*
state funding, public health and prevention, 351–62
  block grants, 1981 Omnibus Reconciliation Act, 354, 355*t*
  braiding, blending, and aligning funding streams, 357
  collaborative, for mental well-being, rural South Carolina, 352–53*b*, 359
  flexibilities, in Medicaid, 356
  flexibilities, in Medicaid, Washington, 356
  flexibilities, in public health funding, 354, 355*t*
  innovations, 354, 355*t*, 356
  innovations: cross-sector integration, 358
  innovations: cross-sector integration, South Carolina, 352–53*b*, 359

innovations: cross-sector integration, Vermont, 359
innovations: cross-sector integration, Virgina, 359
innovations: department-wide change, 357
innovations: department-wide change, Oregon, 358
innovations: no federal change, 360
innovations: no federal change, Louisiana, 360
innovations: no federal change, Rhode Island, 360
innovations: status quo, 357
Minnesota opioid crisis, 353–54*b*
policymaker strategies, potential, 353–54*b*, 361
tightly targeted *vs.* broader funding, 351
State Innovation Models initiative, 170
status quo, state funding, 357
Steven M. Teutsch Prevention Effectiveness Fellowship (PEF), 469
Stewards for Affordable Housing for the Future (SAHF), 335, 336, 338
sticky capital, 366
St. Louis Multimodal Plan, 47, 48*b*
  transportation decision-making, 51*b*
Stoddardt, G., 69–70
Stop Child Abuse Now (SCAN) of Northern Virginia, 317
Strategic Solutions Partners, 28
*Strategies for Reducing the Consumption of Sugar-Sweetened Beverages*, 389–90

structural competency, 458
student programs, public health, 469
student voices, 491–504. *See also* New Voices essay contest
  governing systems, approaches, 491–92
  New Voices essay contest, 491–504
Study Data Tabulation Model (SDTM), 180
Substance Abuse and Mental Health Services Administration (SAMHSA) 42 CFR part 2, 167–68
Substance Misuse and Addiction Framework, 429–30, 430*f*
substance use, Alliance for Health Equity, 275, 277*f*
sugary drink consumption. *See also* Big Soda, fighting at local level
  policy options reducing, 389, 390*t*
suicide risk reduction, Community of Solutions for, 90, 137–47. *See also* Community of Solutions (CoS)
suicide risk reduction, Palo Alto, 142, 145–46
Support for Services at Home (SASH), Vermont, 359
surveillance, opioid crisis, 429
  as primary prevention, 436
surveillance for community outbreak, automation, 177–85
500 Cities Project, 189*b*
asthma, childhood, housing conditions, 185–87*b*

case example,
hypothetical, 177
challenges and future
directions, 184f, 184
data exchange,
179–80b, 185
data models, 179–88b
data transport and
exchange, 182–83b
Digital Bridge project,
183, 184f
electronic case
and laboratory
reporting, 181
electronic health
records, meaningful
use, 179b, 180
history and
background, 177–79
home visit, 187–88b
information age,
177, 179b
sustainability and finance,
325–28. See also
finance
cross-sector
collaboratives,
value-based health
care, 325
health investments,
acquiring and
managing, 325
health investments,
sustaining, 325–26
syringe & needle exchange
programs (SNEPs),
431, 432, 433f

Targeted Rural
Underserved Track
(TRUST), 475
target population,
social screening
programs, 239
Teaching Health
Centers Graduate
Medical Education
(THCGME)
program, 476,
477b
Tennessee, Shelby County,
drug overdose data,
209, 210–13f
chronic disease, 211
Tennessee Medicaid
(TennCare), 40

Texas
Pasadena, building
ties with business
community, 327,
375–81 (see also
business community,
building ties with
(Pasadena, Texas);
Pasadena, Texas)
People's Community
Clinic, 297
Three Pockets of
Prevention
Framework, 410–11
Thriving Communities
Fund, Kaiser
Permanente,
339–40b
Tobacco21 (T21)
Kansas City,
386–87, 448
San Antonio,
416–19
tobacco reforms, San
Antonio, 417
tobacco use, cost to
employers, 64
preventing and
reducing, CDC
strategy, 417–18
training and education.
See also education,
public health
Green & Healthy
Homes Initiative, 38
health equity, 11
medical education,
rural, 474
responsibility for, all
staff, 126
transportation
sector, 50
training and workforce,
453–54
community
partnerships, 453
future, 454
new competencies,
health care and
public health
workforce, 454
Public Health
Accreditation
Board, 454
schools, 453–54 (see
also universities)

students' and residents'
voice, 454
training providers
in population
health, 457–64
community
engagement,
458, 459b
critical thinking, 460
leadership
development,
461, 462b
milestones and
competencies, 457
public health
competencies, 458
transformation, from
innovation, 251, 258
transit-oriented
development, 342
transportation, 78
active, 48, 53t
air quality, 48, 53t
equitable connectivity
and mobility, 48, 53t
interconnected,
47, 48b
noise, 49, 53t
planning, as continuous
process, 49
profession, 47
safety, 48, 53t
Transportation and
Health Tool
(THT), 48–49
transportation sector
actors and
advocates, 47–57
advocacy groups, 50
clarify issue and gather
data, 48b, 50
employers/high-impact
utilizers, 50
identify initiative scope
and focus, 52b,
52, 53t
infrastructure
owners, 49
integrate for impact,
55, 57b
key leverage points,
focus allies on,
55, 56f
partnering for
population health
and equity, 53–54

partnering for
population health
and equity, closest
transportation
sector actor, 54
partnering for
population
health and equity,
established coalition
allies, 53
partnering for
population health
and equity, flexible
blueprint for change,
51b, 54, 56f
planning documents,
publicly available, 50
professional training
and education
associations, 50
regulators and
policymakers, 49–50
service providers, 49
stakeholders, actors,
and influencers, 49
transportation-
health connection,
demonstrating, 48
tribal communities, 327
Trinity Health, loan
fund, 342
Tripe Aim, 103
trust
Accountable
Community for
Health model,
152, 157
building, scaling up
collaboration, 127
sense of, 93, 97b, 97

UCLA Win-Win
Project, 20
umbrella organizations,
national, 336
Unity Accountable
Community for
Health (ACH),
Minnesota,
353–54b, 362
Universal Resource
Identifier
(URI), 182b
universities. See also
training and
education

universities (cont.)
accreditation, Council on Education in Public Health, 466
building population health, 267
digital revolution on, 465
expenditures, large, 366
functions, 465
public health education, 465, 466
University of Arkansas for Medical Sciences (UAMS), 474–75
Upstream Capability Assessment, 80, 81*t*
upstream
determinants, 3–4
philanthropic foundations, 4–5
upstream efforts, 9, 301–12
upstreamists, 12
Upstream Medicine Quality Improvement (QI) Project Matrix, 304
Upstream Strategy Matrix, 80–81, 82*t*
urgent care, 78

value, hospitals and health systems, enhancing, 68
value-based health care, 292
cross-sector collaboratives, 325
value-based payment models, 83, 103–4, 242. *See also* accountable care organizations (ACO)
value-based purchasing, 42

Pay for Success financing with, 42, 43*f*, 44
Value Set Authority Center (VSAC), 180*b*
vending, healthy
advertising campaign, 389, 397*f*
local government support, 393
local legislation, 391
message framing and reframing, 397–98
neighboring governments, 393
newspaper support, 400
Vermont, Blueprint for Health, 359
violence
domestic, breaking cycle of, 305, 306*b*, 306
prevention, health care engagement in, 277*f*
Virginia
Children's Services Act, 359
cross-sector integration, federal funding cuts/changes, 359
Fairfax, suicide epidemic, 137–38
Loudon County, child abuse and neglect, 317
Northern, 315, 316
Northern Virginia Health Foundation, 315–16
One Virginia Foundation, 315–21 (*see also* One Virginia Foundation)
Vita Health & Wellness District, 342–43, 343*f*

voice
community, BUILD Health Challenge, Cleveland, 28
New Voices essay contest, 491–504 (*see also* New Voices essay contest)
student, 491–504 (*see also* student voices)
students' and residents', in training and workforce, 454
Voices for Healthy Kids, 390–91
vulnerable populations, 265

Wald, Lillian, 484
War on Poverty, 332
Washington
Accountable Communities of Health, 356
Medicaid flexibilities, 356
Washington, Wyoming, Alaska, Montana, Idaho (WWAMI) Regional Medical Education model, 475
Rural Integrated Training Experience, 475
Weingart Foundation, 403
Wellness Fund, 149, 156
wellness program, workplace, and stock price performance, 64
Wellness School Assessment Tool (WellSAT), 393
WePLAN 2020, 275

West Side United, 369–70
WHO Alma Ata declaration, 77–78
whole-person systems of care, multisector data, 165*b*, 165
"The Widget Story," 63–64
Win-Win Project, 20
"With Synergy, We Flourish: A Case for Interdisciplinary Collaboration to Improve Health in the United States" (Duncan), 503
workflow
definition, 169
technology adoption on, 169
workforce training, public health, 453–54. *See also* training and workforce
World Health Organization, Commission on Social Determinants, 16
WWAMI Rural Integrated Training Experience (WRITE), 475

zip code improvement, 336–40
cross-sector interest, 338
fundamentals, 336–37
health return on investment and research and partnership opportunities, 337
Zola, Irving, 302